Screening and Treatment of Perinatal Depression and Anxiety

Screening and Treatment of Perinatal Depression and Anxiety

Editor

Francesca Agostini

MDPI • Basel • Beijing • Wuhan • Barcelona • Belgrade • Manchester • Tokyo • Cluj • Tianjin

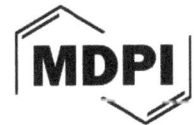

Editor
Francesca Agostini
University of Bologna
Italy

Editorial Office
MDPI
St. Alban-Anlage 66
4052 Basel, Switzerland

This is a reprint of articles from the Special Issue published online in the open access journal *International Journal of Environmental Research and Public Health* (ISSN 1660-4601) (available at: https://www.mdpi.com/journal/ijerph/special_issues/STPDA).

For citation purposes, cite each article independently as indicated on the article page online and as indicated below:

LastName, A.A.; LastName, B.B.; LastName, C.C. Article Title. *Journal Name* **Year**, *Volume Number*, Page Range.

ISBN 978-3-0365-5823-3 (Hbk)
ISBN 978-3-0365-5824-0 (PDF)

Cover image courtesy of Francesca Agostini.

© 2022 by the authors. Articles in this book are Open Access and distributed under the Creative Commons Attribution (CC BY) license, which allows users to download, copy and build upon published articles, as long as the author and publisher are properly credited, which ensures maximum dissemination and a wider impact of our publications.
The book as a whole is distributed by MDPI under the terms and conditions of the Creative Commons license CC BY-NC-ND.

Contents

About the Editor vii

Preface to "Screening and Treatment of Perinatal Depression and Anxiety" ix

Sara Molgora, Emanuela Saita, Maurizio Barbieri Carones, Enrico Ferrazzi and Federica Facchin
Predictors of Postpartum Depression among Italian Women: A Longitudinal Study
Reprinted from: *Int. J. Environ. Res. Public Health* **2022**, *19*, 1553, doi:10.3390/ijerph19031553 ... 1

Grażyna Iwanowicz-Palus, Mariola Mróz, Aleksandra Korda, Agnieszka Marcewicz and Agnieszka Palus
Perinatal Anxiety among Women during the COVID-19 Pandemic—A Cross-Sectional Study
Reprinted from: *Int. J. Environ. Res. Public Health* **2022**, *19*, 2603, doi:10.3390/ijerph19052603 ... 15

Michalina Ilska, Anna Kołodziej-Zaleska, Anna Brandt-Salmeri, Heidi Preis and Marci Lobel
Pandemic Stress and Its Correlates among Pregnant Women during the Second Wave of COVID-19 in Poland
Reprinted from: *Int. J. Environ. Res. Public Health* **2021**, *18*, 11140, doi:10.3390/ijerph182111140 . 29

Francesca Agostini, Erica Neri, Federica Genova, Elena Trombini, Alessandra Provera, Augusto Biasini and Marcello Stella
Depressive Symptoms in Fathers during the First Postpartum Year: The Influence of Severity of Preterm Birth, Parenting Stress and Partners' Depression
Reprinted from: *Int. J. Environ. Res. Public Health* **2022**, *19*, 9478, doi:10.3390/ijerph19159478 ... 41

Hanna Margaretha Heller, Stasja Draisma and Adriaan Honig
Construct Validity and Responsiveness of Instruments Measuring Depression and Anxiety in Pregnancy: A Comparison of EPDS, HADS-A and CES-D
Reprinted from: *Int. J. Environ. Res. Public Health* **2022**, *19*, 7563, doi:10.3390/ijerph19137563 ... 57

Gracia Fellmeth, Siân Harrison, Maria A. Quigley and Fiona Alderdice
A Comparison of Three Measures to Identify Postnatal Anxiety: Analysis of the 2020 National Maternity Survey in England
Reprinted from: *Int. J. Environ. Res. Public Health* **2022**, *19*, 6578, doi:10.3390/ijerph19116578 ... 69

Zuzana Škodová, Ľubica Bánovčinová, Eva Urbanová, Marián Grendár and Martina Bašková
Factor Structure of the Edinburgh Postnatal Depression Scale in a Sample of Postpartum Slovak Women
Reprinted from: *Int. J. Environ. Res. Public Health* **2021**, *18*, 6298, doi:10.3390/ijerph18126298 ... 83

Nichole Fairbrother, Fanie Collardeau, Arianne Albert and Kathrin Stoll
Screening for Perinatal Anxiety Using the Childbirth Fear Questionnaire: A New Measure of Fear of Childbirth
Reprinted from: *Int. J. Environ. Res. Public Health* **2022**, *19*, 2223, doi:10.3390/ijerph19042223 ... 97

Nichole Fairbrother, Arianne Albert, Fanie Collardeau and Cora Keeney
The Childbirth Fear Questionnaire and the Wijma Delivery Expectancy Questionnaire as Screening Tools for Specific Phobia, Fear of Childbirth
Reprinted from: *Int. J. Environ. Res. Public Health* **2022**, *19*, 4647, doi:10.3390/ijerph19084647 . 121

Lavinia De Chiara, Cristina Mazza, Eleonora Ricci, Alexia Emilia Koukopoulos, Georgios D. Kotzalidis, Marco Bonito, Tommaso Callovini, Paolo Roma and Gloria Angeletti
The Relevance of Insomnia in the Diagnosis of Perinatal Depression: Validation of the Italian Version of the Insomnia Symptom Questionnaire
Reprinted from: *Int. J. Environ. Res. Public Health* **2021**, *18*, 12507, doi:10.3390/ijerph182312507 . **141**

Stephen Matthey
Is Validating the Cutoff Score on Perinatal Mental Health Mood Screening Instruments, for Women and Men from Different Cultures or Languages, Really Necessary?
Reprinted from: *Int. J. Environ. Res. Public Health* **2022**, *19*, 4011, doi:10.3390/ijerph19074011 . . . **155**

Archana Raghavan, Veena A. Satyanarayana, Jane Fisher, Sundarnag Ganjekar, Monica Shrivastav, Sarita Anand, Vani Sethi and Prabha S. Chandra
Gender Transformative Interventions for Perinatal Mental Health in Low and Middle Income Countries—A Scoping Review
Reprinted from: *Int. J. Environ. Res. Public Health* **2022**, *19*, 12357, doi:10.3390/ijerph191912357 . **163**

Sarah Kittel-Schneider, Ethel Felice, Rachel Buhagiar, Mijke Lambregtse-van den Berg, Claire A. Wilson, Visnja Banjac Baljak, Katarina Savic Vujovic, Branislava Medic, Ana Opankovic, Ana Fonseca and Angela Lupattelli
Treatment of Peripartum Depression with Antidepressants and Other Psychotropic Medications: A Synthesis of Clinical Practice Guidelines in Europe
Reprinted from: *Int. J. Environ. Res. Public Health* **2022**, *19*, 1973, doi:10.3390/ijerph19041973 . . . **179**

About the Editor

Francesca Agostini

Francesca Agostini, PhD in Clinical Psychology, Psychotherapist, Associate Professor in Dynamic Psychology at Department of Psychology, University of Bologna (Italy). Her general interests regard mental health during childhood and developmental psychopathology in the first years of life. Her main scientific interests focus on perinatal mental health, with qualitative investigations and quantitative research on two main areas. The first one regards the study of the transition to motherhood and fatherhood, including analysis of mental representations, identification of psychosocial risk factors and specific parenting risk contexts (such as severe preterm birth). The second area is represented by the study of perinatal psychopathology, with an emphasis on clinical expressions of perinatal depression and anxiety in women and men and on the development of instruments for the screening and early detection. She currently leads the Developmental Psychodynamic Laboratory and the Clinical services of psychological support for childhood at the Department of Psychology, University of Bologna.

Preface to "Screening and Treatment of Perinatal Depression and Anxiety"

This book aims to deepen the scientific knowledge and clinical understanding of perinatal depression and anxiety, which are internationally recognized as significant mental health problems for both women and men.

Among the perinatal mental disorders, depression and anxiety have received ample attention from research and clinical fields. Specifically, the first disorder, perinatal depression, has been extensively investigated in women over the last 20 years. There is a multitude of relevant research studies showing the clinical evidence of this psychopathological picture, its prevalence across several countries according to different socio-economic and cultural backgrounds, the specificity of its risk and etiological factors, and its potential negative influence at several levels. Indeed, empirical evidence has revealed how perinatal depression can severely impact parental couples' adjustment, early mother–infant interactions, and mother–child relationships; moreover, longitudinal investigations have revealed a significant influence on child development and mental health, even consisting of long-term consequences up to adolescence.

The investigation and description of the clinical characteristics of perinatal anxiety have also become relevant among researchers and clinicians, especially in the last 10 years. Along with this topic, the identification of both perinatal depression and anxiety in the male population is receiving greater interest, highlighting the need to further investigate these issues in the scientific literature.

Based on these premises, the contents of this book offer a glance at the investigation of emerging research areas and those of interest in the context of perinatal depression and anxiety.

The contributions cover a wide range of topics. The first area regards the investigation of the clinical characteristics and predictors of perinatal depression and anxiety, paying special attention to both women and men and the impact of the recent COVID-19 pandemic. A second investigated topic in the book constitutes the analysis of assessment and screening tools for the detection of both perinatal depression and anxiety. The early identification of clinically relevant symptoms is crucial for the implementation of ad hoc tailored interventions. Since the development of the Edinburgh Postnatal Depression Scale (EPDS; Cox et al., 1987), ample research activity has been dedicated to creating new instruments and evaluating their psychometric properties. This section further investigates the characteristics of the pre-existing questionnaires and proposes new tools to be potentially implemented in order to improve the screening processes. The third area focuses more on intervention, including critical reviews on psychosocial and pharmacological interventions for the general improvement of perinatal mental health.

The contents of this book are of interest for all professionals working in the field of perinatal mental health, with the aim of fostering the progress of research knowledge and clinical perspectives.

Francesca Agostini
Editor

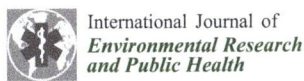

Article

Predictors of Postpartum Depression among Italian Women: A Longitudinal Study

Sara Molgora [1,*], Emanuela Saita [1], Maurizio Barbieri Carones [2], Enrico Ferrazzi [2,3] and Federica Facchin [1]

[1] Department of Psychology, Università Cattolica del Sacro Cuore, 20123 Milan, Italy; emanuela.saita@unicatt.it (E.S.); federica.facchin@unicatt.it (F.F.)
[2] Fondazione IRCCS Cà Granda, Ospedale Maggiore Policlinico, 20122 Milan, Italy; m.barbiericarones@gmail.com (M.B.C.); enrico.ferrazzi@unimi.it (E.F.)
[3] Department of Clinical Science and Community Health, Università degli Studi di Milano, 20122 Milan, Italy
* Correspondence: sara.molgora@unicatt.it; Tel.: +39-0272342347; Fax: +39-0272345962

Abstract: Introduction: Postpartum depression is commonly experienced by mothers worldwide and is associated with anxiety disorders, parenting stress, and other forms of distress, which may lead to a complex illness condition. Several studies have investigated the risk factors for this disorder, including biological and socio-demographic variables, medical and obstetric factors, and psychological and relational dimensions. The present study aimed to describe the psychological status of mothers up to 12 months postpartum, and to investigate the predictors of depressive symptoms at 12 months postpartum, considering obstetric factors along with psychological and relational variables. Methods: A sample of 137 women completed a questionnaire composed of a sheet on anamnestic and obstetric information and the following scales: Wijma Delivery Experience Questionnaire; State-Trait Anxiety Inventory; Edinburgh Postnatal Depression Scale; Parenting Stress Index (Short Form); Dyadic Adjustment Scale; and Multidimensional Scale of Perceived Social Support. Data were collected at four assessment times: 2–3 days, 3 months, 6 months, and 12 months postpartum. Results: Findings showed that the highest percentage of women with clinically significant symptoms of anxiety (state and trait) and depression was found at 12 months postpartum, which indicated that this was the most critical time. The quality of childbirth experience and trait anxiety at three months postpartum emerged as significant predictors of postpartum depression at 12 months. Conclusion: Our findings highlight the importance of providing stable programs (such as educational programs) to mothers in the first year postpartum. Furthermore, because the quality of the childbirth experience is one of the most important predictors of PPD at 12 months postpartum, effort should be made by healthcare professionals to guarantee a positive experience to all women to reduce possible negative long-term consequences of this experience.

Keywords: postpartum depression; predictors; longitudinal study; anxiety; childbirth experience

1. Introduction

The birth of a child significantly impacts a women's psychological well-being and may lead to several forms of diseases, ranging from baby blues to more severe conditions such as anxiety disorders, depression, puerperal psychosis, and post-traumatic stress disorders [1–5].

Postpartum depression (PPD) represents an important clinical problem because it is frequently experienced by mothers worldwide, as demonstrated in several recent meta-analyses (e.g., [6–9]). PPD compromises women's psychological health and, in some instances, may lead to suicidal behaviours [10]; it can also impair the relationship with the partner and the baby, with negative consequences on the child's development [11].

PPD can be associated with anxiety disorders and parenting stress, deriving from a poor perceived ability to cope with the multiple challenges related to the new parental

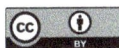

role [12], especially in first-time mothers [1,13–16]. PPD is also predicted by a variety of risk factors, such as biological (e.g., levels of specific hormones) and/or sociodemographic (e.g., socio-economic status) factors [17,18], medical and obstetrics variables related to pregnancy, labor and delivery [19], and psychological variables [20]. For example, complications during pregnancy (e.g., gestational diabetes, preeclampsia, thyroid autoimmunity) are associated with higher levels of PPD [19,21–23], which are also predicted by either elective or emergency caesarean section [24–26], although overall research findings are inconsistent [27]. In addition, mothers of preterm infants are more likely to develop PPD [28]. Most studies have investigated the predictive role of these factors on PPD in the first months postpartum, whereas few studies have examined their long-term impact on PPD. For this reason, PPD and its risk factors 1 year after giving birth remain unclear [20].

Furthermore, there is evidence of a significant association between PPD and previous anxiety or depression disorders, breastfeeding self-efficacy, and low maternal self-efficacy [29–34]. The subjective experience of childbirth can also affect women's postpartum psychological well-being, with a negative experience being associated with higher levels of PPD [35–37].

Regarding relational variables, poor couple relationships and low social support by the formal and the informal network are important risk factors for PPD [29,33,38,39]. Furthermore, maternal violence experiences were significantly associated with an increased risk of developing PPD [38,40].

Moreover, specific contextual variables such as stressful life events are associated with a high prevalence of PPD [41]. The current COVID-19 pandemic can be considered as an additional stressful condition that may affect mothers' psychological well-being [42]. In this regard, an increasing number of studies investigating the psychological impact of the pandemic showed higher levels of anxiety and depressive symptoms among postpartum women during the COVID-19 pandemic compared to similar cohorts assessed before the pandemic [43–46]. These findings can be explained considering both mothers' concerns about the risk of coronavirus for themselves and the baby, and the reduced support received in this period [42].

Many studies on PPD are cross-sectional and focus on the prevalence and the correlates of PPD; prospective studies mainly consider a limited time frame, without including long-term effects of childbirth or the evolution of PPD symptoms over time [47,48]. In this study, we considered a longer postpartum time frame (1 year). Moreover, the longitudinal design allows for a more in-depth understanding of the effects of becoming a mother on women's psychological health, considering childbirth as a complex event [48].

The aims of this study were to: (1) describe the psychological (depression, anxiety, parenting stress) and relational (couple adjustment, perceived social support) status of mothers up to 12 months postpartum; and (2) identify the main predictors of PPD at 12 months postpartum, considering obstetrics factors, and psychological and relational variables. Based on previous studies, we expected that PPD would be predicted by either individual or relational variables, with higher levels of depression associated with lower levels of social support and couple adjustment, and a more negative experience of childbirth. Furthermore, we expected that PPD at 12 months postpartum would be predicted by previous psychological distress, i.e., PPD, anxiety, and parenting stress at 3 months postpartum.

2. Methods

2.1. Procedures and Participants

This was a longitudinal study that comprised 137 Italian postpartum women, recruited between October 2019 and March 2021 in a public hospital located in Northern Italy. Inclusion criteria were being a postpartum women aged ≥18 years and fluent in Italian. Eligible participants received complete information about all the aspects of the research by a member of the research team during postpartum hospitalization. All the women who accepted our invitation to participate in the study provided written informed consent. Ethical approval was received by the Institutional Review Board (approval number 922_2019bis; approval date: 9 October 2019).

Data collection involved four assessment times: 2–3 days after-delivery (Time 1), after 3 months (Time 2), 6 months (Time 3), and 12 months (Time 4). At Time 1, women completed the questionnaires at the hospital, whereas at Time 2, 3, and 4 the questionnaires were completed on the Qualtrics platform following a reminder by email. A total of 323 eligible participants were initially identified. Of these, 2 did not meet the inclusion criteria (age < 18 years) and were excluded from the study. Therefore, 321 women completed the questionnaires at Time 1. Overall, incomplete information (>80% of missing data) was reported by 184 participants, whose data were not used in the final statistical analyses. In total, the questionnaires were returned at all of the four assessment times by 137 participants.

2.2. Measures

At Time 1, women completed a sheet focused on sociodemographic (age, education, employment status, parity) and obstetric information (gestational age, labor induction, mode of delivery, use of epidural analgesia, episiotomy). Women also provided information regarding previous psychological disorders (e.g., depression, anxiety, eating disorders, alcoholism, drug addiction), distressing experiences before pregnancy (such as previous miscarriages), conception (spontaneous or using assisted reproductive technology), and type of pregnancy (including complications during pregnancy and threat of miscarriage). We subsequently collected information about mode of feeding (at Time 2; i.e., "How do you feed your child?", 4 possible responses: exclusive breastfeeding, exclusive artificial milk, mixed, other). Moreover, although the questionnaire was not specifically aimed at investigating the impact of COVID-19 on mothers' psychological health, we included two questions related to the pandemic—(1) To what extent do you think your health and that of your child are threatened by the pandemic? (2) To what extent has the pandemic impacted on your life?—with responses scored on a 0 (Not at all) to 5 (Extremely) Likert scale. Because Time 1 occurred before the COVID-19 outbreak, these two questions were asked at Time 2, 3, and 4.

At Time 1 and 2, women completed the Wijma Delivery Experience Questionnaire-WDEQ(B) [49,50]. The Italian-validated version evaluates the childbirth experience through 14 items on a 6-point Likert scale; the total score ranges from 0 to 70, with a higher score indicating a more negative experience. Internal consistency was good (Cronbach's alpha = 0.86) at Time 1 and very good (Cronbach's alpha = 0.91) at Time 2. We considered a score of 39 as the cut-off value to identify cases of severe fear of childbirth [51].

At Time 2, Time 3 and Time 4, women also completed the following instruments:

- Edinburgh Postnatal Depression Scale—EPDS [52,53]. This instrument is composed of 10 items on a 4-point Likert scale, with a total score ranging from 0 to 30: the higher the score, the higher the depressive symptoms. Internal consistency was good, ranging from 0.84 at Time 2 to 0.88 at Time 4. According to Benvenuti and colleagues [53], a cut-off value of 9 or higher was used to distinguish clinical depression, whereas according to Gibson and colleagues [54] the cut-off value is fixed at 12 or higher.
- State-Trait Anxiety Inventory–STAI, Y form [55,56]. This instrument is composed of 40 items (20 items for trait anxiety and 20 items for state anxiety) on a 4-point Likert scale, with a total score of 20–80: the higher the score, the higher the anxiety symptoms. Internal consistency was very good for both the state (Cronbach's alpha = 0.94 at Time 2, and 0.95 at Time 3 and Time 4) and the trait (Cronbach's alpha = 0.90 at Time 2 and Time 4, and 0.88 at Time 3) subscales. Based on previous studies on similar cohorts, a cut-off score of 40 or higher was used to identify both state and trait clinical anxiety [15,57].
- Parenting Stress Index—PSI [12,58]. This scale is composed of 36 items on a 5-point Likert scale, with a total score ranging from 36 to 180: the higher the score, the higher the perceived level of global parenting stress. Internal consistency was very good,

ranging from 0.92 at Time 3 to 0.95 at Time 2. We considered a score of 90 as the cut-off value to identify high levels of parenting stress [58].
- Dyadic Adjustment Scale—DAS [59,60]. This scale is composed of 32 items, of which 31 are related to couple adjustment, and one item refers to the overall perceived happiness with the relationship. The total score ranges from 0 to 151: the higher the score, the higher the couple adjustment. Internal consistency was very good (Cronbach's alpha ranging from 0.94 at Time 2 to 0.96 at Time 4).
- Multidimensional Scale of Perceived Social Support—MSPSS [61,62]. This instrument is composed of 12 items, with a 12–80 total score range, and measures the perception of social support from three different sources (family, friends, and significant others); the higher the score, the higher the perceived social support. Internal consistency was very good (Cronbach's alpha = 0.93 at all times).

2.3. Statistical Analyses

Statistical analyses were performed using SPSS software, version 27 (IBM, New York, NY, USA). Descriptive statistics were computed to summarize the participant characteristics. Means and standard deviations (SDs) were reported for continuous variables (WDEQ(B), EPDS, STAI, PSI, DAS, MSPSS), and frequencies and percentages for categorical variables. Continuous psychological health outcomes (data collected using the WDEQ(B), the EPDS, the STAI, and the PSI) were also dichotomized using the cut-offs of each scale, to establish the percentage of clinical subsamples for each scale. Normality of distribution was verified at all the assessment times, considering skewness and kurtosis. Values ranging between −2 and +2 indicated that the data distribution was approximately normal [63]. Only the social support (MSPSS) at T4 and couple adjustment (DAS) at T3 and T4 did not have a normal distribution and were excluded from the analyses.

First, we used independent samples t-test and chi-squared test (as appropriate) to compare the women who abandoned the study after Time 1 with those who returned the questionnaires at all the assessment times. The effect of time on the psychological and relational variables was examined using repeated measures ANOVA. To identify the predictors of women's postpartum depression at Time 4, Pearson correlations were performed for continuous variables, whereas univariate ANOVAs were performed for categorial independent variables. Those factors that were significantly related to PPD were subsequently included in a multivariable regression model. All the categorical predictors entered into the regression models were dichotomous (i.e., previous stressful event) or were dichotomized and recoded as dummy variables [64]. For instance, the pandemic-related perceived threat was recoded as low threat (scores between 0 and 3) or high threat (scores from 4 to 5). Statistical significance was set at $p < 0.05$.

3. Results

3.1. Participant Characteristics

Women's age was 34.91 (SD = 4.0; range= 24–44). The 137 women who agreed to participate in the study at all assessment times were more likely to be first-time mothers ($\chi^2(1,137) = 4.75$; $p = 0.029$) and to have a higher level of education ($\chi^2(5,137) = 21.07$; $p = 0.001$) than those who abandoned the study after Time 1. As regards the other socio-demographic, obstetric, and psychological variables, no significant differences emerged between the two groups. The majority of the 137 final participants had an academic degree (55.5%), was employed (67.9%), and was married (63.4%) or cohabiting (36.6%). The mean length of the couple relationship was 8.21 years (SD = 4.5).

Most participants (67.9%) were primiparae, conceived spontaneously (83.9%), and had a vaginal birth (59.9%), vs. 38% of women who had a caesarean section (of which 40.4% had a planned caesarean section, 42.3% had an emergency caesarean section, and 17.3% had an elective caesarean section) and 2.1% who had operative delivery. As regards mode of feeding, 60.2% reported exclusive breastfeeding, 17.2% used artificial milk, and 20.3% used both breast and artificial milk (mixed).

A minority of women (27.2% at T2, 17.3% at T3, and 24.1% at T4) reported a high perceived threat for their own health and that of their child in relation to COVID-19. Considering the impact of the pandemic on women's life, the majority of participants reported a perceived high impact (68.3% at T2, 44.8% at T3, and 61.4% at T4). Further sociodemographic and obstetric information is reported in Table 1.

Table 1. Participants' sociodemographic and obstetric information.

	N (137)	%
SOCIODEMOGRAPHIC INFORMATION		
Level of education		
Professional licensing course	2	1.4
High school	40	29.2
Degree/graduate specialization	76	55.5
PhD/post-graduate specialization	19	13.9
Occupational status		
Self-employed	17	12.4
Employed	93	67.9
Unemployed	9	6.6
Housewife	7	5.1
Student	2	1.4
Other	9	6.6
Distressing experience		
No stressful event	104	75.9
At least one stressful event (economic problems, work-related problems, health problems, bereavement, etc.)	33	24.1
Previous psychological disorders		
No	97	70.8
Yes	40	29.2
OBSTETRIC INFORMATION		
Type of pregnancy		
Single	131	95.6
Twin	6	4.4
Previous miscarriage		
No	103	75.2
Yes	34	24.8
Complications during pregnancy		
No complication	79	57.7
At least one complication (threatened miscarriage, detached placenta, hypertension, gestational diabetes, etc.)	58	42.3
Gestational age		
≤37	24	20.7
≥38	38	79.3
Rupture of membranes		
No	109	80.1
Yes	27	19.9
Induction		
No	72	52.9
Yes	64	47.1
Epidural		
No	41	30.1
Yes	95	69.9
Episiotomy		
No	100	74.6
Yes	34	25.4

3.2. Women's Psychological and Relational Status

Table 2 reports women's scores for all the psychological variables (individual and relational) at all of the four assessment times. Repeated measures ANOVAs showed no differences among the times of assessment, except for trait anxiety, which was significantly higher at Time 4 than the other times (F = 3.9; p = 0.022).

Table 2. Repeated measures ANOVA: differences among times of assessment for the psychological and relational variables.

	Time 1	Time 2	Time 3	Time 4	
	M(SD)	M(SD)	M(SD)	M(SD)	p
WDEQ-B	26.2 (12.7)	27.7 (12.1)	/	/	0.225
EPDS	/	7.7 (5.0)	7.4 (5.0)	7.8 (5.4)	0.708
STAI-State	/	38.0 (10.4)	38.4 (10.7)	40.3 (10.4)	0.171
STAI-Trait	/	37.8 (9.1)	38.2 (8.3)	39.5 (9.2)	0.022
PSI	/	67.2 (19.6)	65.7 (16.6)	66.9 (17.6)	0.600
MSPSS	/	68.4 (12.6)	68.5 (12.0)	/	0.131
DAS	/	118.0 (18.6)	/	/	/

Table 3 shows the percentages of mothers who reported clinically significant symptoms of anxiety and depression, parenting stress, and negative quality of childbirth experience, considering the cut-off scores of the scales. The highest percentage of women with clinically significant symptoms of anxiety (state and trait) and depression was found at Time 4, which indicated that this was the most critical time. Furthermore, 7% and 17% of women—considering a cut-off score of 9 and 12, respectively—reported clinically significant depressive symptoms at all of the three assessment points.

Table 3. Percentage of women above the clinical cut-off for psychological variables across times.

Scale (Cut-Off Core)	Time 1	Time 2	Time 3	Time 4
WDEQ-B (39)	29.7	25.2	/	/
EPDS (12)	/	20.3	21.3	21.9
EPDS (9)	/	40.6	36.0	40.9
STAI-State (40)	/	33.6	35.3	46.0
STAI-Trait (40)	/	35.4	39.0	44.5
PSI (90)	/	10.2	6.1	9.5

The Pearson's correlations reported in Table 4 showed that PPD at 12 months (Time 4) postpartum was positively correlated with the quality of childbirth experience at three months (Time 2), and with anxiety and depression at all assessment times. Conversely, PPD was negatively associated with social support and couple adjustment.

The ANOVAs conducted to detect group differences, based on sociodemographic (parity) and obstetric (type of delivery, mode of conception, complications during pregnancy, epidural analgesia, episiotomy, induction, weeks of gestation) factors in depressive symptoms at 12 months postpartum (Time 4) showed no statistically significant results. In addition, mode of feeding did not have an impact on PPD at 12 months postpartum.

Table 4. Pearson's correlation matrix among psychological and relational variables at all times of assessment.

	WDEQ(B)_t1	WDEQ(B)_t2	STAI_S_t2	STAI_T_t2	EPDS_t2	PSI_t2	DAS_t2	MSPSS_t2	STAI_S_t3	STAI_T_t3	EPDS_t3	PSI_t3	MSPSS_t3	STAI_S_t4	STAI_T_t4	EPDS_t4	PSI_t4
WDEQ(B)_t1	0.77 **	0.18	0.24 *	0.20	0.19	−0.09	−0.23 *	0.09	0.13	0.08	0.11	−0.21 *	0.16	0.26 **	0.18	0.24 *
WDEQ(B)_t2		0.39 **	0.36 **	0.40 **	0.37 **	−0.18	−0.37 **	0.25 **	0.29 **	0.25 **	0.31 **	−0.32 **	0.31 **	0.34 **	0.35 **	0.37 **
STAI_S_t2			0.78 **	0.76 **	0.58 **	−0.51 **	−0.49 **	0.50 **	0.53 **	0.53 **	0.48 **	−0.35 **	0.56 **	0.59 **	0.57 **	0.48 **
STAI_T_t2				0.68 **	0.61 **	−0.61 **	−0.47 **	0.59 **	0.76 **	0.60 **	0.48 **	−0.40 **	0.53 **	0.71 **	0.58 **	0.40 **
EPDS_t2					0.58 **	−0.37 **	−0.43 **	0.40 **	0.48 **	0.59 **	0.52 **	−0.33 **	0.44 **	0.52 **	0.54 **	0.54 **
PSI_t2						−0.49 **	−0.42 **	0.40 **	0.41 **	0.42 **	0.72 **	−0.34 **	0.35 **	0.36 **	0.38 **	−0.26 **
DAS_t2							0.35 **	−0.37 **	−0.49 **	−0.36 **	−0.41 **	0.29 **	−0.37 **	−0.47 **	−0.38 **	−0.29 **
MSPSS_t2								−0.16	−0.27 **	−0.13	−0.34 **	0.63 **	−0.16 *	−0.26 **	−0.25 **	−0.29 **
STAI_S_t3									0.78 **	0.53 **	0.50 **	−0.33 **	0.56 **	0.60 **	0.57 **	0.48 **
STAI_T_t3										0.72 **	0.49 **	−0.39 **	0.61 **	0.75 **	0.56 **	0.52 **
EPDS_t3											0.48 **	−0.19 *	0.51 **	0.53 **	0.57 **	0.46 **
PSI_t3												−0.40 **	0.40 **	0.40 **	0.36 **	0.70 **
MSPSS_t3													−0.23 **	−0.35 **	−19 *	−0.36 **
STAI_S_t4														0.79 **	0.77 *	0.55 **
STAI_T_t4															0.69 **	0.57 **
EPDS_t4																0.50 **
PSI_t4																

* $p < 0.01$, ** $p < 0.001$.

Women who had experienced one or more stressful events (e.g., economic problems, work problems, own illness, or illness of a significant person, etc.) during pregnancy or in the postpartum (Time 1) reported greater depressive symptoms at 12 months postpartum (Time 4; F = 8.53; p = 0.004). Furthermore, women who reported a high perceived threat related to COVID-19 at three months postpartum (Time 2) showed greater depressive symptoms at 12 months postpartum (Time 4; F = 4.29; p = 0.043). Finally, the quality of childbirth experience at three months (Time 2) had a significant impact on PPD, with women reporting a critical or even traumatic experience (cut-off score above 39) showing higher levels of depressive symptoms at 12 months postpartum (Time 4; F = 12.64; p = 0.001). In particular, the chi-squared test showed that women who had a negative experience of childbirth at three months postpartum (Time 2) were more likely to report clinically significant depressive symptoms at 12 months postpartum (Time 4; $\chi^2(1,111)=13.60$; p = 0.000).

We subsequently performed a linear regression, including previous stressful event (assessed at Time 1), perception of COVID-19 threat at three months, quality of childbirth experience at three months, anxiety (state and trait), depression and parenting stress at three months, couple adjustment, and social support at three months as predictors of PPD at 12 months. The findings of this analysis are reported in Table 5 and showed statistically significant results for two predictors: the quality of childbirth experience and trait anxiety. Conversely, the other variables did not significantly predict postpartum depression at one year. The model (F $_{(8,36)}$ = 4.42; p < 0.001) explains 38% of the total variance of the dependent variable (R_2 = 0.38).

Table 5. Multiple linear regression: Effect of previous stressful events, WDEQ(B), STAI (state and trait), PSI, MSPSS, DAS and perception of threat related to COVID-19 at 3 months on EPDS at 12 months.

Predictors	b	SE b	β	t	p
Stressful event_t1	0.191	1.707	0.014	0.112	0.912
WDEQ(B)_t1	0.172	0.064	0.387	2.705	0.010
STAI_S_t1	0.024	0.107	0.053	0.228	0.821
STAI_T_t1	0.341	0.121	0.643	2.822	0.008
PSI_t1	−0.039	0.046	−0.164	−0.849	0.401
MSPSS_t1	0.114	0.065	0.289	1.759	0.087
DAS_t1	−0.036	0.059	−0.110	−0.606	0.548
Covid_Threat_t1	0.253	1.612	0.020	0.157	0.876

4. Discussion

Because the birth of a child represents a critical and potentially stressful experience with possible negative consequences on women's mental health [1–5], the primary aim of this study was to describe the psychological status of mothers up to 12 months postpartum. Indeed, this longitudinal framework, which is broader than that of other longitudinal studies or cross-sectional studies, allows more in-depth analysis of the psychological impact of transitioning to parenthood, also considering that women's psychological status in the postpartum period can change over time.

Our findings showed that trait anxiety was significantly higher at 12 months postpartum; furthermore, the highest percentage of women with clinically significant symptoms of state and trait anxiety and depression was found at 12 months postpartum. These results interestingly confirmed the findings of another recent study [65], in which the highest levels of depression were detected at 9–12 months postpartum, and suggest that approximately one year after birth represents one of the most critical and challenging time windows in the postpartum period (this is a useful information, also considering the paucity of research investigating women's psychological health 12 months after childbirth). In another study on fathers' trajectories of postpartum depression, the men participants reported the highest percentage of depressive symptoms at one year postpartum [48]. We can speculate that this is a critical time because in Italy it usually coincides with the end of maternity leave and the return to work, with the concomitant admission of the child to the kindergarten. For these reasons, it may represent a complex time for women who have to manage both work and family commitments. These findings also underline the importance of longitudinal studies to examine the psychological wellbeing of new parents over time, which may also highlight the possible long-term consequences of the transition to parenthood.

Furthermore, our findings showed higher percentages of women with clinically significant psychological symptoms (considering all of the four assessment times) compared with those reported in the pre-pandemic literature on similar cohorts, which suggests that in our sample the experience of motherhood was also shaped by pandemic-related factors [42], especially the pandemic-related perceived threat. The overall estimated prevalence of anxiety disorders/symptoms in this population was around 10–15% before the pandemic [66]; in our sample, the percentage of women above the clinical cut-off score was more than double at 3 and 6 months postpartum, and approximately more than triple at 12 months postpartum. These percentages are in line with those of a previous study carried out during the first lockdown of the pandemic [42]. At the same time, in our sample, the percentage of women with clinically significant symptoms of depression was higher than those reported in the pre-pandemic literature [67–69]. For up to the 17% of the participants who reported clinically significant symptoms of depression, the levels of depression were clinically significant at all of the three assessment points, which indicated a stable but critical situation. These findings confirm those of previous studies that identified a high-risk trajectory, with relevant depressive symptoms at all assessment points [70–72], and provide useful information for clinical intervention, underlining the importance of continuous support for postpartum women. However, the highest percentage of stable high-risk women found in this study highlights the significant impact of the pandemic on mothers' well-being, which further underlines the importance of offering supportive interventions not only immediately after childbirth, but also throughout the following year. Regarding the childbirth experience, approximately one-third of women reported a very negative experience, emphasizing how the experience of childbirth during the pandemic was negative for many women, as highlighted in a previous study [73].

Finally, the presence of multiple correlations between the psychological and the relational variables included in the study indicates a complex condition of psychological distress that cannot be reduced to depressive symptoms alone. In this scenario, relational variables can play a protective role, as has been well documented in both the pre-pandemic and pandemic literature [44,74].

Regarding the main predictors of PPD at 12 months postpartum (the second aim of our study), our findings showed significant associations with the quality of childbirth experience and trait anxiety. This result only partially confirms our hypothesis. As expected, PPD was predicted by the quality of childbirth experience and anxiety at three months, which is in line with findings of previous studies. Specifically, several studies found an association between a negative subjective experience of childbirth and maternal depression [36,37,75–79], which highlights the importance of improving the quality of the childbirth experience to reduce its possible negative consequences on women's well-being, and on the relationship with the baby and the baby's development [80,81].

Furthermore, the significant predictive role of trait anxiety on PPD at 12 months indicates that "structural" rather than situational factors have an impact on depressive symptoms. This result confirms those from previous studies that underlined the continuity of psychological distress across the transition to parenthood [82]. Surprisingly, in our study, PPD at previous assessment times did not affect PPD at 12 months. Taken together, these findings may suggest that an initial condition of anxiety in mothers, if untreated, may lead to long-term negative consequences including PPD.

On the contrary, neither couple adjustment nor social support were found to be predictive of PPD, although they were negatively correlated with PPD. Therefore, although relational variables can have a protective role in mothers' psychological adjustment, PPD is directly predicted by individual variables related to psychological dimensions, and especially to the quality of childbirth experience.

The current study has some limitations. First, more than half of the participants abandoned the study. Second, two scales (DAS and MSPSS) did not have a normal distribution and for this reason they were not included in all the analyses conducted. Third, mothers' well-being was investigated using only self-report instruments, exposed to social desirability bias. Future studies could investigate mothers' psychological health using qualitative designs based on in-depth interviews, to better understand the subjective experience of the transition to parenthood. Finally, although this study was not originally focused on motherhood experience during the pandemic, this unexpected event inevitably had an impact on our research, so that some questions related to COVID-19 needed to be included.

Despite these limitations, the longitudinal design of our study allows a longer period of time to be covered compared with other studies, and can provide useful information to plan specific support interventions for postpartum women. For instance, although antenatal classes are routinely offered to Italian expectant mothers, it may be useful to provide stable programs (such as educational programs) to mothers in the first year postpartum. Because the quality of the childbirth experience is the most important predictor of PPD, effort should be made by healthcare professionals to guarantee a positive experience to all women.

5. Conclusions

Investigating women's psychological status in the postpartum period is essential to understand how we can support women through targeted interventions based on their specific needs. In this regard, our findings may usefully contribute to research and clinical practice by showing that the quality of the childbirth experience has long-term effects on women's psychological well-being. The fact that the whole first year represents a window of vulnerability, rather than only the first months after giving birth, should be considered by healthcare professionals in clinical practice with mothers.

Author Contributions: Conceptualization, S.M., E.S., M.B.C., E.F. and F.F.; Methodology, S.M. and F.F.; Formal Analysis, S.M.; Investigation, S.M., M.B.C. and F.F.; Data Curation, S.M., M.B.C. and F.F.; Writing—Original Draft Preparation, S.M.; Writing—Review and Editing, S.M., E.S. and F.F.; Project Administration, S.M., E.S., M.B.C., E.F. and F.F. All authors have read and agreed to the published version of the manuscript.

Funding: This research received no external funding.

Institutional Review Board Statement: The project was approved by the Hospital Institutional Review Board (922_2019bis, 9 October 2019).

Informed Consent Statement: Informed consent was obtained from all subjects involved in the study.

Data Availability Statement: Data are available on request contacting the authors.

Conflicts of Interest: The authors declare no conflict of interest.

References

1. Meltzer-Brody, S.; Maegbaek, M.L.; Medland, S.E.; Miller, W.C.; Sullivan, P.; Unk-Olsen, T. Obstetrical, pregnancy and socioeconomic predictors for new-onset severe postpartum psychiatric disorders in primiparous women. *Psycholgical Med.* **2017**, *47*, 1427–1441. [CrossRef] [PubMed]
2. Mohamied, F. Postpartum psychosis and management: A case study. *Br. J. Midwifery* **2019**, *27*, 77–84. [CrossRef]
3. Paulson, J.F.; Bazemore, S.D. Prenatal and postpartum depression in fathers and its association with maternal depression: A meta-analysis. *JAMA* **2010**, *303*, 1961–1969. [CrossRef] [PubMed]
4. Pellowski, J.A.; Bengtson, A.M.; Barnett, W.; DiClemente, K.; Koen, N.; Zar, H.J.; Stein, D.J. Perinatal depression among mothers in a South African birth cohort study: Trajectories from pregnancy to 18 months postpartum. *J. Affect. Disord.* **2019**, *259*, 279–287. [CrossRef]
5. Rezaie-Keikhaie, K.; Arbabshastan, M.E.; Rafiemanesh, H.; Amirshahi, M.; Ostadkelayeh, S.M.; Arbabisarjou, A. Systematic Review and Meta-Analysis of the Prevalence of the Maternity Blues in the Postpartum Period. *J. Obstet. Gynecol. Neonatal. Nurs.* **2020**, *49*, 127–136. [CrossRef] [PubMed]

6. Falah-Hassani, K.; Shiri, R.; Dennis, C.-L. The prevalence of antenatal and postnatal co-morbid anxiety and depression: A meta-analysis. *Psychol. Med.* **2017**, *47*, 2041–2053. [CrossRef] [PubMed]
7. Karaçam, Z.; Çoban, A.; Akbaş, B.; Karabulut, E. Status of postpartum depression in Turkey: A meta-analysis. *Health Care Women Int.* **2018**, *39*, 821–841. [CrossRef] [PubMed]
8. Shorey, S.; Chee, C.Y.I.; Ng, E.D.; Chan, Y.H.; Tam, W.W.S.; Chong, Y.S. Prevalence and incidence of postpartum depression among healthy mothers: A systematic review and meta-analysis. *J. Psychiatr. Res.* **2018**, *104*, 235–248. [CrossRef]
9. Zeleke, T.A.; Getinet, W.; Tadesse Tessema, Z.; Gebeyehu, K. Prevalence and associated factors of post-partum depression in Ethiopia. A systematic review and meta-analysis. *PLoS ONE.* **2021**, *16*, e0247005. [CrossRef]
10. Ghaedrahmati, M.; Kazemi, A.; Kheirabadi, G.; Ebrahimi, A.; Bahrami, M. Postpartum depression risk factors: A narrative review. *J. Educ. Health Promot.* **2017**, *6*, 60.
11. Lubotzky-Gete, S.; Ornoy, A.; Grotto, I.; Calderon-Margalit, R. Postpartum depression and infant development up to 24 months: A nationwide population-based study. *J. Affect. Disord.* **2021**, *285*, 136–143. [CrossRef]
12. Abidin, R.R. *Manual for the Parenting Stress Index*; Pediatric Psychology Press: Charlottesville, VA, USA, 1995.
13. Ali, E. Women's experiences with postpartum anxiety disorders: A narrative literature review. *Int. J. Women's Health* **2018**, *10*, 237–249. [CrossRef] [PubMed]
14. Rollè, L.; Prino, L.E.; Sechi, C.; Vismara, L.; Neri, E.; Polizzi, C.; Trovato, A.; Volpi, B.; Molgora, S.; Fenaroli, V.; et al. Parenting stress, mental health, dyadic adjustment: A structural equation model. *Front. Psychol.* **2017**, *8*, 839. [CrossRef]
15. Vismara, L.; Rollè, L.; Agostini, F.; Sechi, C.; Fenaroli, V.; Molgora, S.; Neri, E.; Prino, L.E.; Odorisio, F.; Trovato, A.; et al. Perinatal parenting stress, anxiety, and depression outcomes in first-time mothers and fathers: A 3-to 6-months postpartum follow-up study. *Front. Psychol.* **2016**, *7*, 938. [CrossRef] [PubMed]
16. Yim, I.S.; Stapleton, L.R.T.; Guardino, C.M.; Hahn-Holbrook, J.; Schetter, C.D. Biological and psychosocial predictors of postpartum depression: Systematic review and call for integration. *Annu. Rev. Clin. Psychol.* **2015**, *11*, 99–137. [CrossRef] [PubMed]
17. Aishwarya, S.; Rajendiren, S.; Kattimani, S.; Dhiman, P.; Haritha, S.; Narayanan, P.H.A. Homocysteine and serotonin: Association with postpartum depression. *Asian J. Psychiatry* **2013**, *6*, 473–477. [CrossRef]
18. Alshikh Ahmad, H.; Alkhatib, A.; Luo, J. Prevalence and risk factors of postpartum depression in the Middle East: A systematic review and meta-analysis. *BMC Pregnancy Childbirth* **2021**, *21*, 542. [CrossRef]
19. Abdollahpour, S.; Heydari, A.; Ebrahimipour, H.; Faridhoseini, F.; Heidarian Miri, H.; Khadivzadeh, T. Postpartum depression in women with maternal near miss: A systematic review and meta-analysis. *J. Matern. Fetal Neonatal Med.* **2021**, *15*, 1–7. [CrossRef]
20. Hutchens, B.F.; Kearney, J. Risk Factors for Postpartum Depression: An Umbrella Review. *J Midwifery Women's Health* **2020**, *65*, 96–108. [CrossRef]
21. Azami, M.; Badfar, G.; Soleymani, A.; Rahmati, S. The association between gestational diabetes and postpartum depression: A systematic review and meta-analysis. *Diabetes Res. Clin. Pract.* **2019**, *149*, 147–155. [CrossRef]
22. Caropreso, L.; De Azevedo Cardoso, T.; Eltayebani, M.; Frey, B.N. Preeclampsia as a risk factor for postpartum depression and psychosis: A systematic review and meta-analysis. *Arch. Women's Ment. Health* **2020**, *24*, 493–505. [CrossRef]
23. Minaldi, E.; D'Andrea, S.; Castellini, C.; Martorella, A.; Francavilla, F.; Francavilla, S.; Barbonetti, A. Thyroid autoimmunity and risk of post-partum depression: A systematic review and meta-analysis of longitudinal studies. *J. Endocrinol. Investig.* **2020**, *43*, 271–277. [CrossRef] [PubMed]
24. Bahadoran, P.; Oreizi, H.R.; Safari, S. Meta-analysis of the role of delivery mode in postpartum depression (Iran 1997–2011). *J. Educ. Health Promot.* **2014**, *3*, 118. [PubMed]
25. Moameri, H.; Ostadghaderi, M.; Khatooni, E.; Doosti-Irani, A. Association of postpartum depression and cesarean section: A systematic review and meta-analysis. *Clin. Epidemiol. Glob. Health* **2019**, *7*, 471–480. [CrossRef]
26. Nam, J.Y.; Park, E.C.; Cho, E. Does Urinary Incontinence and Mode of Delivery Affect Postpartum Depression? A Nationwide Population-Based Cohort Study in Korea. *Int. J. Environ. Res. Public Health* **2021**, *18*, 437. [CrossRef] [PubMed]
27. Eckerdal, P.; Kollia, N.; Karlsson, L.; Skoog-Svanberg, A.; Wikström, A.K.; Högberg, U.; Skalkidou, A. Epidural Analgesia During Childbirth and Postpartum Depressive Symptoms: A Population-Based Longitudinal Cohort Study. *Anesth. Analg.* **2020**, *130*, 615–624. [CrossRef]
28. De Paula Eduardo, J.A.F.; De Rezende, M.G.; Menezes, P.R.; Del-Ben, C.M. Preterm birth as a risk factor for postpartum depression: A systematic review and meta-analysis. *J. Affect. Disord.* **2019**, *259*, 393–403. [CrossRef]
29. Edwards, L.M.; Le, H.N.; Garnier-Villarreal, M. A systematic review and meta-analysis of risk factors for postpartum depression among Latinas. *Matern. Child Health J.* **2021**, *25*, 554–564. [CrossRef]
30. Grigoriadis, S.; Graves, L.; Peer, M.; Mamisashvili, L.; Tomlinson, G.; Vigod, S.N.; Cindy-Lee, D.; Steiner, M.; Brown, C.; Cheung, A.; et al. A systematic review and meta-analysis of the effects of antenatal anxiety on postpartum outcomes. *Arch. Women's Ment. Health* **2019**, *22*, 543–556. [CrossRef]
31. Lee, D.T.; Yip, A.S.; Leung, T.Y.; Chung, T.K. Identifying women at risk of postnatal depression: Prospective longitudinal study. *Hong Kong Med. J.* **2000**, *6*, 349–354.
32. Mercan, Y.; Selcuk, K.T. Association between postpartum depression level, social support level and breastfeeding attitude and breastfeeding self-efficacy in early postpartum women. *PLoS ONE.* **2021**, *16*, e0249538. [CrossRef] [PubMed]
33. Qi, W.; Zhao, F.; Liu, Y.; Li, Q.; Hu, J. Psychosocial risk factors for postpartum depression in Chinese women: A meta-analysis. *BMC Pregnancy Childbirth* **2021**, *21*, 174. [CrossRef] [PubMed]

34. Van Der Zee-Van Den Berg, A.I.; Boere-Boonekamp, M.M.; Groothuis-Oudshoorn, C.G.M.; Reijneveld, S.A. Postpartum depression and anxiety: A community-based study on risk factors before, during and after pregnancy. *J Affect. Disord.* **2021**, *286*, 158–165. [CrossRef] [PubMed]
35. Bell, A.F.; Andersson, E. The birth experience and women's postnatal depression: A systematic review. *Midwifery* **2016**, *39*, 112–123. [CrossRef] [PubMed]
36. MacKinnon, A.L.; Yang, L.; Feeley, N.; Gold, I.; Hayton, B.; Zelkowitz, P. Birth setting, labour experience, and postpartum psychological distress. *Midwifery* **2017**, *50*, 110–116. [CrossRef]
37. Molgora, S.; Fenaroli, V.; Saita, E. The association between childbirth experience and mother's parenting stress: The mediating role of anxiety and depressive symptoms. *Women Health* **2020**, *60*, 341–351. [CrossRef]
38. Desta, M.; Memiah, P.; Kassie, B.; Ketema, D.B.; Amha, H.; Getaneh, T.; Sintayehud, M. Postpartum depression and its association with intimate partner violence and inadequate social support in Ethiopia: A systematic review and meta-analysis. *J. Affect. Disord.* **2021**, *279*, 737–748. [CrossRef]
39. Hutchens, B.F.; Holland, M.L.; Tanner, T.; Kennedy, H.P. Does perceived quality of care moderate postpartum depression? A secondary analysis of a two-stage survey. *Matern. Child Health J.* **2021**, *25*, 613–625. [CrossRef]
40. Zhang, S.; Wang, L.; Yang, T.; Chen, L.; Qiu, X.; Wang, T.; Chen, L.; Zhao, L.; Ye, Z.; Zheng, Z.; et al. Maternal violence experiences and risk of postpartum depression: A meta-analysis of cohort studies. *Eur. Psychiatry* **2019**, *55*, 90–101. [CrossRef]
41. Peng, S.; Lai, X.; Du, Y.; Meng, L.; Gan, Y.; Zhang, X. Prevalence and risk factors of postpartum depression in China: A hospital-based cross-sectional study. *J. Affect. Disord.* **2021**, *282*, 1096–1100. [CrossRef]
42. Molgora, S.; Accordini, M. Motherhood in the time of coronavirus: The impact of the pandemic emergency on expectant and postpartum women's psychological well-being. *Front. Psychol.* **2020**, *11*, 567155. [CrossRef] [PubMed]
43. Ceulemans, M.; Foulon, V.; Ngo, E.; Panchaud, A.; Winterfeld, U.; Pomar, L.; Lambelet, V.; Cleary, B.; O'Shaughnessy, F.; Passier, A.; et al. Mental health status of pregnant and breastfeeding women during the COVID-19 pandemic—multinational cross-sectional study. *Acta Obstet. Et Gynecol. Scand.* **2021**, *100*, 1219–1229. [CrossRef] [PubMed]
44. Lebel, C.; MacKinnon, A.; Bagshawe, M.; Tomfohr-Madsen, L.; Giesbrecht, G. Elevated depression and anxiety symptoms among pregnant individuals during the COVID-19 pandemic. *J. Affect. Disord.* **2020**, *277*, 5–13. [CrossRef] [PubMed]
45. Liu, C.H.; Erdei, C.; Mittal, L. Risk factors for depression, anxiety, and PTSD symptoms in perinatal women during the COVID-19 Pandemic. *Psychiatry Res.* **2021**, *295*, 113552. [CrossRef] [PubMed]
46. Patabendige, M.; Gamage, M.M.; Weerasinghe, M.; Jayawardane, A. Psychological impact of the COVID-19 pandemic among pregnant women in Sri Lanka. *Int. J. Gynecol. Obstet.* **2020**, *151*, 150–153. [CrossRef] [PubMed]
47. Fenaroli, V.; Molgora, S.; Malgaroli, M.; Saita, E. The transition to motherhood and fatherhood: Trajectories of wellbeing and emotional disease. *G. Ital. Di Psicol.* **2017**, *2*, 407–424.
48. Molgora, S.; Fenaroli, V.; Malgaroli, M.; Saita, E. Trajectories of Postpartum Depression in Italian First-Time Fathers. *Am. J. Men's Health* **2017**, *11*, 880–887. [CrossRef] [PubMed]
49. Wijma, K.; Wijma, B.; Zar, M. Psychometric aspects of the W-DEQ; A new questionnaire for the measurement of fear of childbirth. *J. Psychosom. Obstet. Gynaecol.* **1998**, *19*, 84–97. [CrossRef] [PubMed]
50. Fenaroli, V.; Saita, E. Fear of childbirth: A contribution to the validation of the Italian version of the Wijma Delivery Expectancy/Experience Questionnaire (WDEQ). *TPM—Test. Psychom. Methodol. Appl. Psychol.* **2013**, *20*, 131–154.
51. Molgora, S.; Fenaroli, V.; Prino, L.E.; Rollé, L.; Sechi, C.; Trovato, A.; Vismara, L.; Volpi, B.; Brustia, P.; Lucarelli, L.; et al. Fear of childbirth in primiparous Italian pregnant women: The role of anxiety, depression, and couple adjustment. *Women Birth* **2018**, *31*, 117–123. [CrossRef]
52. Cox, J.L.; Holden, J.M.; Henshaw, C. *Perinatal Mental Health: The Edinburg Postnatal Depression Scale (EPDS) Manual*; RCPsych: London, UK, 2014.
53. Benvenuti, P.; Ferrara, M.; Niccolai, C.; Valoriali, V.; Cox, J.L. The Edinburgh Postnatal Depression Scale: Validation for an Italian sample. *J. Affect. Disord.* **1999**, *53*, 137–141. [CrossRef]
54. Gibson, J.; McKenzie-McHarg, K.; Shakespeare, J.; Price, J.; Gray, R. A systematic review of studies validating the Edinburgh Postnatal Depression Scale in antepartum and postpartum women. *Acta Psychiatr. Scand.* **2009**, *119*, 350–364. [CrossRef] [PubMed]
55. Spielberger, C.D.; Gorsuch, R.L.; Lushene, R.; Vagg, P.R.; Jacobs, G.A. *Manual for the State-Trait Anxiety Inventory*; Consulting Psychologists Press: Palo Alto, CA, USA, 1983.
56. Pedrabissi, L.; Santinello, M. *Inventario per l'ansia di Stato e di Tratto: Nuova Versione Italiana dello STAI-Forma*; Organizzazioni Speciali: Firenze, Italy, 1989.
57. Giardinelli, L.; Innocenti, A.; Benni, L.; Stefanini, M.C.; Lino, G.; Lunardi, C.; Svelto, V.; Afshar, S.; Bovani, R.; Castellini, G.; et al. Depression and anxiety in perinatal period: Prevalence and risk factors in an Italian sample. *Arch. Women Ment. Health* **2012**, *15*, 21–30. [CrossRef] [PubMed]
58. Guarino, A.; di Blasio, P.; D'Alessio, M.; Camisasca, E.; Serantoni, G. *Parenting Stress Index—Short Form*; Giunti Organizzazioni Speciali: Firenze, Italy, 2008.
59. Spanier, G. Measuring dyadic adjustment: New scales for assessing the quality of marriage and similar dyads. *J. Marriage Fam.* **1976**, *38*, 15–28. [CrossRef]
60. Gentili, P.; Contreras, L.; Cassaniti, M.; D'Arista, F. La Dyadic Adjustment Scale: Una misura dell'adattamento di coppia. *Minerva Psichiatr.* **2002**, *43*, 107–116.

61. Zimet, G.D.; Dahlem, N.W.; Zimet, S.G.; Farley, G.K. The Multidimensional Scale of Perceived Social Support. *J. Personal. Assess.* **1988**, *52*, 30–41. [CrossRef]
62. Prezza, M.; Principato, M.P. *La Rete Sociale e il Sostegno Sociale*; Il Mulino: Bologna, Italy, 2002.
63. Bonanomi, A.; Facchin, F.; Id, S.B.; Villani, D. Prevalence and health correlates of Online Fatigue: A cross-sectional study on the Italian academic community during the COVID-19 pandemic. *PLoS ONE* **2021**, *16*, e0255181. [CrossRef]
64. Frazier, P.; Tix, A.; Barron, K. Testing moderator and mediator effects in counseling psychology research. *J. Couns. Psychol.* **2004**, *51*, 115–134. [CrossRef]
65. Rosander, M.; Berlin, A.; Frykedal, K.F.; Barimani, M. Maternal depression symptoms during the first 21 months after giving birth. *Scand. J. Public Health* **2021**, *49*, 606–615. [CrossRef]
66. Dennis, C.L.; Falah-Hassani, K.; Shiri, R. Prevalence of antenatal and postnatal anxiety: Systematic review and meta-analysis. *Br. J. Psychiatry* **2017**, *210*, 315–323. [CrossRef]
67. Zaers, S.; Waschke, M.; Ehlert, U. Depressive symptoms and symptoms of post-traumatic stress disorder in women after childbirth. *J. Psychosom. Obstet. Gynecol.* **2008**, *29*, 61–71. [CrossRef] [PubMed]
68. Pampaka, D.; Papatheodorou, S.I.; AlSeaidan, M.; Al Wotayan, R.; Wright, R.J.; Buring, J.E.; Dockery, D.W.; Christophi, C.A. Depressive symptoms and comorbid problems in pregnancy—Results from a population based study. *J. Psychosom. Res.* **2018**, *112*, 53–58. [CrossRef] [PubMed]
69. Sunnqvist, C.; Sjöström, K.; Finnbogadóttir, H. Depressive symptoms during pregnancy and postpartum in women and use of antidepressant treatment—A longitudinal cohort study. *Int. J. Women's Health* **2018**, *11*, 109–117. [CrossRef]
70. Luoma, I.; Korhonen, M.; Salmelin, R.K.; Helminen, M.; Tamminen, T. Long-term trajectories of maternal depressive symptoms and their antenatal predictors. *J. Affect. Disord.* **2015**, *170*, 30–38. [CrossRef]
71. Cent, R.; Diamantopoulou, S.; Hudziak, J.J.; Hofman, A.; Jaddoe, V.; Verhulst, F.C.; Lambregtse-Van Den Berg, M.P.; Tiemeier, H. Trajectories of maternal depressive symptoms predict child problem behaviour: The Generation R Study. *Psychol. Med.* **2013**, *43*, 13–25.
72. Van Der Waerden, L.; Galera, C.; Saurel-Cubizolles, M.; Sutter-Dallay, A.L.; Melchior, M. Predictors of persistent maternal depression trajectories in early childhood: Results from the EDEN mother-child cohort study in France. *Psychol. Med.* **2015**, *45*, 1999–2012. [CrossRef] [PubMed]
73. Aydin, E. Giving birth in a Pandemic: Women's Birth Experiences in England during COVID-19. *medRxiv* **2021**. [CrossRef]
74. Biaggi, A.; Conroy, S.; Pawlby, S.; Pariante, C.M. Identifying the women at risk of antenatal anxiety and depression: A systematic review. *J. Affect. Disord.* **2016**, *191*, 62–77. [CrossRef]
75. Coo, S.; García, M.I.; Mira, A. Examining the association between subjective childbirth experience and maternal mental health at six months postpartum. *J. Reprod. Infant Psychol.* **2021**. [CrossRef]
76. Dikmen-Yildiz, P.; Ayers, S.; Phillips, L. Longitudinal trajectories of post-traumatic stress disorder (PTSD) after birth and associated risk factors. *J. Affect. Disord.* **2018**, *229*, 377–385. [CrossRef]
77. Garthus-Niegel, S.; Knoph, C.; Von Soest, T.; Nielsen, C.S.; Eberhard-Gran, M. The role of labor pain and overall birth experience in the development of posttraumatic stress symptoms: A longitudinal cohort study. *Birth* **2014**, *41*, 108–115. [CrossRef] [PubMed]
78. Gürber, S.; Baumeler, L.; Grob, A.; Surbek, D.; Stadlmayr, W. Antenatal depressive symptoms and subjective birth experience in association with postpartum depressive symptoms and acute stress reaction in mothers and fathers: A longitudinal path analysis. *Eur. J. Obstet. Gynecol. Reprod. Biol.* **2017**, *215*, 68–74. [CrossRef] [PubMed]
79. Horak, T.A. The psychology of labour. *Obstet. Gynaecol. Forum* **2017**, *27*, 4–10.
80. Choi, K.W.; Sikkema, K.J.; Vythilingum, B.; Geerts, L.; Faure, S.C.; Watt, M.H.; Roos, A.; Stein, D.J. Maternal childhood trauma, postpartum depression, and infant outcomes: Avoidant affective processing as a potential mechanism. *J. Affect. Disord.* **2017**, *211*, 107–115. [CrossRef]
81. Simpson, M.; Catling, C. Understanding psychological traumatic birth experiences: A literature review. *Women Birth* **2016**, *29*, 203–207. [CrossRef] [PubMed]
82. Molgora, S.; Fenaroli, V.; Saita, E. Psychological distress profiles in expectant mothers: What is the association with pregnancy-related and relational variables? *J. Affect. Disord.* **2020**, *262*, 83–89. [CrossRef] [PubMed]

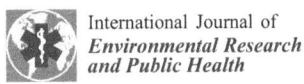

Article

Perinatal Anxiety among Women during the COVID-19 Pandemic—A Cross-Sectional Study

Grażyna Iwanowicz-Palus [1], Mariola Mróz [1,*], Aleksandra Korda [2], Agnieszka Marcewicz [1] and Agnieszka Palus [3]

[1] Chair of Obstetrics Development, Faculty of Health Sciences, Medical University of Lublin, 4-6 Staszica Str., 20-081 Lublin, Poland; spupalus@gmail.com (G.I.-P.); agnieszkamarcewicz@umlub.pl (A.M.)
[2] Students' Scientific Circle at the Chair of Obstetrics Development, Faculty of Health Sciences, Medical University of Lublin, 20-081 Lublin, Poland; kordaaleksandra050@gmail.com
[3] Medical Doctor in Medical Center in NowyDwór Mazowiecki, Faculty of Medicine, Warsaw Medical University, 02-091 Warsaw, Poland; aga1906@gmail.com
* Correspondence: mariolamroz2015@gmail.com; Tel.: +48-81-448-6840

Abstract: Introduction: The COVID-19 pandemic has changed the way prenatal education and obstetric care are provided. Pandemic-related anxiety, restrictions, limitations in perinatal care, and the inability to be accompanied by a loved one can have negative psychological consequences for future parents and their child. The aim of this study was to analyze the determinants and assess the anxiety of pregnant women in individual trimesters, as well as to learn about the sources of support and medical personnel proceeding methods. Materials and Methods: This research was conducted as a diagnostic survey, using the State-Trait Anxiety Inventory (STAI), Childbirth Anxiety Questionnaire (CAQ), and a standardized interview questionnaire, on 534 pregnant women in Poland. Resultsand Conclusions: The pregnant women, regardless of the trimester of pregnancy, are characterized by: increased anxiety level influenced by the current epidemiological situation, psychophysical condition, previous maternal experiences, participation in classes preparing for childbirth, organization of perinatal care, their relationship with a partner, and the presence of a loved one during childbirth. A negative correlation was shown between the level of childbirth anxiety and maternal experience, as well as the support of a doctor and midwife.

Keywords: childbirth anxiety; anxiety in pregnancy; COVID-19; SARS-CoV-2; pandemic; support; perinatal care; pregnancy; childbirth school

Citation: Iwanowicz-Palus, G.; Mróz, M.; Korda, A.; Marcewicz, A.; Palus, A. Perinatal Anxiety among Women during the COVID-19 Pandemic—A Cross-Sectional Study. *IJERPH* **2022**, *19*, 2603. https://doi.org/10.3390/ijerph19052603

Academic Editor: Francesca Agostini

Received: 19 January 2022
Accepted: 22 February 2022
Published: 24 February 2022

Publisher's Note: MDPI stays neutral with regard to jurisdictional claims in published maps and institutional affiliations.

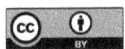

Copyright: © 2022 by the authors. Licensee MDPI, Basel, Switzerland. This article is an open access article distributed under the terms and conditions of the Creative Commons Attribution (CC BY) license (https://creativecommons.org/licenses/by/4.0/).

1. Introduction

When faced with situations threatening life or health, negative emotions appear. One of these is anxiety. When it is only moderate, it can increase the motivation to take action. However, as it worsens, it becomes a type of pathological emotion that has a negative impact on the person's psyche and health [1].

Perinatal anxiety has a significant influence on the health situation of the mother and the development of the child. It is a common problem, as one in ten mothers experience symptoms of anxiety in pregnancy and postpartum [2].

Due to their situation, pregnant women constitute a special group with regard to anxiety over their own health and that of their child. In each of the three trimesters of pregnancy, there are different stress factors thatchange or evolve over the course of the pregnancy. A particular stressor is the approach to childbirth, which is associated with perinatal anxiety. Moreover, a high level of anxiety is also associated with a decrease in the effectiveness of coping strategies [3–5].

Stress and anxiety in pregnancy can have a catastrophic effect both on the course of the pregnancy and on the condition of the child. Stress-induced pregnancy complications are a significant cause of morbidity and mortality in mothers and newborns [6,7].

Infants of mothers experiencing perinatal anxiety have a greater risk of developing negative effects. In this group of children, disorders of sleep, interaction with the mother, emotional development, and social relationships are more often observed. The consequences for the mother may be difficulties in breastfeeding and preterm labor [8].

Accurate identification of factors influencing the risk of perinatal anxiety may significantly contribute to the detection of disorders even before pregnancy. Early diagnosis reduces the severity and recurrence of symptoms [9].

Perinatal care in Poland is based on the Standard of Perinatal Care guidelines. This document discusses, inter alia, prenatal education and childbirth procedure. It emphasizes the importance of social, emotional, and informational support for the pregnant woman. It also guarantees the pregnant woman the choice of the place for giving birth, the opportunity of a family midwife, and the benefit of the support of a loved one [10].

The rapid progress of the SARS-CoV-2 pandemic has been a challenge for healthcare systems and has contributed to changes in the manner of delivering prenatal education and maternity care while safeguarding mother and child. Unfortunately, due to the pandemic and prevailing restrictions, access to prenatal education has become difficult. Moreover, there is only limited data on the effects coronavirus has on the pregnant woman and her baby [11,12]. The lack of such important information can also contribute to an increase in uneasiness and perinatal anxiety of pregnant women. In addition, factors such as pandemic-related anxiety, a time of isolation, restrictions, limitations on the process of childbirth and perinatal care, and the impossibility of being accompanied by a loved one have been associated with negative psychological consequences for future parents and their children [13,14].

Available empirical reports have shownthat the COVID-19 pandemic had a significant impact on the mental health of pregnant women. Perinatal anxiety was significantly higher during the pandemic period than before it. Moreover, the previous analyses indicate social support both from relatives and medical staff as a protective factor. The exact determinants of this phenomenon remain a subject of research [15–17].

The analysis of determinants of social anxiety in the context of health care system activities-perinatal care and antenatal education was an innovative aspect of our study. An important issue seems to be the assessment of psychophysical condition and its determinants, as well as the determination of correlations between psychological and physical condition and the level of anxiety experienced by pregnant women. Results presented inprevious studies have not determined the relationship between patients' expectations about labour and care provided by medical staff and perinatal anxiety, so we included this issue in our manuscript.

Due to the importance of the problem of fear of childbirth and the complexity of the topic resulting from the special situation caused by the COVID-19 pandemic, it is very important to assess the determinants of the phenomenon in pregnant women. Obtaining knowledge on the determinants of labour fear in the context of the COVID-19 pandemic might set new directions in psychopreventive actions in the population of pregnant women. Understanding the characteristics and identification of vulnerable groups of women will enable the implementation of appropriate psychoprophylactic interventions. As a result, it might contribute to reducing the risk of sequelae in the form of emotional disorders in the perinatal period.

The main aim of the study was to evaluate perinatal anxiety in pregnant women during the first wave of the COVID-19 pandemic.

Specific objectives:

- Learning about respondents' opinions on the support received from medical personnel and relatives.
- Assessment of received social support impact on the perinatal anxiety level.
- Assessment of perinatal care and education and its impact on experienced perinatal anxiety level.

- Analysis of the relation between psychological condition and experienced perinatal anxiety level.
- Assessment of the influence of selected obstetric factors on the experienced perinatal anxiety occurrence.

2. Materials and Methods

We declare that all procedures performed in studies involving human participants were in accordance with the ethical standards of the institutional and/or national research committee (the Bioethics Committee of the Medical University of Lublin: KE-0254/30-2019) and with the 1964 Helsinki declaration and its later amendments or comparable ethical standards. Informed consent was obtained from all individual participants included in the study.

2.1. Study Design and Participants

The study was conducted from 1 March 2020 to 2 June 2020, among women in the first (119), second (170), and third (245) trimesters of pregnancy, availing themselves of check-up visits to an OB-GYN and prenatal education conducted by a midwife or a family school in the territory of the Voivodeship of Lublin (eastern Poland).

The sample size was of a non-probalistic character. The study was conducted in selected medical centers providing free medical care for women under health insurance which is available to all pregnant women in Poland, regardless of their income level. From the beginning of a pregnancy, women in Poland are entitled to physician's care or midwife care (although in practice this is more rarely chosen). From the twenty-first week of the pregnancy, they can take advantage of free visits to a midwife for prenatal education.

Qualification criteria for the study were: agreement to participate in the diagnostic survey, being at least 18 years of age, and diagnosed with a single pregnancy. Persons undergoing psychotherapy or psychiatric treatment were excluded from the study.

In determining the sample size, we took into consideration the number of births from the beginning of 2020 to the moment of our project's implementation (January–February 2020). The number of births during this period was 3120, so the minimum number of respondents was calculated at 342 (with a maximum error of 5% and a confidence level of 95%). The respondents were informed that participation in the study was voluntary and anonymous and that the results would be used only for scientific purposes. The course and purpose of the study as well as the method of filling in the questionnaire were discussed with the respondents. Each participant received a questionnaire and an informed consent form. In order to preserve participants' anonymity, the questionnaires and consent forms were deposited into a ballot-type box, which was opened after the end of the study.

The original goal of the project was to study perinatal anxiety in women in the individual trimesters of pregnancy. Due to the pandemic, which occurred at the same time, the study was adapted to the epidemiological situation and this final version is the one presented in the manuscript. The first complete questionnaires, taking into account aspects of the epidemiological situation, were received on 20 March 2020, and are included in the study.There was a total of 556 participants in the study, out of which four persons did not give consent to participate in the diagnostic survey, plus 18 questionnaires were incomplete or filled in incorrectly. Therefore, 534 questionnaires qualified for statistical analysis. The efficiency ratio of the obtained data was 96.04% (Figure 1).

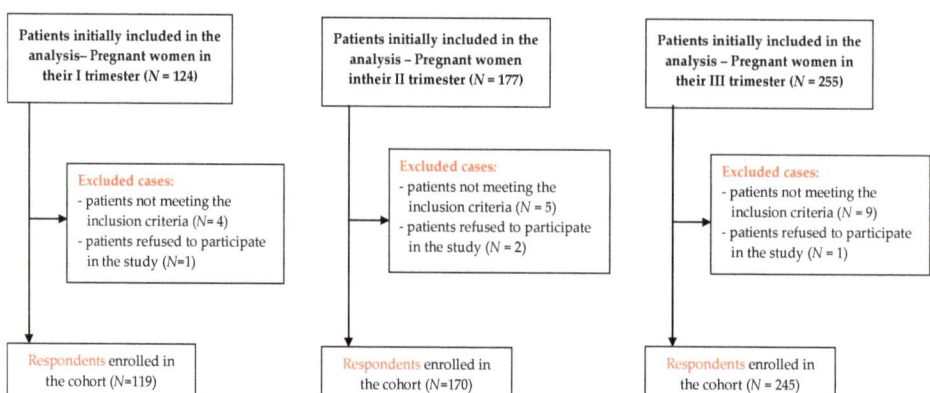

Figure 1. Recruitment process flowchart.

The study was conducted by diagnostic survey method, with the use of a questionnaire. The research tool was a questionnaire consisting of three sections:

- The State-Trait Anxiety Inventory (STAI) is a tool comprising two scales. The first part of the STAI (x-1) examines the level of anxiety as a current emotional state. It consists of 20 statements, for each of which the respondent chooses one of four possible answers (definitely, probably, probably not, definitely not). The responses to these statements describe the respondent's feelings while filling out the questionnaire. The second part (x-2) concerns anxiety understood as a personality trait. It also consists of 20 statements that the respondent can answer, using a four-point scale (almost never, sometimes, often, almost always). The responses for this second part provide a picture of how the respondent usually feels [18,19]. The Cronbach's alpha coefficient for the questionnaire for the studied group was 0.908 (x-1) and 0.869 (x-2), (Supplementary File).
- The Childbirth Anxiety Questionnaire (CAQ): a tool for gaining information on emotions associated with upcoming childbirth. The CAQ is made up of nine statements to which the respondent answers by choosing one of four categories (definitely, probably, probably not, definitely not) to which numerical values are assigned. The higher the score, the greater severity of childbirth anxiety [20]. The Cronbach's alpha reliability coefficient for the research group was 0.824, (Supplementary File).
- The questionnaire specially prepared for this study takes into consideration the characteristics of the women being researched as well as questions concerning the research topic. The respondents answered on a five-point Likert scale (1—definitely not, 5—definitely yes) on the topics of determinants of childbirth anxiety they felt and healthcare conditions in the time of the SARS-CoV-2 virus pandemic.

2.2. Statistical Analysis

SPSS software (IBM SPSS 25 Statistic, Chicago, IL, USA) was used in the data analysis. The analysis of descriptive statistics, chi-square tests of independence, analyses of Pearson's and rho Spearman's r correlation, Student's *t*-tests for independent samples, Mann–Whitney's tests, one-way ANOVA, and Kruskal–Wallis tests were performed with its help. The level of statistical significance was $p < 0.05$.

3. Results

Table 1 presents the characteristics of the women participating in the diagnostic survey, broken down according to the trimester of their pregnancy. Participating in the study were 534 women aged 18 to 48 years old (average age: 27.47 ± 3.92 years), of whom 119 (22.3%) were in their first trimester (1–13 weeks), 170 (31.8%) in the second trimester (14–26 weeks), and 245 (45.9%) in their third trimester (27–40 weeks) of pregnancy (Table 1).

Table 1. Participants' baseline characteristics.

Participants' Characteristics		I Trimester % (n)	II Trimester % (n)	III Trimester % (n)	Total
Age	<20	2.5 (3)	0.6 (1)	2.4 (6)	1.9 (10)
	20–29	78.2 (93)	64.1 (109)	61.2 (150)	65.9 (352)
	30–39	19.3 (23)	33.5 (57)	34.3 (84)	30.7 (164)
	≥40	-	1.8 (3)	2.0 (5)	1.5 (8)
Residence	urban—province capital	36.1 (43)	38.8 (66)	41.2 (101)	39.3 (210)
	other cities	40.3 (48)	37.6 (64)	33.5 (82)	36.3 (194)
	rural	23.5 (28)	23.5 (40)	25.3 (62)	24.3 (130)
Education	university	63.9 (76)	64.2 (109)	60.0 (147)	62.2 (332)
	other educational stages	36.1 (43)	35.8 (61)	40.0 (98)	37.8 (202)
Professional activity	currently does not work	18.5 (22)	65.9 (112)	81.2 (199)	68.2 (364)
	does not work professionally at all	44.5 (53)	13.5 (23)	6.1 (15)	11.2 (60)
	(she) works	37.0 (44)	20.6 (35)	12.7 (31)	20.8 (110)
Relationship status	married/informal relationship	89.1 (106)	90.0 (153)	92.7 (227)	91.0 (486)
	single	10.9 (13)	10.0 (17)	7.3 (18)	9.0 (48)
Self-reported financial standing	good	73.9 (88)	74.7 (127)	73.1 (179)	73.8 (394)
	bad	26.1 (31)	25.3 (43)	26.9 (66)	26.2 (140)
Having children	no, it's the first pregnancy	58.8 (70)	63.5 (108)	69.4 (170)	65.2 (348)
	one child	26.9 (32)	28.8 (49)	23.7 (58)	26.0 (139)
	two or more children	14.3 (17)	7.7 (13)	6.9 (17)	8.8 (47)
The person providing care	doctor	67.2 (80)	73.5 (125)	66.9 (164)	69.1 (369)
	midwife	5.9 (7)	1.2 (2)	0.4 (1)	1.9 (10)
	doctor and midwife	25.2 (30)	24.1 (41)	31.8 (78)	27.9 (149)
	she was not under the care of a doctor/midwife	1.7 (2)	1.2 (2)	0.8 (2)	1.1 (6)
Participation in Childbirth Classes	yes—face-to-face meeting with the midwife	30.3 (36)	18.8 (32)	31.8 (78)	27.3 (146)
	yes—video- and teleconferences	0.8 (1)	10.0 (17)	12.3 (30)	9.0 (48)
	no, she did not have the opportunity/possibility	5.9 (7)	14.1 (24)	25.7 (63)	17.6 (94)
	no, she was not interested	12.6 (15)	23.5 (40)	24.1 (59)	21.3 (114)
	has not participated yet but would like to	50.4 (60)	33.5 (57)	6.1 (15)	24.7 (132)

(n)—number, %—percentage.

The respondents were dominated by women residing in places within the voivodeship (39.3%), persons with higher education (62.2%), not working during their pregnancy (68.2%), in a married or informal relationship (91.0%), recognizing their material situation as good (73.8%), and not having maternal experience (65.2%). They were also mostly people whose current pregnancy was being attended by an OB-GYN (69.1%), as well as women preparing for childbirth through education, in direct contact with a midwife (27.3%) (Table 1).

In the first stage of the study, the level of anxiety of the respondents was assessed with regard to the stage of pregnancy. The women participating in the study, regardless of pregnancy trimester, were characterized by elevated, high, or very high degrees of anxiety. Most of the women in their second trimester (82.9%) obtained this result, whereas the women in their first (57.2%) or third (58.0%) trimester had very similar anxiety levels. More than half the women stated that their current pregnancy taking place in this epidemiological situation contributes to the anxiety they feel before childbirth (I: 57.2%; II: 56.5%; III: 60.0%). Women in their third semester agreed the most with this opinion ($p = 0.008$). Statistical analysis showed that respondents declaring that their pregnancy concluding in accordance with their previous ideas or plans would not reduce their feelings of anxiety represent a higher level of anxiety ($p = 0.004$), as compared to pregnant women who believe the opposite or who do not have an opinion on this topic (Table 2).

Table 2. Anxiety levels of the pregnant women according to pregnancy trimester.

Pregnancy Trimester	Childbirth Anxiety			
	Anxiety as a State		Anxiety as a Trait	
	M	SD	M	SD
I trimester	40.97	8.46	40.97	8.77
II trimester	41.12	9.24	42.35	8.63
III trimester	42.40	8.42	42.20	8.75
Statistic	$F = 1.58\ p = 0.207\ \eta^2 = 0.01$		$F = 1.03\ p = 0.35\ \eta^2 = <0.01$	

Anxiety Level	Pregnancy Trimester		
	I % (n)	II % (n)	III % (n)
Low	42.8 (51)	37 (63)	42 (103)
Elevated	11.8 (14)	16.5 (28)	15.5 (38)
High	15.1 (18)	25.2 (30)	14.7 (36)
Very High	30.3 (36)	41.20 (49)	27.8 (68)
Statistic	$Chi^2 = 2.6868\ p = 0.846\ C = 0.07$		

Pregnancy in the current epidemiological situation contributes to increased feelings of anxiety	I % (n)	II % (n)	III %(n)
Yes	57.2 (68)	56.5 (96)	60 (147)
No Opinion	11.8 (14)	13.5 (23)	17.1 (42)
No	31.1 (37)	30.0 (51)	22.9 (56)
Statistic	$Chi^2 = 43.5963\ p = 0.008\ C = 0.2747$		

Completion of the pregnancy in accord with prior ideas/plans would lessen feelings of anxiety.	Opinion					
	Yes		No Opinion		No	
	Average Rank	Me	Average Rank	Me	Average Rank	Me
Childbirth Anxiety	351.05	15.00	246.56	14.00	265.72	18.00
Statistic	$p = 0.004$					

(Me)—median, (M)—mean, (SD)—standard deviation.

An assessment was made of the attitude of pregnant women regarding support from their loved ones and from medical personnel in the current epidemiological situation. Their responses show that the vast majority of them consider the support of their OB-GYN to be sufficient (I: 76.5%, II: 79.4%, III: 75.5%). Women in their third trimester (42.4%) cited support from the midwife as adequate, while the respondents in the first (52.9%) and second trimester (52.9%) did not have an opinion on this matter. The respondents stated that the support of their loved ones (partner, relatives, friends) is important (I: 95.8%; II: 100%; III: 99.2%, $p = 0.0260$) and, in the current situation, they find it to be adequate (I: 91.6%; II: 90.6%; III: 89.4%). The majority of respondents also gave positive answers to a question about the influence of their relationship with their partner (I: 86.5%; II: 91.8%; III: 93.5%) and the presence of a loved one during childbirth (I: 77.3%; II: 78.2%; III: 78.8%) have on their level of childbirth anxiety (Table 3).

Table 3. Opinions of the respondents on specific sources of support and methods of treatment, by pregnancy trimester.

Source of Support/Factors	Pregnancy Trimester	Yes % (n)	No Opinion/ Not Applicable % (n)	No % (n)	Statistic
In the current epidemiological situation, the support of the doctor in charge of the pregnancy was appropriate	I II III	76.5 (91) 79.4 (135) 75.5 (185)	16.8 (20) 7.6 (13) 9.8 (24)	6.7 (8) 12.9 (22) 14.7 (36)	$Chi^2 = 10.2185$ $p = 0.036$ $C = 0.1370$
In the current epidemiological situation, the support of the midwife providing prenatal education was appropriate	I II III	42.0 (50) 31.2 (53) 42.4 (104)	52.9 (63) 52.9 (90) 34.7 (85)	5.0 (6) 15.8 (27) 22.8 (56)	$Chi^2 = 28.9580$ $p = 7.972$ $C = 0.2268$
The support of loved ones (partner, family, friends) is important	I II III	95.8 (114) 100 (170) 99.2 (243)	3.4 (4) - 0.8 (2)	0.8 (1) - -	$Chi^2 = 11.0432$ $p = 0.026$ $C = 0.1423$
I am receiving sufficient support from my loved ones	I II III	91.6 (109) 90.6 (154) 89.4 (219)	3.4 (4) 2.9 (5) 2.4 (6)	5.0 (6) 6.5 (11) 8.2 (20)	$Chi^2 = 1.5008$ $p = 0.826$ $C = 0.0529$
My marital/partnership relations have an influence on the level of childbirth anxiety	I II III	86.5 (103) 91.8 (156) 93.5 (229)	7.6 (9) 4.1 (7) 2.0 (5)	5.9 (7) 4.1 (7) 4.5 (11)	$Chi^2 = 7.1569$ $p = 0.127$ $C = 0.1150$
The presence of a companion during childbirth helps to lessen perinatal anxiety	I II III	77.3 (92) 78.2 (133) 78.8 (193)	13.4 (16) 18.8 (32) 13.9 (34)	9.2 (12) 3.0 (5) 7.3 (18)	$Chi^2 = 10.0701$ $p = 0.089$ $C = 0.1360$
Birthing school/prenatal education prepares you for childbirth physically	I II III	61.4 (73) 56.5 (96) 47.3 (116)	25.2 (30) 33.5 (57) 29.4 (72)	13.4 (16) 10.0 (17) 23.3 (57)	$Chi^2 = 16.5734$ $p = 0.002$ $C = 0.1734$
Birthing school/prenatal education prepares you for childbirth psychologically	I II III	71.4 (85) 72.4 (123) 69.3 (170)	21.0 (25) 22.9 (39) 21.6 (53)	7.5 (9) 4.7 (8) 8.9 (22)	$Chi^2 = 2.7928$ $p = 0.593$ $C = 0.0721$
The subject of childbirth anxiety was brought up during meetings with the midwife/in birthing school	I II III	33.6 (40) 34.7 (59) 45.7 (112)	55.5 (66) 58.2 (99) 42.9 (105)	10.9 (13) 7.1 (12) 11.5 (28)	$Chi^2 = 11.9339$ $p = 0.017$ $C = 0.1478$
Birthing school/prenatal education helps for coping with perinatal anxiety	I II III	55.5 (66) 57.0 (97) 57.9 (140)	32.8 (39) 34.1 (58) 33.1 (81)	11.8 (14) 8.9 (15) 9.8 (24)	$Chi^2 = 0.7100$ $p = 0.950$ $C = 0.0364$
The subject of SARS-CoV-2 (coronavirus) was brought up during meetings/teleconferences with the family midwife or in classes at the birthing school	I II III	16.8 (20) 17.6 (30) 36.7 (90)	77.3 (92) 75.9 (129) 53.5 (131)	9.36 (7) 13.37 (11) 19.27 (24)	$Chi^2 = 31.9594$ $p = 0.001$ $C = 0.2376$
The current epidemiological situation was discussed during meetings/video conferences with the family midwife or in classes at the birthing school	I II III	17.6 (21) 18.2 (31) 38.8 (95)	78.2 (98) 75.3 (128) 53.1 (130)	1.7 (5) 1.8 (11) 4.1 (20)	$Ch^2 = 33.8456$ $p < 0.001$ $C = 0.2441$
Perinatal care has an influence on feelings of childbirth anxiety	I II III	73.1 (87) 78.8 (134) 79.2 (194)	21.0 (25) 18.8 (32) 12.7 (31)	5.8 (7) 2.4 (4) 8.1 (20)	$Chi^2 = 10.4824$ $p = 0.033$ $C = 0.1387$
Knowing about the standards of perinatal care helps in coping with anxiety	I II III	58.8 (70) 75.2 (128) 79.2 (194)	31.1 (37) 15.9 (27) 13.1 (32)	10.1 (12) 8.9 (15) 7.7 (19)	$Chi^2 = 18.2418$ $p = 0.001$ $C = 0.1817$
Concluding the pregnancy by means of Cesarean section would lessen anxiety	I II III	31.1 (37) 26.4 (45) 23.3 (57)	14.3 (17) 22.4 (38) 19.2 (47)	54.6 (65) 51.2 (87) 57.5 (141)	$Chi^2 = 5.0353$ $p = 0.283$ $C = 0.0966$

About half of the respondents considered birthing schools or individual prenatal education provided by a midwife to be helpful in preparing physically (I: 61.4%, II: 56.5%, III: 47.3%, $p = 0.002$) and psychologically (I: 71.4%, II: 72.4%, III: 69.3%, $p < 0.05$) for childbirth. According to women in the third trimester of pregnancy (45.7%), childbirth anxiety during the current epidemiological situation was also discussed during the classes, while other respondents did not have an opinion on this subject ($p = 0.017$). When asked whether the topic of coronavirus (I: 77.3%, II: 75.9%, III: 53.5) and childbirth in the current epidemiological situation (I: 78.2%, II: 75.3%, III: 53.1%) were discussed during meetings/videoconferences with a family midwife or in birthing school, most of the respondents answered that they did not have an opinion on this subject because they had not had the opportunity to take advantage of such forms of prenatal education or were not interested in them. Regardless of their stage of pregnancy, the respondents were of the opinion that birthing school and perinatal education are helpful in coping with perinatal anxiety (I: 55.5%, II: 57.0%, III: 57.9%) (Table 3).

The pregnant women taking part in the study were asked to give their opinion on factors that might lower childbirth anxiety. Respondents in all three trimesters said that perinatal care (I: 73.1%, II: 78.8%, III: 79.2%) and familiarity with perinatal care standards (I: 58.8%, II: 75.2%, III: 79.2%) had an effect on feelings of anxiety before childbirth ($p < 0.05$). On the other hand, the respondents did not agree with the statement that concluding the pregnancy by Cesarean section would mitigate anxiety (I: 54.6%, II: 51.2%, III: 57.5%) (Table 3).

In the next stage of the study, we looked at the opinions on social support and factors influencing the level of childbirth anxiety. The results were also statistically significant ($p < 0.05$).

Respondents more highly valuing the support of loved ones, their attending physician, and the midwife providing prenatal education agreed more with the statement that they are in good psychological condition ($p = 0.001$). In turn, the pregnant women saying they considered the support of medical personnel as sufficient assessed their physical condition as good to a greater extent (Table 4).

Table 4. Differences in respondents' opinions on social support and factors influencing childbirth anxiety.

Psychological Condition	Sources of Support					
	Loved Ones		Attending Physician		Family Midwife Providing Prenatal Education	
	Average Rank	Me	Average Rank	Me	Average Rank	Me
Bad	208.04	4.00	228.13	4.00	226.22	3.00
Good	283.64	5.00	278.19	4.00	278.70	3.00
Statistic	Z = −5.16	p = 0.001	Z = −3.27	p = 0.001	Z = −3.40	p = 0.001

Physical Condition	Loved Ones		Attending Physician		Family midwife providing prenatal education	
	Average Rank	Me	Average Rank	Me	Average Rank	Me
Bad	261.43	4.00	249.70	4.00	241.72	3.00
Good	272.42	5.00	281.92	4.00	288.38	3.00
Statistic	Z = −0.91	p = 0.363	Z = −2.56	p = 0.011	Z = −3.67	p < 0.001

Manner of pregnancy conclusion	Factors Affecting Childbirth Anxiety					
	Perinatal care and Birthing school		Pregnancy in the current epidemiological situation contributes to increased feelings of anxiety		Concluding the pregnancy by means of Cesarean section would lessen anxiety	
	M	SD	M	SD	M	SD
Not Applicable	22.69	3.50	3.65	1.20	2.48	1.31
Delivery without Complications	22.15	4.24	3.17	1.37	2.01	1.21
Delivery with Complications	22.25	3.96	3.50	1.33	3.12	1.48
Statistic	F = 1.09	p = 0.336	F = 5.34	p = 0.005	F = 19.95	p < 0.001

Participation in Childbirth Classes	Perinatal care and Birthing school		Pregnancy in the current epidemiological situation contributes to increased feelings of anxiety		Concluding the pregnancy by means of Cesarean section would lessen anxiety	
	M	SD	M	SD	M	SD
Yes	24.13	3.76	3.58	1.25	2.46	1.39
No	21.60	3.37	3.49	1.29	2.58	1.38
Statistic	T = 7.98	p < 0.001	T = 0.80	p = 0.426	T = −0.95	p = 0.341

(Me)—median, (M)—mean, (SD)—standard deviation.

The statement that their current pregnancy contributes to an increase in anxiety was most strongly agreed to by women who are first-time mothers (M = 3.65) and, to a lesser degree, by respondents whose previous delivery was uneventful (M = 3.17, $p = 0.005$). Furthermore, compared to women in their first pregnancy (M = 2.48) and respondents who had given birth without complications (M = 2.01), pregnant women who had had a delivery burdened with complications (M = 3.12) stated significantly more often that concluding their pregnancy by Cesarean section would reduce feelings of anxiety.

It was also shown that the respondents participating in childbirth preparation classes (M = 24.13) significantly more often ($p < 0.001$) stated that the organization of perinatal care and prenatal education/birthing school reduced childbirth anxiety, compared to those who did not use such activities (M = 21.60), (Table 4).

Tables 5 and 6 present results of analysis between childbirth anxiety and specific factors: psychophysical condition, maternal experience, manner of conclusion of a previous pregnancy, participation in childbirth preparation classes, and support of medical staff. The data obtained indicate significant relationships among the selected variables ($p < 0.05$).

It has been shown that pregnant women in poor mental ($p < 0.001$) or physical ($p < 0.001$) condition are exposed to a higher level of anxiety as a state and anxiety as a trait than women assessing their psychophysical condition as good (Table 5).

This analysis indicated a statistically significant effect for anxiety as a trait ($p = 0.019$): the women not participating in childbirth preparation classes are characterized by a greater severity of anxiety as a personality trait than are women receiving prenatal education (Table 5).

Table 5. Differences in assessment of childbirth anxiety and factors influencing it.

Psychological Condition	Childbirth Anxiety			
	Anxiety as a State		Anxiety as a Trait	
	M	SD	M	SD
Bad	48.75	7.38	49.23	6.46
Good	39.75	8.03	40.00	8.20
Statistic	T = 10.80	$p < 0.001$	T = 12.72	$p < 0.001$
Physical Condition	Anxiety as a State		Anxiety as a Trait	
	M	SD	M	SD
Bad	44.13	8.57	44.95	8.30
Good	39.68	8.32	39.55	8.31
Statistic	T = 6.05	$p < 0.001$	T = 7.48	$p < 0.001$
The course of the previous birth	Anxiety as a State		ANXIETY AS A Trait	
	M	SD	M	SD
Not Applicable	41.57	8.42	42.12	8.67
Delivery without Complications	41.79	8.62	41.76	8.78
Delivery with Complications	41.84	9.52	41.77	8.86
Statistic	F = 0.05	$p = 0.948$	F = 0.10	$p = 0.901$
Participation in Childbirth Classes	Anxiety as a State		Anxiety as a Trait	
	M	SD	M	SD
Yes	41.21	9.04	40.80	8.77
No	41.94	8.52	42.64	8.63
Statistic	T = −0.92	$p = 0.356$	T = −2.35	$p = 0.019$

(M)—mean, (SD)—standard deviation.

Analysis of the research showed a statistically significant ($p < 0.05$) negative correlation between the level of childbirth anxiety as a state and anxiety as a trait, as well as the support of an attending OB-GYN(respectively: r = −0.15, r = −0.17) and a family midwife providing prenatal education (r = −0.13, r = −0.18), (Table 6).

Table 6. Analysis of the correlation between childbirth anxiety and the assessment of support from medical personnel and maternal experience.

Factors		Anxiety as a State	Anxiety as a Trait
Support during the current epidemiological situation from the OB-GYN treating the pregnancy	r	−0.15	−0.17
	p	<0.001	<0.001
Support during the current epidemiological situation from a family midwife providing prenatal education	r	−0.13	−0.18
	p	0.002	<0.001
Maternal experience	rho	0.01	−0.02
	p	0.882	0.628
Number of pregnancies	rho	0.02	−0.01
	p	0.653	0.860

r—Pearson's correlation coefficient, rho—Spearman's rho.

The design of the research questionnaire also allowed respondents to freely express themselves about perinatal care, in particular childbirth during the SARS-CoV-2 virus pandemic. Several women in the second or third trimester of pregnancy shared their opinions; a few selected statements are presented below:

"I am worried about the current epidemiological situation and the impossibility of family members being present for the delivery; even more, I am stressed about giving birth by myself."

"I have brief attacks of hysteria, but they pass quickly."

"The current epidemic greatly increases my anxiety before giving birth. My husband has promised to be with me for the delivery, our due-date is the end of September. Knowing that having family members at the delivery has still not been restored yet at the hospitals in my region causes additional, senseless anxiety and panic. And to what purpose? I am not afraid of a virus, I am afraid of trauma and post-partum depression caused by having my rights, peace, and dreams taken away. I cannot imagine being alone in such a difficult situation as giving birth to my first child."

Analysis of the responses shows that for women who had made long efforts to become pregnant and had a difficult gynecological examination, anxiety associated with labor and delivery was concerned more with the health of the child than with their own psychophysical comfort regarding support and help from their loved ones, including being accompanied by their partner:

"The long years of fighting infertility have certainly influenced my perception of anxiety and childbirth, because I know that I may not have a second chance, so I am more afraid. And now this epidemic . . . "

"More than labor and delivery, I am afraid about successfully carrying the pregnancy, due to an earlier miscarriage and long, in my opinion, attempts to have a baby. My desire for a child is so great that I am not interested in the fact that I will feel pain, I am ready for anything, just to give birth successfully, especially in this situation with coronavirus."

4. Discussion

In the perinatal period, as a result of the psychological and physiological changes taking place, a woman is particularly exposed to an increased risk of anxiety. The difficult epidemiological situation of the COVID-19 pandemic and the restrictions associated with it, as well as fluctuating socio-economic changes, can additionally increase the spread of psychological problems among perinatal women [21,22].

Women who were pregnant during the first wave of the COVID-19 pandemic, regardless of trimester, were characterized by at least an elevated level of perinatal anxiety.

In our analysis, conducted during the first wave of COVID-19 pandemic, the majority of pregnant women were characterized by at least an elevated level of perinatal anxiety.

The respondents claimed that pregnancy in the current epidemiological situation contributes to increased feelings of anxiety. The level of perinatal anxiety experienced by the respondents was also influenced by maternal experience, the course of the previous delivery, and the psychophysical condition. Social support and perinatal care were important for the occurrence of labour anxiety.

In their study, Ahmad et al. observed that during the pandemic the level of anxiety in pregnant women increased in comparison with the period before the epidemic [21].

The findings of this review suggest that the respondents, regardless of which trimester of pregnancy, were characterized by elevated, high, or even very high levels of anxiety. In contrast, Shrestha's research showed that manifestation of anxiety symptoms was more intense in women in the first trimester of pregnancy [23]. On the other hand, other reports show that the highest level of anxiety was shown by pregnant women in the third trimester of pregnancy [24]. Kahyaoglu, in turn, showed no correlation between the week of pregnancy and the severity of perinatal anxiety [25].

The results obtained by our own research indicate that pregnant women assess the support received by their loved ones as important. A statistically significant relationship was found between the mental condition of pregnant women and the support they received from their loved ones during the COVID-19 pandemic. The effects we present correspond to the reports of Naz et al., which demonstrate a strong relationship between family support received by pregnant women and reduction of their feelings of childbirth anxiety. Women who received support from their loved ones declared milder feelings of childbirth anxiety. In turn, respondents who did not receive this kind of support felt a significantly higher level of anxiety [26].

The results of our analysis indicate a relationship between the support received by pregnant women from medical staff and anxiety of the pregnant women. The available research confirms that pregnant women have a particular need for support from medical personnel. This is very relevant during the COVID-19 pandemic. The support provided them reduces stress and anxiety, increasing their quality-of-life assessment. It has a positive effect on psychophysical well-being, reducing the anxiety associated with hospitalization [27–29]. According to reports by other authors, the support of medical staff was not able to compensate for the lack of a loved one. This absence caused a feeling of helplessness and intensified perinatal anxiety [30]. The social distancing in force everywhere can constitute a serious problem resulting in psychological discomfort, as social support is of particular importance in buffering the negative effects of stress and anxiety [31].

Our findings indicate that pregnant women attending birthing schools showed less severe anxiety as a personality trait than women not choosing to participate in prenatal education. The outcomes of analyses by Aksoy et al. concur with these results [12]. Other researchers have observed particularly helpful effects from participating in birthing schools among first-time mothers. This group feels great stress in adapting to the role of motherhood. Prenatal education makes possible the preparation of young mothers for a new situation. Moreover, positive effects can be seen in the collaboration of the first-time mother with the obstetric team during childbirth. Thanks to the emotional support of other women in the same situation, a significant reduction of perinatal anxiety comes from the exchange of experiences in organized group activities [32].

Karlström et al. explain the limited effects of participation in childbirth classes among multiparous women by the stronger influence of previous obstetric experiences, which have formed the pregnant woman's attitude regarding the next birth [33].

Results of research by Swift et al. demonstrated that women who had expressed feelings of childbirth anxiety declared a decrease in them under the influence of participation in birthing school classes [34]. Kuciel et al., conducting research during the COVID-19 pandemic, showed that the knowledge acquired by respondents in prenatal education did not affect their level of perinatal anxiety [35]. Hassanzadeh, guided by the positive effect of studies on the benefits of participation in prenatal classes, suggests implementing participation in birthing training as part of standard prenatal care [36].

Research studies have sought evidence of the influence of the ordering of pregnancies on the mother's mental health and related factors. Farewell et al. indicated moderate or severe intensification of perinatal anxiety symptoms in more than half of the respondents who were in their first pregnancy [37]. In the group we studied, women in their first pregnancies agreed to the greatest degree with the statement that their current pregnancy was contributing to increased anxiety. This similarity of the results may be related to the natural tendency to fear the unknown, or to an intensified conviction that childbirth is associated with medical intervention.

Our probe showed that pregnant women are not of the opinion that having a Cesarean section eases perinatal anxiety. An analysis conducted by Mehdizadehkashi was dominated by respondents characterized by a high level of anxiety, of whom as many as 39% asked for an elective Cesarean section. In this same group, 86.4% of respondents felt frustrated because of the COVID-19 pandemic [38]. In the reports byMortazavi et al., the main predictor of pregnancy being concluded by Cesarean section was the pregnant woman's fear of childbirth and the pain associated with it [39]. Research conducted by Størksen also shows that the main reason for a woman choosing Cesarean section without clear medical indication is fear of childbirth [40]. Despite increasingly frequent study results which indicate a growing number of patients awaiting elective Cesarean section, Malhotra demonstrates in his analyses that during the first year of the COVID-19 pandemic, the number of Cesarean sections in New York remained at a level similar to that recorded in the preceding years [41].

The existing research analysis shows how important it is to properly adjust the perinatal care system to the current epidemiological situation. It shows the importance of proper care implementation, despite the difficulties related to, inter alia, restrictions, as well as support from medical staff. Bearing in mind the potential negative psychological consequences of social isolation during the COVID-19 pandemic, there is a need to conduct further research on the determinants of perinatal anxiety and to identify protective factors, the knowledge of which will enable the provision of appropriate care to pregnant women.

Strengths and Limitations of the Study

The presented results come from an analysis based on a subjective assessment of Level of COVID-19 Anxiety in pregnant women. Although we used scales that are considered sensitive research tools, they are based on subjective feelings and do not include objective criteria of clinical symptoms.It is worth conducting a study where the same analysis for pandemic and non-pandemic situations could be performed to better understand which factor has a greater influence on the level of anxiety (pregnancy, preparation, social support or the pandemic situation itself). Moreover, the study did not include the assessment of individual and sociodemographic characteristics (e.g., low-risk pregnancies, high-risk pregnancies, education, place of residence, self-reported financial standing). This is a cross-sectional study, so no claims can be made about causality.

The advantage of our work is the size of the study group (534 people), and the fact that our questionnaire was delivered to each respondent in person. It should also be emphasized that the study utilized a standardized tool, which allows other authors studying the issue to compare research results and explore the subject.

Despite certain limitations, our study can constitute a reference point for further exploration of the problem of COVID-19-related childbirth anxiety. Moreover, it can make possible a rapid initiation of appropriate psychoprophylactic interventions in a given epidemiological situation.

Supplementary Materials: The following supporting information can be downloaded at: https://www.mdpi.com/article/10.3390/ijerph19052603/s1, Supplementary File: The Childbirth Anxiety Questionnaire.

Author Contributions: Conceptualization, G.I.-P. and M.M.; methodology, G.I.-P. and M.M.; formal analysis, M.M. and A.K.; investigation, G.I.-P. and A.K.; resources, A.K.; data curation, A.K.; writing–original draft preparation, G.I.-P., M.M., A.P. and A.M.; writing–review and editing, G.I.-P., M.M., A.P. and A.M.; supervision, G.I.-P. and M.M.; project administration, G.I.-P. All authors have read and agreed to the published version of the manuscript.

Funding: This research received no external funding.

Institutional Review Board Statement: We declare that all procedures performed in studies involving human participants were in accordance with the ethical standards of the institutional and/or national research committee (the Bioethics Committee of the Medical University of Lublin: KE-0254/30-2019) and with the 1964 Helsinki declaration and its later amendments or comparable ethical standards.

Informed Consent Statement: Informed consent was obtained from all subjects involved in the study.

Data Availability Statement: Data are available upon reasonable request.

Acknowledgments: The authors are deeply grateful to all patients participating in this study.

Conflicts of Interest: The authors declare no conflict of interest.

References

1. Kef, K. COVID-19: The Level of Knowledge, Anxiety and Symptom Presentation. *Psychol. Res. Behav. Manag.* **2021**, *14*, 541–548. [CrossRef] [PubMed]
2. Stojanov, J.; Stankovic, M.; Zikic, O.; Stankovic, M.; Stojanov, A. The risk for nonpsychotic postpartum mood and anxiety disorders during the COVID-19 pandemic. *Int.J. Psychiatry Med.* **2021**, *56*, 228–239. [CrossRef] [PubMed]
3. Bayrampour, H.; Ali, E.; McNeil, D.; Benzies, K.; MacQueen, G.; Tough, S. Pregnancy-related anxiety: A concept analysis. *Int. J. Nurs. Stud.* **2016**, *55*, 115–130. [CrossRef]
4. Nechita, D.; Nechita, F.; Motorga, R. A review of influence the anxiety exerts on humanlife. *Rom. J. Morphol. Embryol.* **2018**, *59*, 1045–1051. [PubMed]
5. Dennis, C.L.; Falah-Hassani, K.; Shiri, R. Prevalence of antenatal and postnatal anxiety: Systematic review and meta-analysis. *Br. J. Psychiatry* **2017**, *210*, 315–323. [CrossRef] [PubMed]
6. Cardwell, M.S. Stress: Pregnancy considerations. *Obstet. Gynecol. Surv.* **2013**, *68*, 119–129. [CrossRef]
7. Mah, B.L.; Pringle, K.G.; Weatherall, L.; Keogh, L.; Schumacher, T.; Eades, S.; Brown, A.; Lumbers, E.R.; Roberts, C.T.; Diehm, C.; et al. Pregnancy stress, healthy pregnancy and birth outcomes-the need for early preventative approaches in pregnant Australian Indigenous women: A prospective longitudinal cohort study. *J. Dev. Orig. Health Dis.* **2019**, *10*, 31–38. [CrossRef]
8. Polte, C.; Junge, C.; von Soest, T.; Seidler, A.; Eberhard-Gran, M.; Garthus-Niegel, S. Impact of maternal perinatal anxiety on social-emotional development of 2-year-olds, a prospective study of Norwegian mothers and their offspring: The impact of perinatal anxiety on child development. *Matern. Child Health J.* **2019**, *23*, 386–396. [CrossRef]
9. Noonan, M.; Jomeen, J.; Doody, O. A review of the involvement of partners and family members in psychosocial interventions for supporting women at risk of or experiencing perinatal depression and anxiety. *Int. J. Environ. Res. Public Health* **2021**, *18*, 5396. [CrossRef]
10. Rozporządzenie Ministra Zdrowia z dnia 16 Sierpnia 2018 r. w Sprawie Standardu Organizacyjnego Opieki Okołoporodowej. Dz.U. 1756. 2018. Available online: https://isap.sejm.gov.pl/isap.nsf/download.xsp/WDU20180001756/O/D20181756.pdf (accessed on 16 December 2021).
11. Wang, C.L.; Liu, Y.Y.; Wu, C.H.; Wang, C.Y.; Wang, C.H.; Long, C.Y. Impact of COVID-19 on pregnancy. *Int. J. Med. Sci.* **2021**, *18*, 763–767. [CrossRef]
12. Derya, Y.A.; Altiparmak, S.; AkÇa, E.; GÖkbulut, N.; Yilmaz, A.N. Pregnancy and birth planning during COVID-19. The effects of tele-education offered to pregnant women on prenatal distress and pregnancy-related anxiety. *Midwifery* **2021**, *92*, 102877. [CrossRef]
13. Polizzi, C.; Burgio, S.; Lavanco, G.; Alesi, M. Parental Distress and perception of children's executive functioning after the first COVID-19 lockdown in Italy. *J. Clin. Med.* **2021**, *10*, 4170. [CrossRef] [PubMed]
14. Karaçam, Z.; Ançel, G. Depression, anxiety and influencing factors in pregnancy: A study in a Turkish population. *Midwifery* **2009**, *25*, 344–356. [CrossRef] [PubMed]
15. Basu, A.; Kim, H.H.; Basaldua, R.; Choi, K.W.; Charron, L.; Kelsall, N.; Hernandez-Diaz, S.; Wyszynski, D.F.; Koenen, K.C. A cross-national study of factors associated with women's perinatal mental health and wellbeing during the COVID-19 pandemic. *PLoS ONE* **2021**, *16*, e0249780. [CrossRef]
16. Zhang, J.; Yu, H.; Gao, Y.; Xu, Q.; Yin, Y.; Zhou, R. Prevalence of Anxiety and Depression among Pregnant Women during the COVID-19 Pandemic: A Systematic Review and Meta-Analysis. 2020. Available online: https://assets.researchsquare.com/files/rs-87129/v1/7c0115bb_a955_417c-a457-2725e9eff1ab.pdf?c=1631857548 (accessed on 18 January 2022). [CrossRef]

17. Vacaru, S.; Beijers, R.; Browne, P.D. The risk and protective factors of heightened prenatal anxiety and depression during the COVID-19 lockdown. *Sci. Rep.* **2021**, *11*, 20261. [CrossRef]
18. Liu, K.; Chen, Y.; Wu, D.; Lin, R.; Wang, Z.; Pan, L. Effects of progressive muscle relaxation on anxiety and sleep quality in patients with COVID-19. *Complement. Ther. Clin. Pract.* **2020**, *39*, 101132. [CrossRef]
19. Janik, K.; Cwalina, U.; Iwanowicz-Palus, G.; Cybulski, M. An assessment of the level of COVID-19 anxiety among pregnant women in Poland: A cross-sectional study. *J. Clin. Med.* **2021**, *10*, 5869. [CrossRef]
20. Putyński, L.; Paciorek, M. Kwestionariusz lęku porodowego (KLP II) wersja zrewidowana–konstrukcja i właściwości psychometryczne. *Acta Univ. Lodziensis. Folia Psychol.* **2008**, *12*, 129–133.
21. Ahmad, M.; Vismara, L. The psychological impact of COVID-19 pandemic on women's mental health during pregnancy: A rapid evidence review. *Int. J. Environ. Res. Public Health* **2021**, *18*, 7112. [CrossRef]
22. Brooks, S.K.; Webster, R.K.; Smith, L.E.; Woodland, L.; Wessely, S.; Greenberg, N.; Rubin, G.J. The psychological impact of quarantine and how to reduce it: Rapid review of the evidence. *Lancet* **2020**, *395*, 912–920. [CrossRef]
23. Shrestha, S.; Pun, K.D. Anxiety on primigravid women attending antenatal care: A hospital based cross-sectional study. *Kathmandu Univ. Med. J. (KUMJ)* **2018**, *16*, 23–27.
24. Chan, C.Y.; Lee, A.M.; Lam, S.K.; Lee, C.P.; Leung, K.Y.; Koh, Y.W.; Tang, C.S.K. Antenatal anxiety in the first trimester: Risk factors and effects on anxiety and depression in the third trimester and 6-week postpartum. *Open J. Psychiatry* **2013**, 301–310. [CrossRef]
25. Kahyaoglu, S.H.; Kucukkaya, B. Anxiety, depression, and related factors in pregnant women during the COVID-19 pandemic in Turkey: A web-based cross-sectional study. *Perspect. Psychiatr. Care* **2021**, *57*, 860–868. [CrossRef] [PubMed]
26. Naz, S.; Muhammad, D.; Ahmad, A. Pregnant women perceptions regarding their husbands and in-laws' support during pregnancy: A qualitative study. *Pan. Afr. Med. J.* **2021**, *39*, 229. [CrossRef]
27. Iwanowicz-Palus, G.; Mróz, M.; Bień, A.; Jurek, K. Social support and subjective assessment of psychophysical condition, health, and satisfaction with quality of life among women after pregnancy loss. *BMC Pregnancy Childbirth* **2021**, *21*, 750. [CrossRef] [PubMed]
28. Bäckström, C.; Thorstensson, S.; Pihlblad, J.; Forsman, A.C.; Larsson, M. Parents' experiences of receiving professional support through extended home visits during pregnancy and early childhood-A Phenomenographic study. *Front. Public Health* **2021**, *9*, 578917. [CrossRef]
29. Brooks, S.K.; Weston, D.; Greenberg, N. Psychological impact of infectious disease outbreaks on pregnant women: Rapid evidence review. *Public Health* **2020**, *189*, 26–36. [CrossRef]
30. Baran, J.; Leszczak, J.; Baran, R.; Biesiadecka, A.; Weres, A.; Czenczek-Lewandowska, E.; Kalandyk-Osinko, K. Prenatal and Postnatal Anxiety and Depression in Mothers during the COVID-19 Pandemic. *J. Clin. Med.* **2021**, *10*, 3193. [CrossRef]
31. Reid, K.M.; Taylor, M.G. Social support, stress, and maternal postpartum depression: A comparison of supportive relationships. *Soc. Sci. Res.* **2015**, *54*, 246–262. [CrossRef]
32. Hassanzadeh, R.; Abbas-Alizadeh, F.; Meedya, S.; Mohammad-Alizadeh-Charandabi, S.; Mirghafourvand, M. Primiparous women's knowledge and satisfaction based on their attendance at childbirth preparation classes. *Nurs. Open* **2021**, *8*, 2558–2566. [CrossRef]
33. Karlström, A.; Nystedt, A.; Johansson, M.; Hildingsson, I. Behind the myth–few women prefer caesarean section in the absence of medical or obstetrical factors. *Midwifery* **2011**, *27*, 620–627. [CrossRef] [PubMed]
34. Swift, E.M.; Zoega, H.; Stoll, K.; Avery, M.; Gottfreðsdóttir, H. Enhanced antenatal care: Combining one-to-one and group Antenatal Care models to increase childbirth education and address childbirth fear. *Women Birth* **2021**, *34*, 381–388. [CrossRef] [PubMed]
35. Kuciel, N.; Sutkowska, E.; Biernat, K.; Hap, K.; Mazurek, J.; Demczyszak, I. Assessment of the level of anxiety and pain in women who do and do not attend childbirth classes during the SARS-CoV-2 pandemic. *Risk Manag. Healthc Policy* **2021**, *14*, 4489–4497. [CrossRef] [PubMed]
36. Hassanzadeh, R.; Abbas-Alizadeh, F.; Meedya, S.; Mohammad-Alizadeh-Charandabi, S.; Mirghafourvand, M. Fear of childbirth, anxiety and depression in three groups of primiparous pregnant women not attending, irregularly attending and regularly attending childbirth preparation classes. *BMC Womens Health* **2020**, *20*, 180. [CrossRef]
37. Farewell, C.V.; Jewell, J.; Walls, J.; Leiferman, J.A. A Mixed-Methods Pilot Study of Perinatal Risk and Resilience During COVID-19. *J. Prim. Care Community Health* **2020**, *11*, 2150132720944074. [CrossRef] [PubMed]
38. Mehdizadehkashi, A.; Chaichian, S.; Haghighi, L.; Eshraghi, N.; Bordbar, A.; Hashemi, N.; Derakhshan, R.; Mirgalobayat, S.; Rokhgireh, S.; Tahermanesh, K. The Impact of COVID-19 Pandemic on Stress and Anxiety of Non-infected Pregnant Mothers. *J. Reprod. Infertil.* **2021**, *22*, 125–132. [CrossRef] [PubMed]
39. Mortazavi, F.; Mehrabadi, M. Predictors of fear of childbirth and normal vaginal birth among Iranian postpartum women: A cross-sectional study. *BMC Pregnancy Childbirth* **2021**, *21*, 316. [CrossRef]
40. Størksen, H.T.; Garthus-Niegel, S.; Adams, S.S.; Vangen, S.; Eberhard-Gran, M. Fear of childbirth and elective caesarean section: A population-based study. *BMC Pregnancy Childbirth* **2015**, *15*, 221. [CrossRef]
41. Malhotra, Y.; Miller, R.; Bajaj, K.; Sloma, A.; Wieland, D.; Wilcox, W. No change in cesarean section rate during COVID-19 pandemic in New York City. *Eur. J. Obstet. Gynecol. Reprod. Biol.* **2020**, *253*, 328–329. [CrossRef]

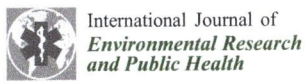

Article

Pandemic Stress and Its Correlates among Pregnant Women during the Second Wave of COVID-19 in Poland

Michalina Ilska [1,*], Anna Kołodziej-Zaleska [1], Anna Brandt-Salmeri [1], Heidi Preis [2] and Marci Lobel [2]

1. Institute of Psychology, University of Silesia in Katowice, Grażyńskiego Street 53, 40-126 Katowice, Poland; anna.kolodziej-zaleska@us.edu.pl (A.K.-Z.); anna.brandt-salmeri@us.edu.pl (A.B.-S.)
2. Department of Psychology, Stony Brook University, Stony Brook, NY 11794, USA; heidi.preis@stonybrook.edu (H.P.); marci.lobel@stonybrook.edu (M.L.)
* Correspondence: michalina.ilska@us.edu.pl

Abstract: **Background:** The ongoing COVID-19 pandemic has created numerous stressful conditions, especially for vulnerable populations such as pregnant women. Pandemic-related pregnancy stress consists of two dimensions: stress associated with feeling unprepared for birth due to the pandemic (Preparedness Stress), and stress related to fears of perinatal COVID-19 infection (Perinatal Infection Stress). The purpose of our study was to elucidate the association between various factors—sociodemographic, obstetric, pandemic-related, and situational—and pandemic stress in its two dimensions during the second wave of the COVID-19 pandemic in Polish pregnant women. **Methods:** A cross-sectional study with a total of 1119 pregnant women recruited during the second wave of the COVID-19 pandemic in Poland (between November 2020 and January 2021). Participants were recruited via social media to complete an online study questionnaire that included sociodemographic, obstetric, situational, and COVID-19 pandemic factors, as well as the Pandemic-Related Pregnancy Stress Scale (PREPS). **Results:** Nearly 38.5% of participants reported high Preparedness Stress; 26% reported high Perinatal Infection Stress. Multivariate analyses indicated that lack of COVID-19 diagnosis, higher compliance with safety rules and restrictions, and limited access to outdoor space were independently associated with moderate to severe levels of Infection Stress. Current emotional or psychiatric problems, nulliparity, limited access to outdoor space, and alterations to obstetric visits were independently associated with moderate to severe Preparedness Stress. **Conclusion:** Study findings suggest that particular attention should be focused on the groups of pregnant women who are most vulnerable to pandemic-related stress and therefore may be more prone to adverse outcomes associated with prenatal stress.

Keywords: pregnancy; COVID-19; pandemic stress; correlates of stress; infection; preparedness

Citation: Ilska, M.; Kołodziej-Zaleska, A.; Brandt-Salmeri, A.; Preis, H.; Lobel, M. Pandemic Stress and Its Correlates among Pregnant Women during the Second Wave of COVID-19 in Poland. *IJERPH* **2021**, *18*, 11140. https://doi.org/10.3390/ijerph182111140

Academic Editor: Francesca Agostini

Received: 12 September 2021
Accepted: 19 October 2021
Published: 23 October 2021

Publisher's Note: MDPI stays neutral with regard to jurisdictional claims in published maps and institutional affiliations.

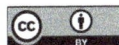

Copyright: © 2021 by the authors. Licensee MDPI, Basel, Switzerland. This article is an open access article distributed under the terms and conditions of the Creative Commons Attribution (CC BY) license (https://creativecommons.org/licenses/by/4.0/).

1. Introduction

The 2019 coronavirus disease (COVID-19) pandemic is a global health threat, and by far the largest outbreak of an infectious illness in modern history. The COVID-19 pandemic constitutes a significant source of distress for all people but may be particularly stressful for vulnerable groups [1]. Pregnant women are a high-risk population due to the potential dual impact on mother and fetus [2]. Pregnancy is a particularly critical period for women's mental health [3,4]. Depression and anxiety are some of the most prevalent pregnancy morbidities that have increased since the start of the COVID-19 pandemic [5–7]. Tomfohr-Madsen et al. [5] observed higher anxiety prevalence in pregnant women, which is potentially linked to exposure to pandemic chronic stressors and ongoing uncertainty. These authors point out that rates of antenatal depression and anxiety are significantly elevated during the COVID-19 pandemic compared to historical pre-pandemic norms, for example [8]. Other reports on the mental health of pregnant women during the pandemic confirm these trends. Researchers highlight the prevalence of anxiety symptoms [2,9,10], severe pandemic stress [9,11,12], and depression [2,13,14] and also indicate that expectant and postpartum women have higher levels of anxiety and depression compared to similar cohorts assessed before the outbreak [15–18]. Studies of the determinants of anxiety and depression in pregnancy conducted during the COVID-19 pandemic have confirmed the importance of risk factors described previously as well as stressors related to pandemic circumstances [19,20].

The COVID-19 pandemic is a danger to reproductive and perinatal health both directly, through infection itself, and indirectly, as a consequence of changes in health care, social policy, and social and economic circumstances [21]. The pandemic has introduced widespread chronic fear of infection and, in pregnant women, fear for the health of the fetus in the face of the spreading virus [11,22]. Pandemic stress as a consequence of these circumstances includes infection stress and stress related to preparing for childbirth [22]. Previous studies indicate that prenatal stress (including pandemic stress) and fear of childbirth are factors that may disrupt preparation for delivery and the course of the delivery itself and increase the likelihood of adverse birth outcomes including low birth weight and preterm delivery [23–25]. Moreover, recent research indicates that pandemic-related stress is a powerful construct that can affect the mental health of pregnant women, including an increase in symptoms of depression and anxiety [9,20].

A growing body of evidence confirms the harmful consequences of COVID-19 for perinatal physical and mental health. A review carried out by Chmielewska et al. [15] showed that global maternal and fetal outcomes have worsened during the COVID-19 pandemic, with an increase in maternal deaths, stillbirths, ruptured ectopic pregnancies, and maternal depression. Pregnant women are among those who are most worried and concerned about spreading or becoming infected by SARS-CoV-2 [26,27]. Numerous factors may have intensified the worries of pregnant women, including the diverse range of symptoms and complications caused by the disease, limited scientific knowledge about its impact on fetal well-being, confinement, changes in daily routine, transformations of social life, financial problems, and interruptions of prenatal care [2,28].

The pandemic unfolded in a wave-like manner. The outbreak of COVID-19 in Poland began at the end of March 2020 and reached its first peak during March and April 2020, with few infections and a small number of deaths. The first lockdown was introduced at this time as a preventive measure, which limited the possibility of movement, medical care (canceled or rescheduled medical appointments, introduction of telephone consultations), and the functioning of maternity wards and delivery rooms (suspension of appointments, births without a companion) [29,30]. The following months saw a slow return to normalcy, along with the re-opening of the economy, and a gradual lifting of restrictions in maternity care (e.g., accompanied births resumed, and a less restrictive protocol was adopted for the treatment of mothers infected with the virus).

The second wave of the pandemic in Poland, which started in November 2020 and lasted until January 2021, differed from the first in many respects. A sharp increase was observed in incidence of the coronavirus, with numerous deaths and hospitalizations of people suffering from severe COVID-19. A second lockdown was introduced along with shutdown of the economy, schools, and the return of restrictions relating to travel [31]. Constraints in medical care were reintroduced, including maternity care (suspension of accompanied labor, uncertainty about place of delivery, and total ban on hospital visitors). The second wave was also accompanied by changes in the public mood. Although the second wave was objectively more threatening than the first, there was less adherence to preventive measures. Research conducted by Chodkiewicz and colleagues [32] suggests that after initial mobilization in the first wave, stress became chronic and resilience mechanisms were increasingly ineffective, leading to psychological burnout. Additional studies have documented fatigue, burnout, loneliness, and a rise in anxiety, depression, and post-traumatic stress disorder [33–36].

Therefore, the aim of this study was to investigate the magnitude of pandemic stress in pregnant women during the second wave of the pandemic in Poland and identify its sociodemographic, obstetric, and situational correlates, including pandemic conditions.

2. Materials and Methods

From November 2020 to January 2021, we recruited a sample of 1119 pregnant women through social media (i.e., Facebook, pregnancy and birth forums, the Polish Childbirth with Dignity Foundation). A cross-sectional study design with non-random sampling was used. Research assistants posted study advertisements on pregnancy-related social media that directed women to a link with the study questionnaire. The online questionnaire was completed through LimeSurvey, an online survey system. Inclusion criteria were Polish speaking women over 18 years of age who were pregnant during completion of the survey. The research procedure was approved by the Ethics Committee of Silesian University in Katowice (KEUS.43/05.2020).

2.1. Methods

COVID-19-related stress. The Pandemic-Related Pregnancy Stress Scale (PREPS [22]; Polish adaptation [11]) is a novel instrument that assesses prenatal stress during the pandemic. The PREPS has been translated into several languages and has been found to have good psychometric properties in different populations [12,19,20]. The PREPS includes a subscale that assesses stress related to preparation for birth and the postpartum period due to the pandemic (PREPS-Preparedness; PREPS-PS) and a second subscale that assesses stress involving concerns about infection of oneself or one's fetus/baby (PREPS-Infection; PREPS-IS). Both scales were internally consistent (PREPS-PS α = 0.83; PREPS-IS α = 0.79). A third PREPS subscale assessing positive appraisal was not pertinent to this study and therefore not used. Scores for each PREPS scale are calculated as mean item response on a scale from 1 = Very little to 5 = Very much.

Sociodemographic characteristics included maternal age (coded younger < 35/older $\geq$ 35), financial status (below average/average/above average), relationship status (some or no relationship/married or cohabiting), and level of education (high school/bachelor/postgrad).

Obstetric factors included unplanned pregnancy (no/yes), nullipara (no/yes), gestational age (in weeks and coded by trimester), high-risk pregnancy (no/yes/unsure), chronic medical conditions (no/yes), fertility treatments (no/yes), and length of time trying to conceive (up to a year/one year or more).

Situational predictors. Four factors were assessed with dichotomous questions (no/yes): experience of lifetime abuse, current emotional or psychiatric problems, major life events while pregnant, and feelings of discrimination or harassment because of race, sexuality, gender, or body size.

COVID-19-related conditions included loss of income because of COVID-19 (no/yes), COVID-19 tests in the last 2 months (no/yes), COVID-19 diagnosis in the last 2 months (no/yes), suspected COVID-19 infection without being medically diagnosed (no/yes/unsure), obstetric visit canceled or rescheduled because of COVID-19 (no/yes), telemedicine (no/yes, but only during COVID/yes, in the past), access to outdoor space (yes, whenever I want/sometimes/rarely), and compliance with safety rules and restrictions (not much or a little/average or a lot).

2.2. Statistical Analysis

Mean differences in the continuous PREPS-IS and PREPS-PS stress score for women with different sociodemographic characteristics, obstetric factors, situational factors, and COVID-19-related conditions were evaluated using Independent Sample t-tests or ANOVA as appropriate. Following these steps, all variables that exhibited significant associations with the continuous PREPS-IS and PREPS-PS stress score in bivariate analyses were entered into a binary logistic regression model to calculate unadjusted and adjusted odds for high levels of PREPS-IS and PREPS-PS. Cut-off scores ($\geq$4 on the 1–5 response scale) were used to identify women experiencing moderate or severe levels of stress [37]. The criterion for statistical significance was $p < 0.05$ for all analyses.

3. Results

Participants were on average 29.79 ± 3.81 years old, with an average gestational age of 25 weeks (25.43 ± 9.73). Almost half of the participants were nulliparas (n = 494, 44.1%). Sixty-three women (5.6%) reported being diagnosed with COVID-19 during pregnancy, and one-quarter (n = 253, 22.6%) thought they might have contracted COVID-19 during pregnancy but were not diagnosed. Other participant characteristics are displayed in Table 1.

Approximately a quarter (26.1%) and more than a third (38.5%) of the women scored a 4 or higher on the PREPS-IS subscale and PREPS-PS subscale, respectively, indicating high levels of COVID-19-related pregnancy stress.

Table 1. Sample characteristics and mean differences in PREPS-IS and PREPS-PS scale score based on sociodemographic characteristics, obstetric factors, and other predictors (N = 1119).

Sociodemographic Characteristics		N (%)	PREPS-IS	PREPS-PS
Age (years)			$t = -0.18$	$t = -0.55$
	Younger (< 35)	986 (88.1)	3.11 ± 1.04	3.55 ± 0.88
	Older ($\geq$ 35)	133 (11.9)	3.13 ± 0.96	3.51 ± 0.77
Relationship status			$t = -0.02$	$t = -0.86$
	Some or no relationship	38 (3.4)	3.12 ± 1.01	3.67 ± 0.98
	Married or cohabiting	1077 (96.2)	3.12 ± 1.03	3.54 ± 0.86
Financial status			$F = 0.51$	$F = 8.69$ ***
	Below average	65 (5.8)	3.03 ± 1.10	3.60 ± 0.90 [a,b]
	Average	701 (62.6)	3.14 ± 1.03	3.62 ± 0.85 [a]
	Above average	353 (31.5)	3.09 ± 1.00	3.39 ± 0.86 [b]
Education			$F = 1.04$	$F = 0.29$
	High school	129 (11.5)	3.03 ± 1.13	3.56 ± 0.97
	Bachelor	108 (9.7)	3.03 ± 1.09	3.61 ± 0.86
	Postgrad	882 (78.8)	3.14 ± 1.00	3.54 ± 0.85
Obstetric Factors		N (%)	PREPS-IS	PREPS-PS
Unplanned pregnancy			$t = 0.47$	$t = 0-1.18$
	Yes	894 (79.9)	3.12 ± 1.02	3.58 ± 0.86
	No	225 (20.1)	3.09 ± 1.07	3.61 ± 0.87
Nullipara			$t = -0.87$	$t = 2.57$ *
	Yes	494 (44.1)	3.14 ± 1.02	3.62 ± 0.89
	No	614 (54.9)	3.11 ± 1.02	3.48 ± 083
Trimester			$F = 0.52$	$F = 2.74$
	1st	181 (16.2)	3.18 ± 1.00	3.42 ± 0.87
	2nd	384 (34.3)	3.11 ± 1.06	3.60 ± 0.86
	3rd	554 (49.5)	3.09 ± 1.02	3.55 ± 0.86
High-risk pregnancy			$F = 4.03$ *	$F = 2.62$
	Yes	127 (11.3)	3.32 ± 1.00 [a]	3.68 ± 0.83
	No	934 (83.5)	3.08 ± 1.03 [b]	3.52 ± 0.87
	Unsure	58 (5.2)	3.29 ± 1.05 [a,b]	3.70 ± 0.84
Chronic medical conditions			$F = 1.26$	$F = 1.71$
	Yes	332 (29.7)	3.19 ± 1.03	3.62 ± 0.85
	No	779 (69.6)	3.08 ± 1.02	3.52 ± 0.87
	Unsure	8 (0.7)	3.05 ± 1.38	3.66 ± 1.04
Fertility treatments			$t = -0.19$	$t = 0.91$
	Yes	64 (5.7)	3.14 ± 1.04	3.55 ± 0.86
	No	1055 (94.2)	3.11 ± 1.03	3.45 ± 0.91
Length of time trying to conceive			$t = -2.38$ *	$t = -2.84$ **
	Up to a year	987 (88.2)	3.09 ± 1.04	3.52 ± 0.87
	One year or more	132 (11.8)	3.30 ± 0.94	3.75 ± 0.79

Table 1. Cont.

Situational Predictors		N (%)	PREPS-IS	PREPS-PS
Lifetime abuse			t = −0.99	t = −0.25
	Yes	59 (5.3)	2.98 ± 1.05	3.52 ± 0.89
	No	1060 (94.7)	3.12 ± 1.03	3.55 ± 0.86
Current emotional or psychiatric problems			t = 2.08 *	t = 4.11 ***
	Yes	194 (10.4)	3.25 ± 1.01	3.78 ± 0.81
	No	925 (89.6)	3.09 ± 1.03	3.50 ± 0.87
Major life event while pregnant			t = 0.62	t = 2.82 **
	Yes	282 (25.2)	3.15 ± 1.03	3.67 ± 0.81
	No	837 (74.8)	3.10 ± 1.03	3.51 ± 0.88
Felt discriminated against			t = 2.03 *	t = 3.73 ***
	Yes	53 (4.7)	3.38 ± 0.96	3.98 ± 0.74
	No	1066 (95.3)	3.10 ± 1.03	3.53 ± 0.86

Note: * $p < 0.05$; ** $p < 0.01$; *** $p < 0.001$. Means with different superscripts are significantly different at $p < 0.05$ in a post hoc Scheffé test.

We investigated the association of PREPS factors with sociodemographic variables (age, relationship status, financial status, education), obstetric characteristics (unplanned pregnancy, nullipara, trimester, high-risk pregnancy, chronic medical conditions, fertility treatment, length of time trying to conceive), and situational factors (lifetime abuse, current emotional or psychiatric problems, major life event while pregnant, discrimination) (Table 1). We also examined associations with COVID-19-related conditions (income lost, COVID-19 test, diagnosis and perceived risk of COVID-19, prenatal care appointment alteration, telemedicine during COVID-19, access to outdoor space, safety rule restrictions) (Table 2).

Table 2. Sample characteristics and mean differences in PREPS-IS and PREPS-PS scale score based on COVID-19-related conditions (N = 1119).

COVID-19-Related Conditions		N (%)	PREPS-IS	PREPS-PS
Loss of income because of COVID-19			t = −0.31	t = −2.77 **
	Yes	259 (23.1)	3.13 ± 1.08	3.68 ± 0.87
	No	860 (76.9)	3.11 ± 1.01	3.51 ± 0.86
COVID-19 test			t = −1.73	t = 0.78
	Yes	165 (14.7)	2.99 ± 0.95	3.58 ± 0.91
	No	954 (85.3)	3.14 ± 1.04	3.54 ± 0.86
COVID-19 diagnosis			t = −2.61 **	t = −0.83
	Yes	63 (5.6)	2.79 ± 0.84	3.46 ± 0.89
	No	1056 (94.4)	3.13 ± 1.03	3.55 ± 0.86
Suspected COVID-19 infection			F = 4.11 *	F = 3.45 *
	Yes	148 (13.2)	2.93 ± 1.01 [a]	3.62 ± 0.90
	No	718 (64.2)	3.11 ± 1.04 [a,b]	3.50 ± 0.87
	Unsure	253 (22.6)	3.23 ± 1.00 [b]	3.65 ± 0.80
Obstetric visit lost or rescheduled			t = −2.74 **	t = −2.84 **
	Yes	161 (14.4)	3.32 ± 0.98	3.82 ± 0.72
	No	958 (85.6)	3.08 ± 1.03	3.50 ± 0.88
Telemedicine			F = 3.04 *	F = 5.04 **
	No	859 (76.8)	3.07 ± 1.04	3.51 ± 0.88 [a]
	Yes, but only during COVID	223 (19.9)	3.23 ± 1.00	3.71 ± 0.80 [b]
	Yes, in the past	37 (3.3)	3.34 ± 0.77	3.44 ± 0.85 [a,b]
Access to outdoor space			F = 7.59 **	F = 11.04 ***
	Yes, whenever I want	945 (84.5)	3.06 ± 1.03 [a]	3.50 ± 0.86 [a]
	Sometimes	142 (12.7)	3.41 ± 0.95 [b]	3.84 ± 0.81 [b]
	Rarely	32 (2.9)	3.32 ± 1.18 [a,b]	3.81 ± 0.88 [a,b]
Compliance with safety rules and restrictions			t = 6.71 ***	t = 2.11 *
	not much or a little	72 (6.4)	2.34 ± 1.10	3.29 ± 1.06
	average or a lot	1047 (93.6)	3.17 ± 1.00	3.57 ± 0.85

Note: * $p < 0.05$; ** $p < 0.01$; *** $p < 0.001$; Means with different superscripts are significantly different at $p < 0.05$ in a post hoc Scheffé test.

In the bivariate analyses, PREPS-IS was related to some of the obstetric factors, namely, high-risk pregnancy and length of time trying to conceive. PREPS-IS was also associated with current emotional or psychiatric problems and discrimination (see Table 1). As shown in Table 2, PREPS-IS was also associated with all but one of the COVID-19-related variables. The omnibus F-test was significant for telemedicine during pregnancy; however, the post hoc analysis showed no significant differences.

PREPS-PS was associated with financial status, nullipara, and length of time trying to conceive. PREPS-PS was also related to current emotional or psychiatric problems, major life events during pregnancy, and discrimination (see Table 1). As shown in Table 2, PREPS-PS was also associated with all but one of the COVID-19-related variables (see Table 2). The omnibus F-test was significant for suspected COVID-19 infection; however, the post hoc analysis showed no significant differences. Two logistic regression analyses were carried out to calculate the adjusted odds ratio (AOR) for those who reported the highest level of PREPS-IS and PREPS-PS. As shown in Table 3, the model predicting high levels of Perinatal Infection Stress incorporated variables that exhibited significant bivariate associations with a continuous PREPS-IS score. This regression model predicted 4% of the variance in PREPS-IS, with COVID-19 diagnosis (AOR 4.02, $p < 0.01$), compliance with the safety rules and restrictions (AOR 3.05, $p < 0.01$), and limited access to outdoor space (AOR 1.49, $p < 0.05$), uniquely increasing the odds of high perinatal infection stress.

Table 3. Binary multivariate logistic regression predicting high levels of Infection Stress—PREPS-IS ($N = 1119$).

	PREPS-IS	
	AOR	95% CI
Obstetric factors		
High-risk [†]	1.3	0.87, 1.96
Length of time trying to conceive	1.09	0.72, 1.65
Situational factors		
Emotional or psychiatric problems	1.15	0.81, 1.64
Discrimination	1.14	0.62, 2.11
COVID-19-related factors		
No COVID diagnosis	4.02 **	1.69, 9.56
Perceived risk of having had COVID-19 [†]	1.06	0.79, 1.41
Appointment altered	1.35	0.91, 1.99
Telemedicine obstetrician [†]	1.19	0.84, 1.67
Limited access to outdoor space [†]	1.49 *	1.04, 2.1
Compliance with safety rules and restrictions	3.05 **	1.44, 6.48
	$R^2 = 0.04$	

* $p < 0.05$, ** $p < 0.01$. AOR—Adjusted Odds Ratio; CI—Confidence Interval. [†] Women who reported being high-risk and those who were unsure were grouped together. Women who reported perceived risk of having COVID-19 and those who were unsure were grouped together. Women who reported no telemedicine obstetrician during COVID-19 and those who reported it before the pandemic were grouped together. Women who reported sometimes or rarely having access to outdoor space were grouped together.

As shown in Table 4, the model predicting high levels of Preparedness Stress incorporated variables that exhibited significant bivariate associations with the continuous PREPS-PS score. The regression model included sociodemographic, obstetric, situational, and COVID-19-related variables, which predicted 8% of the variance in PREPS-PS, with nulliparity (AOR 1.51, $p < 0.05$), current emotional or psychiatric problems (AOR 1.52, $p < 0.05$), income lost because of COVID-19 (AOR 1.36, $p < 0.05$), obstetric visits canceled or rescheduled (AOR 1.52, $p < 0.05$), and limited access to outdoor space (AOR 2.21, $p < 0.001$) uniquely increasing the odds of high perinatal Preparedness Stress.

Table 4. Binary multivariate logistic regression predicting high levels of Preparedness Stress ($N = 1119$).

	PREPS-PS	
	AOR	95% CI
Sociodemographic factors		
Financial status [†]	0.93	0.54, 1.62
Obstetric factors		
Nulliparity	1.51 **	1.17, 1.95
Length of time trying to conceive	1.21	0.82, 1.78
Situational factors		
Discrimination	1.63	0.91, 2.94
Emotional or psychiatric problems	1.52 *	1.09, 2.14
Major life event	1.12	0.84, 1.51
COVID-19-related factors		
Income lost	1.36 *	1.01, 1.83
Perceived risk of having had COVID-19 [†]	1.17	0.90, 1.52
Appointment altered	1.52 *	1.06, 2.17
Telemedicine obstetrician [†]	1.28	0.93, 1.76
Limited access to outdoor space [†]	2.21 ***	1.57, 3.11
Compliance with the safety rules and restrictions	1.12	0.67, 1.88
	$R^2 = 0.08$	

* $p < 0.05$, ** $p < 0.01$, *** $p < 0.001$. AOR—Adjusted Odds Ratio; CI—Confidence Interval. [†] Women who reported below average or average financial status were grouped together. Women who reported perceived risk of having COVID-19 and those who were unsure were grouped together. Women who reported no telemedicine obstetrician during COVID-19 and those who reported it before the pandemic were grouped together. Women who reported sometimes or rarely having access to outdoor space were grouped together.

4. Discussion

The COVID-19 pandemic has pervasive consequences for society including death, economic uncertainty, and strained health care systems. Moreover, the pandemic has triggered a wide variety of psychiatric problems, including anxiety and depression, especially in sensitive populations such as pregnant women [5,38,39]. Additional factors related to pandemic conditions and resulting pandemic stress also threaten maternal mental health.

The current study identified the magnitude and correlates of pandemic-related pregnancy stress during the second wave of COVID-19 in Poland. Nearly a third of pregnant women experienced elevated levels of stress related to feeling unprepared for birth or being worried about perinatal infection. The present research is consistent with other studies carried out in Poland, including those devoted to the COVID-19 pandemic's negative impact on various dimensions of mental health in pregnant women [40,41].

Sociodemographic, obstetric, and situational factors including pandemic conditions were important correlates of this stress. Most of these factors were specific to one of the two dimensions of pandemic-related prenatal stress, but some—in particular, the pandemic conditions—were associated with both stress about perinatal infection and about feeling unprepared for birth. These common pandemic-related correlates of stress included uncertainty about being ill with COVID-19, limited access to outdoor space, cancelation or postponement of obstetric appointments, and compliance with safety rules and restrictions. Similarly, trying to conceive for more than a year, as well as feeling discriminated against and experiencing emotional and psychiatric problems, were associated with higher levels of pandemic stress of both types.

Although a more limited number of factors distinguished women who were experiencing moderate or severe levels of stress, pandemic conditions were the only factors associated with moderate or severe infection stress; similarly, pandemic conditions constituted a majority of the factors associated with moderate or severe birth preparation stress. Notably, limited access to outdoor space was the only pandemic-related factor significantly associated with high levels of both types of stress. These results parallel those of comparable studies conducted in the US, Germany, and Switzerland during the first wave of the pandemic [9,12]. It is instructive that alterations of obstetric appointments were associated with maternal stress, for the pandemic disrupted normal ways of preparing for childbirth, including the regularity of obstetric appointments according to an established schedule, the availability of medical care in situations that threaten the health of the mother or baby, and participation in antenatal classes. Research from the first wave of the pandemic in Poland also showed that prenatal care appointment cancelation or rescheduling was associated with pandemic stress in pregnant women [10]. The availability, stability, and continuity of medical care during pregnancy are crucial for a sense of security in pregnancy. The pandemic has highlighted pre-existing challenges related to the delivery of standard, high quality, and accessible prenatal care in Poland [42,43]. These findings reinforce the urgent need to prioritize safe, accessible, and equitable maternity care within the strategic response to this pandemic, and in future health crises.

Study findings also suggest that during the pandemic, close attention should be focused on particular groups of pregnant women, similarly identified by prior research as vulnerable to high maternal stress [12,23,37]: women pregnant for the first time, those with a high-risk pregnancy, women who have been trying to conceive for a long time, women who feel discriminated against for various reasons, those who have experienced major life events during pregnancy, and those with other emotional and psychiatric difficulties. These groups experience a higher level of pandemic-related pregnancy stress and therefore may be more prone to complications associated with prenatal stress, including preterm birth, low birthweight, and other outcomes that are well-recognized consequences of high maternal stress during pregnancy [44,45]. For these women, early intervention and the provision of psychological support tailored to their needs may also prevent the development or aggravation of psychopathology.

A higher level of pandemic-related pregnancy stress was also associated with women's sense of uncertainty around contracting COVID-19. It should be noted that during the second wave of the pandemic in Poland, there was very limited availability of tests, and thus individuals had little knowledge about their possible SARS-CoV-2 infection. A small percentage of women were tested for SARS-CoV-2, and the percentage of pregnant women who knew they had already had COVID-19 was also low. However, almost one-third suspected that they had contracted COVID-19. These women experienced higher pandemic stress of both types: related to infection fear and to lack of preparation for birth. Thus, increasing access to testing would likely help alleviate maternal stress. Research reports that appeared during this time showed that having COVID-19 provides basic immunity against recurrence and reduces the risk of serious complications in the event of another infection [46,47]. This message was widespread in the media and online and is the likely reason why women who reported a prior infection experienced lower stress. Moreover, a stress exposure mechanism may also be at play, reflecting confidence about the ability to manage stress related to the virus among those who were ill and recovered [48].

Interestingly, we found that greater compliance with safety rules and restrictions was associated with higher pandemic-related stress. In other studies, higher anxiety related to COVID-19 has been associated with a tendency to comply with safety rules during the pandemic [49], or with undertaking various protective behaviors [50]. The association that we uncovered between compliance and stress may thus reflect greater cautiousness among pregnant women harboring fears and concerns about infection and birth. However, it is also possible that vigilance with recommended activities designed for safety and health may reinforce or activate fears related to the pandemic and thus intensify pandemic-related stress [48,51]. More in-depth, longitudinal research may be able to untangle these possibilities and distinguish levels of compliance that are healthy and protective from hypervigilance or extreme behaviors that suggest underlying pathology.

4.1. Implications for Practice and/or Policy

Given the pandemic context and the vulnerability of pregnant women, it is imperative to recognize distress signals in order to prevent the development or aggravation of psychopathology. Such observations should be made continuously, at various stages of the pandemic, making it possible to understand the dynamics of these changes and respond with adequate interventions, tailoring support to specific needs.

4.2. Limitations and Strengths

One of the limitations of this study is the recruitment method, which excluded women who had no access to the internet or social media. As a consequence, the results may not be widely generalizable. Another limitation is the cross-sectional nature of the research, which prevents us from ascertaining whether study variables are predictors or consequences of pandemic-related pregnancy stress. Some may have bidirectional associations with stress. Furthermore, because data were collected exclusively by self-report, we cannot confirm their accuracy.

Another study limitation stems from the online recruitment method, which can introduce bias into the sample. During the pandemic, conducting face-to-face research was difficult or impossible. Future research should consider interview-based assessments and medical chart data to replicate and extend these findings.

Nevertheless, this research also possesses a number of strengths. The use of a well-validated instrument to assess pandemic-related stress and its correlates in a large sample of women pregnant during a time of national emergency provides critical information that can be used to protect the health of childbearing women and their offspring, and these data offer a foundation to examine longer-term effects of the pandemic on this vulnerable population.

5. Conclusions

The COVID-19 pandemic and its multiple waves have created numerous conditions that generate stress for pregnant women related to the possibility of infection of themselves or their baby, and stress related to their preparation for childbirth. This study contributes to our understanding of pregnant women's experiences during an especially dangerous period of the COVID-19 pandemic in Poland and extends the literature on stress during pregnancy. Findings highlight which women are at the greatest risk of elevated stress and offer insight into how this stress might be reduced.

Author Contributions: Conceptualization, M.I., A.B.-S., A.K.-Z., H.P. and M.L.; Data curation, M.I., A.B.-S. and A.K.-Z.; Formal analysis, M.I., A.B.-S. and A.K.-Z.; Investigation M.I., A.B.-S. and A.K.-Z.; Methodology M.I., A.B.-S., A.K.-Z., H.P. and M.L.; Project administration M.I.; Resources M.I., A.B.-S. and A.K.-Z.; Software M.I., A.B.-S. and A.K.-Z.; Visualization M.I., Writing—review and editing A.B.-S., A.K.-Z., M.I., A.B.-S., A.K.-Z., H.P. and M.L., Supervision H.P. and M.L. All authors have read and agreed to the published version of the manuscript.

Funding: This research received no external funding.

Institutional Review Board Statement: The study was conducted according to the guidelines of the Declaration of Helsinki, and the research procedure was approved by the Ethics Committee of Silesian University in Katowice (KEUS.43/05.2020).

Informed Consent Statement: Informed consent was obtained from all subjects involved in the study.

Data Availability Statement: The datasets used and/or analyzed during the current study are available from the corresponding author upon request.

Acknowledgments: We would like to thank the excellent research assistants who helped in carrying out this project: Joanna Bojdys, Marta Buchenfeld, Małgorzata Gabryś, Emilia Maciak, Adrianna Małek, Dominika Serzysko, Magdalena Twardowska. Special thanks to Fundacja "Rodzić po Ludzku", Jagoda Sikora, Agnieszka Stążka-Gawrysiak, Alicja Kost, Magdalena Komsta, Dawid Serafin for their invaluable support in conducting this research.

Conflicts of Interest: The authors declare no conflict of interest.

References

1. Pakpour, A.H.; Griffiths, M.D. The fear of COVID-19 and its role in preventive behaviors. *J. Councurrent Disord.* **2020**, *2*, 58–63.
2. López-Morales, H.; del Valle, M.V.; Canet-Juric, L.; Andrés, M.L.; Galli, J.I.; Poó, F.; Urquijo, S. Mental health of pregnant women during the COVID-19 pandemic: A longitudinal study. *Psychiatry Res.* **2021**, *295*, 113567. [CrossRef]
3. Darvill, R.; Skirton, H.; Farrand, P. Psychological factors that impact on women's experiences of first-time motherhood: A qualitative study of the transition. *Midwifery* **2010**, *26*, 357–366. [CrossRef]
4. Ilska, M.; Brandt-Salmeri, A.; Kołodziej-Zaleska, A. Effect of prenatal distress on subjective happiness in pregnant women: The role of prenatal attitudes towards maternity and ego-resiliency. *Pers. Individ. Differ.* **2020**, *163*, 110098. [CrossRef]
5. Tomfohr-Madsen, L.M.; Racine, N.; Giesbrecht, G.F.; Lebel, C.; Madigan, S. Depression and anxiety in pregnancy during COVID-19: A rapid review and meta-analysis. *Psychiatry Res.* **2021**, *300*, 113912. [CrossRef] [PubMed]
6. Underwood, L.; Waldie, K.; D'Souza, S.; Peterson, E.R.; Morton, S. A review of longitudinal studies on antenatal and postnatal depression. *Arch. Women's Ment. Health* **2016**, *19*, 711–720. [CrossRef] [PubMed]
7. Fawcett, E.J.; Fairbrother, N.; Cox, M.L.; White, I.; Fawcett, J.M. The Prevalence of Anxiety Disorders During Pregnancy and the Postpartum Period: A Multivariate Bayesian Meta-Analysis. *J. Clin. Psychiatry* **2019**, *80*, 18r12527. [CrossRef]
8. Dennis, C.-L.; Falah-Hassani, K.; Shiri, R. Prevalence of antenatal and postnatal anxiety: Systematic review and meta-analysis. *Br. J. Psychiatry* **2017**, *210*, 315–323. [CrossRef] [PubMed]
9. Preis, H.; Mahaffey, B.; Heiselman, C.; Lobel, M. Pandemic-related pregnancy stress and anxiety among women pregnant during the coronavirus disease 2019 pandemic. *Am. J. Obstet. Gynecol. MFM* **2020**, *2*, 100155. [CrossRef]
10. Ilska, M.; Brandt-Salmeri, A.; Kołodziej-Zaleska, A.; Preis, H.; Rehbein, E.; Lobel, M. Anxiety in Pregnant Women during the First Wave of the COVID-19 Pandemic in Poland. Unpublished Manuscript.
11. Ilska, M.; Kołodziej-Zaleska, A.; Brandt-Salmeri, A.; Preis, H.; Lobel, M. Pandemic-related pregnancy stress assessment–Psychometric properties of the Polish PREPS and its relationship with childbirth fear. *Midwifery* **2021**, *96*, 102940. [CrossRef]
12. Schaal, N.K.; La Marca-Ghaemmaghami, P.; Preis, H.; Mahaffey, B.; Lobel, M.; Castro, R.A. The German version of the pandemic-related pregnancy stress scale: A validation study. *Eur. J. Obstet. Gynecol. Reprod. Biol.* **2021**, *256*, 40–45. [CrossRef]
13. Salehi, L.; Rahimzadeh, M.; Molaei, E.; Zaheri, H.; Esmaelzadeh-Saeieh, S. The relationship among fear and anxiety of COVID-19, pregnancy experience, and mental health disorder in pregnant women: A structural equation model. *Brain Behav.* **2020**, *10*, e01835. [CrossRef] [PubMed]
14. Perzow, S.E.; Hennessey, E.-M.P.; Hoffman, M.C.; Grote, N.K.; Davis, E.P.; Hankin, B.L. Mental health of pregnant and postpartum women in response to the COVID-19 pandemic. *J. Affect. Disord. Rep.* **2021**, *4*, 100123. [CrossRef] [PubMed]
15. Chmielewska, B.; Barratt, I.; Townsend, R.; Kalafat, E.; van der Meulen, J.; Gurol-Urganci, I.; O'Brien, P.; Morris, E.; Draycott, T.; Thangaratinam, S.; et al. Effects of the COVID-19 pandemic on maternal and perinatal outcomes: A systematic review and meta-analysis. *Lancet Glob. Health* **2021**, *9*, e759–e772. [CrossRef]
16. Ceulemans, M.; Hompes, T.; Foulon, V. Mental health status of pregnant and breastfeeding women during the COVID-19 pandemic: A call for action. *Int. J. Gynecol. Obstet.* **2020**, *151*, 146–147. [CrossRef]
17. Lebel, C.; MacKinnon, A.; Bagshawe, M.; Tomfohr-Madsen, L.; Giesbrecht, G. Elevated depression and anxiety symptoms among pregnant individuals during the COVID-19 pandemic. *J. Affect. Disord.* **2020**, *277*, 5–13. [CrossRef]
18. Liu, X.; Chen, M.; Wang, Y.; Sun, L.; Zhang, J.; Shi, Y.; Wang, J.; Zhang, H.; Sun, G.; Baker, P.N.; et al. Prenatal anxiety and obstetric decisions among pregnant women in Wuhan and Chongqing during the COVID-19 outbreak: A cross-sectional study. *BJOG Int. J. Obstet. Gynaecol.* **2020**, *127*, 1229–1240. [CrossRef]
19. Colli, C.; Penengo, C.; Garzitto, M.; Driul, L.; Sala, A.; Degano, M.; Preis, H.; Lobel, M.; Balestrieri, M. Prenatal Stress and Psychiatric Symptoms During Early Phases of the COVID-19 Pandemic in Italy. *Int. J. Women's Health* **2021**, *13*, 653–662. [CrossRef]
20. Yirmiya, K.; Yakirevich-Amir, N.; Preis, H.; Lotan, A.; Atzil, S.; Reuveni, I. Women's Depressive Symptoms during the COVID-19 Pandemic: The Role of Pregnancy. *Int. J. Environ. Res. Public Health* **2021**, *18*, 4298. [CrossRef] [PubMed]
21. Kotlar, B.; Gerson, E.; Petrillo, S.; Langer, A.; Tiemeier, H. The impact of the COVID-19 pandemic on maternal and perinatal health: A scoping review. *Reprod. Health* **2021**, *18*, 10. [CrossRef]
22. Preis, H.; Mahaffey, B.; Lobel, M. Psychometric properties of the Pandemic-Related Pregnancy Stress Scale (PREPS). *J. Psychosom. Obstet. Gynecol.* **2020**, *41*, 191–197. [CrossRef]
23. Ibrahim, S.M.; Lobel, M. Conceptualization, measurement, and effects of pregnancy-specific stress: Review of research using the original and revised Prenatal Distress Questionnaire. *J. Behav. Med.* **2020**, *43*, 16–33. [CrossRef]
24. Molgora, S.; Accordini, M. Motherhood in the Time of Coronavirus: The Impact of the Pandemic Emergency on Expectant and Postpartum Women's Psychological Well-Being. *Front. Psychol.* **2020**, *11*, 567155. [CrossRef] [PubMed]
25. Preis, H.; Mahaffey, B.; Lobel, M. The role of pandemic-related pregnancy stress in preference for community birth during the beginning of the COVID-19 pandemic in the United States. *Birth* **2021**, *48*, 242–250. [CrossRef]
26. Brooks, S.; Weston, D.; Greenberg, N. Psychological impact of infectious disease outbreaks on pregnant women: Rapid evidence review. *Public Health* **2020**, *189*, 26–36. [CrossRef] [PubMed]
27. Mirzadeh, M.; Khedmat, L. Pregnant women in the exposure to COVID-19 infection outbreak: The unseen risk factors and preventive healthcare patterns. *J. Matern. Neonatal Med.* **2020**, *2020*, 1749257. [CrossRef] [PubMed]
28. Mortazavi, F.; Agah, J. Childbirth Fear and Associated Factors in a Sample of Pregnant Iranian Women. *Oman Med. J.* **2018**, *33*, 497–505. [CrossRef] [PubMed]

29. Zimmer, M. Rekomendowana Ścieżka Postępowania dla Kobiet w Ciąży COVID-19 | PTGiP. Available online: https://www.ptgin.pl/rekomendowana-sciezka-postepowania-dla-kobiet-w-ciazy-covid-19 (accessed on 4 October 2021).
30. Zimmer, M.; Czajkowski, K. Stanowisko PTGiP i Konsultanta Krajowego w Sprawie Porodów Rodzinnych w Obliczu COVID-19 | PTGiP. Available online: https://www.ptgin.pl/stanowisko-ptgip-i-konsultanta-krajowego-w-sprawie-porodow-rodzinnych-w-obliczu-covid-19 (accessed on 4 October 2021).
31. The Council of Ministers. Regarding the Establishment of Certain Restrictions and Prohibitions in Relation to the Onset of an Epidemic. *Polish J. Laws* **2020**, *2020*, 1758.
32. Chodkiewicz, J.; Miniszewska, J.; Krajewska, E.; Biliński, P. Mental Health during the Second Wave of the COVID-19 Pandemic—Polish Studies. *Int. J. Environ. Res. Public Health* **2021**, *18*, 3523. [CrossRef]
33. Morgul, E.; Bener, A.; Atak, M.; Akyel, S.; Aktaş, S.; Bhugra, D.; Ventriglio, A.; Jordan, T.R. COVID-19 pandemic and psychological fatigue in Turkey. *Int. J. Soc. Psychiatry* **2020**, *67*, 128–135. [CrossRef]
34. Torales, J.; O'Higgins, M.; Castaldelli-Maia, J.M.; Ventriglio, A. The outbreak of COVID-19 coronavirus and its impact on global mental health. *Int. J. Soc. Psychiatry* **2020**, *66*, 317–320. [CrossRef]
35. Bartoszek, A.; Walkowiak, D.; Bartoszek, A.; Kardas, G. Mental Well-Being (Depression, Loneliness, Insomnia, Daily Life Fatigue) during COVID-19 Related Home-Confinement—A Study from Poland. *Int. J. Environ. Res. Public Health* **2020**, *17*, 7417. [CrossRef] [PubMed]
36. Rajkumar, R.P. COVID-19 and mental health: A review of the existing literature. *Asian J. Psychiatry* **2020**, *52*, 102066. [CrossRef]
37. Preis, H.; Mahaffey, B.; Heiselman, C.; Lobel, M. Vulnerability and resilience to pandemic-related stress among U.S. women pregnant at the start of the COVID-19 pandemic. *Soc. Sci. Med.* **2020**, *266*, 113348. [CrossRef]
38. Hessami, K.; Romanelli, C.; Chiurazzi, M.; Cozzolino, M. COVID-19 pandemic and maternal mental health: A systematic review and meta-analysis. *J. Matern. Neonatal Med.* **2020**, 1–8. [CrossRef] [PubMed]
39. Yan, H.; Ding, Y.; Guo, W. Mental Health of Pregnant and Postpartum Women During the Coronavirus Disease 2019 Pandemic: A Systematic Review and Meta-Analysis. *Front. Psychol.* **2020**, *11*, 617001. [CrossRef] [PubMed]
40. Mikolajkow, A.; Małyszczak, K. Stress level and general mental state in Polish pregnant women during COVID-19 pandemic. *J. Reprod. Infant Psychol.* **2021**, 1–18. [CrossRef]
41. Nowacka, U.; Kozlowski, S.; Januszewski, M.; Sierdzinski, J.; Jakimiuk, A.; Issat, T. COVID-19 Pandemic-Related Anxiety in Pregnant Women. *Int. J. Environ. Res. Public Health* **2021**, *18*, 7221. [CrossRef]
42. Adamska-Sala, I.; Baranowska, B.; Doroszewska, A.; Piekarek, M.; Pietrusiewicz, J. Perinatal Care in Poland in the Light of Women's Experiences. 2018. Available online: www.rodzicpoludzku.pl (accessed on 19 October 2021).
43. Węgrzynowska, M.; Doroszewska, A.; Witkiewicz, M.; Baranowska, B. Polish maternity services in times of crisis: In search of quality care for pregnant women and their babies. *Health Care Women Int.* **2020**, *41*, 1335–1348. [CrossRef]
44. Lobel, M.; DeVincent, C.J.; Kaminer, A.; Meyer, B.A. The impact of prenatal maternal stress and optimistic disposition on birth outcomes in medically high-risk women. *Health Psychol.* **2000**, *19*, 544–553. [CrossRef]
45. Ding, X.; Liang, M.; Wu, Y.; Zhao, T.; Qu, G.; Zhang, J.; Zhang, H.; Han, T.; Ma, S.; Sun, Y. The impact of prenatal stressful life events on adverse birth outcomes: A systematic review and meta-analysis. *J. Affect. Disord.* **2021**, *287*, 406–416. [CrossRef] [PubMed]
46. Ripperger, T.J.; Uhrlaub, J.L.; Watanabe, M.; Wong, R.; Castaneda, Y.; Pizzato, H.A.; Thompson, M.R.; Bradshaw, C.; Weinkauf, C.C.; Bime, C.; et al. Orthogonal SARS-CoV-2 Serological Assays Enable Surveillance of Low-Prevalence Communities and Reveal Durable Humoral Immunity. *Immunity* **2020**, *53*, 925–933.e4. [CrossRef] [PubMed]
47. Chandrashekar, A.; Liu, J.; Martinot, A.J.; Mcmahan, K.; Mercado, N.B.; Peter, L.; Tostanoski, L.H.; Yu, J.; Maliga, Z.; Nekorchuk, M.; et al. SARS-CoV-2 infection protects against rechallenge in rhesus macaques. *Science* **2020**, *369*, 812–817. [CrossRef] [PubMed]
48. Clark, D.A.; Beck, A.T. Cognitive theory and therapy of anxiety and depression: Convergence with neurobiological findings. *Trends Cogn. Sci.* **2010**, *14*, 418–424. [CrossRef] [PubMed]
49. Kowalczuk, I.; Gębski, J. Impact of Fear of Contracting COVID-19 and Complying with the Rules of Isolation on Nutritional Behaviors of Polish Adults. *Int. J. Environ. Res. Public Health* **2021**, *18*, 1631. [CrossRef]
50. Tkhostov, A.; Rasskazova, E. Psychological Contents of Anxiety and the Prevention in an Infodemic Situation: Protection against Coronavirus or the "Vicious Circle" of Anxiety? *Couns. Psychol. Psychother.* **2020**, *28*, 70–89. [CrossRef]
51. Thwaites, R.; Freeston, M.H. Safety-Seeking Behaviours: Fact or Function? How Can We Clinically Differentiate Between Safety Behaviours and Adaptive Coping Strategies across Anxiety Disorders? *Behav. Cogn. Psychother.* **2005**, *33*, 177–188. [CrossRef]

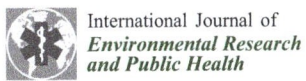

International Journal of
Environmental Research and Public Health

Article

Depressive Symptoms in Fathers during the First Postpartum Year: The Influence of Severity of Preterm Birth, Parenting Stress and Partners' Depression

Francesca Agostini [1,*], Erica Neri [1], Federica Genova [1], Elena Trombini [1], Alessandra Provera [1], Augusto Biasini [2] and Marcello Stella [3]

1. Department of Psychology "Renzo Canestrari", University of Bologna, 40127 Bologna, Italy; erica.neri4@unibo.it (E.N.); federica.genova@unibo.it (F.G.); elena.trombini@unibo.it (E.T.); alessandra.provera3@unibo.it (A.P.)
2. Donor Human Milk Bank Italian Association (AIBLUD), 20126 Milan, Italy; augustoclimb@gmail.com
3. Pediatric and Neonatal Intensive Care Unit, Maurizio Bufalini Hospital, 47521 Cesena, Italy; marcello.stella@auslromagna.it
* Correspondence: f.agostini@unibo.it

Abstract: Although preterm birth constitutes a risk factor for postpartum depressive symptomatology, perinatal depression (PND) has not been investigated extensively in fathers of very low (VLBW) and extremely low birth weight (ELBW) infants. This study explored paternal depression levels at 3, 9, and 12 months of infant corrected age, investigating also the predictive role played by the severity of prematurity, maternal and paternal PND levels, and parenting stress. We recruited 153 fathers of 33 ELBW, 42 VLBW, and 78 full-term (FT) infants, respectively. Depression was investigated by the Edinburgh Postnatal Depression Scale (EPDS) and distress by the Parenting Stress Index-Short Form-PSI-SF (Total and subscales: Parental Distress, Parent–Child Dysfunctional Interaction, and Difficult Child). ELBW fathers showed a significant decrease (improvement) in EPDS, total PSI-SF, and Parental Distress mean scores after 3 months. Paternal EPDS scores at 12 months were significantly predicted by VLBW and FT infants' birth weight categories, fathers' EPDS scores at 3 and 9 months, Parent–Child Dysfunctional Interaction subscale at 3 months, and Difficult Child subscale at 9 months. This study strengthens the relevance of including early routine screening and parenting support for fathers in perinatal health services, with particular attention to fathers who might be more vulnerable to mental health difficulties due to severely preterm birth.

Keywords: perinatal depression; fathers; preterm birth; severity of prematurity; ELBW; VLBW; parenting stress; partner's influence

1. Introduction

Preterm birth occurs when infants are born before the 37th gestational week [1] and constitutes an important risk factor for both the survival, health, and development of the newborn. The risk of negative sequelae especially emerges when preterm delivery occurs in "extreme" conditions, such as when gestational age is lower than 32 weeks (very preterm, VPT), or birth weight is less than 1500 g (very low birth weight, VLBW) or even less than 1000 g (extremely low birth weight, ELBW) [2,3].

Prematurity represents a stressful and potentially traumatic event for parents, who might experience feelings of grief, guilt, anxiety, hopelessness, and persistent concerns about their infant's condition [4]. For this reason, the transition to parenthood after a preterm birth can be complex for both mothers and fathers, and challenges (e.g., parental post-traumatic stress reactions, difficulties in parent–infant bonding, concerns related to preterm infants' atypical appearance) might also continue after infant discharge [5].

Many studies have focused on the description of main psychological reactions in terms of distress, adjustment difficulties, depression, anxiety, and trauma-related symptoms [6–8]

Among these, depressive symptomatology represents one of the most frequent expressions of emotional difficulties after preterm birth.

Depressive symptoms may interfere with the ability of the parent to be emotionally available and sensitive to the infant's needs, therefore there is an increased risk of negative consequences on the parent–infant relationship and preterm infant's development [9,10].

Several studies have investigated the presence of depressive symptoms in parents after preterm birth, mostly in mothers [11,12]. The systematic review and meta-analysis by de Paula Eduardo et al. [13] highlighted a higher risk for postnatal depression (PND) among mothers of preterm infants in assessments up to 24 weeks after birth and especially in the early postpartum period, even if some methodological discrepancies were recognized among the studies, (e.g., poor control of confounding variables, lack of control group). However, no similar reviews exist for postnatal depression in preterm infants' fathers. Particularly, perinatal depressive symptoms in fathers may increase anxiety and feelings of inadequacy related to the assumption of the parental role, hostility, outbursts of rage and aggressive behaviors, social isolation, compromising their ability to support their partner, and the infant [14]. Therefore, it is relevant to deepen the knowledge of paternal affective states after preterm birth. To our knowledge, only some studies have assessed the levels and rates of depressive symptoms in fathers, other than related risk factors, considering different time periods of assessment and heterogeneous samples of preterm infants [15,16].

Regarding the first postpartum weeks, which often correspond to the period of infant hospitalization, Petersen and Quinlivan [12] found no differences in depression scores between 928 full-term (FT) and 72 preterm (PT) fathers at 6 weeks postpartum, even if their PT sample did include different degrees of prematurity (both lower/upper than 2500 g). Cajiao-Nieto et al. [15] assessed at 3 and 20 days after birth depressive symptoms in 51 PT fathers and 33 FT fathers, finding that PT fathers had higher depression scores only at 3 days and that infant's appearance and behavior and parental role alteration (the perception of having a fragile and less responsive infant, as well as having more barriers to participate to care activities and to assuming paternity, respectively) were the most critical aspects contributing to a higher risk of depression. Nevertheless, the preterm sample included together moderate and late preterm babies (ranging from 32 to 36 gestational weeks). These emerging findings seem to suggest that the first days after a preterm birth represent the most critical period for fathers' psychological adaptation. Within this research line, Candelori et al. [16] investigated the rates of depression in 32 couples of PT infants' parents, between 10–20 days after birth; the preterm sample included all the infants under 37 gestational weeks (of which 15.6% ELBW and 25% VLBW). Results showed that the prevalence of parents above the risk threshold for depression was high both for mothers (68.5%) and fathers (37.5%). Helle et al. [17] analyzed one month postpartum the prevalence, risk, and predictors for postnatal depression (PND) in a sample of 230 families, of which 119 FT babies' parents and 111 VLBW preterm infants' parents. Results showed a significantly higher risk for PND in VLBW mothers compared to FT ones; VLBW fathers showed a similar trend, even if scores were overall lower compared to VLBW mothers. In sum, the birth of a VLBW infant resulted to be the most relevant risk factor for PND. Finally, Winter et al. [18] assessed 237 VPT babies' fathers at 38 days after birth for depression, while their babies were still hospitalized and found a depression rate of 16.9%, with no control group included. These studies seem to confirm an increased risk for the occurrence of PND in fathers in the first weeks after preterm birth.

Globally, these findings, given the differences among the studies in terms of research design and methodology (such as preterm samples including different grades of prematurity), as well as the paucity of research on fathers, call for further confirmation.

Very few studies have further explored the depressive symptomatology in preterm infants' fathers across the first postpartum year. Specifically, two studies have considered the first 6 months after birth. Pace et al. [19] longitudinally investigated depression trajectories in VPT infants' parents (113 mothers, 101 fathers) compared to FT parents (117 mothers, 110 fathers), with assessments every 2 weeks for the first 12 weeks after birth and at 6 months postpartum. Both VPT mothers and fathers showed a reduction in mean scores and rates of depression symptoms across the first 12 weeks; however, they continued to show higher rates compared to FT parents both shortly after birth (mothers: 40% vs. 6%; fathers: 36% vs. 5%) and at 6 months postpartum (mothers: 14% vs. 5%; fathers: 19% vs. 6%). Ouwendijk et al. [20] investigated mental health in parents (57 mothers, 51 fathers) of VPT infants, at 3 and 6 months of corrected age. VPT infants' mothers were more likely to experience symptoms and be at risk for a clinical depression disorder than mothers of a reference group from a Dutch population, while preterm infants' fathers did not manifest an increased risk for symptoms of depression.

Three other studies longitudinally assessed paternal depressive symptomatology up to 12 months after birth. McMahon et al. [21] explored depression trajectories in 100 fathers of 125 VPT infants shortly after birth, at 3, 6, and 12 months postpartum: while 82% of VPT fathers showed persistently low symptoms across the first year, 18% of them exhibited high depressive symptoms which persisted over time. The authors concluded that being a father of a VPT infant increases the risk for a chronic course of depressive symptoms. Vriend et al. [22] investigated levels of depression at 1 and 12 months in VPT infants' parents, finding that rates with high symptoms tended to decrease across time in both mothers and fathers; regarding the latter, the rate of depressive symptoms decreased from 9% to 4% from 1 month to 12 months. Additionally, Genova et al. [11] longitudinally explored PND trajectories, specifically at 3, 9, and 12 months postpartum, but they compared different conditions of the severity of prematurity and FT: 38 parental couples of ELBW, 56 for VLBW, and 83 FT ones. At 3 months, ELBW parents showed higher PND levels compared to FT and VLBW parents; at the same time, they showed a greater symptom reduction over the first year. Regarding parental role, ELBW mothers, but not fathers, exhibited higher depressive symptoms at 3 months and a higher reduction in symptomatology compared to VLBW and FT groups.

According to those few studies, it emerges that depressive symptoms in preterm infants' fathers have been poorly investigated over the first postpartum year. This trend is consistent with the more general literature on perinatal psychopathology on normative samples, that has extensively investigated maternal psychological states, while only recently showing a growing interest in the exploration of fathers' emotional issues [23]. Given the paucity of the literature, a need comes to light to further investigate fathers' depressive symptoms in the long-term by also considering specific contexts, such as preterm birth. Moreover, as the few mentioned studies focused only on VPT or VLBW conditions, research should make an effort to better explore the influence of the severity of prematurity and the role of potential influencing variables.

In this sense, one of the psychological dimensions experienced by parents after preterm birth, and that could be related to depressive symptomatology, is a high level of stress (i.e., often referred to as psychological distress, parental stress, parenting stress, etc.). Several studies have indeed found a moderate–high amount of stress experienced by preterm babies' mothers and fathers during baby hospitalization and also after discharge [24–27]. A systematic review highlighted that significant sources of high stress in fathers in NICU are represented by alteration of the parental role (e.g., limited or denied access to infant's care, impaired opportunities to establish emotional bonding), infant appearance (e.g., perception of the infant as fragile, less responsive, more irritable), characteristics of NICU environment (e.g., intensity of sights and sounds of the NICU), staff communication (e.g., unsatisfying access to regular information about infant's health and care) [28]. Additionally, a higher level of stress was related to the severity of prematurity (such as VPT, ELBW) [25,26,29]. Among all these factors, the meta-analysis by Caporali et al. [30] seems to confirm that, during infant hospitalization, the biggest source of stress for both mothers and fathers is represented by parental role alteration, partially independent of the baby's characteristics, birth weight, gestational age at birth and newborn comorbidities. That would mean that it is the traumatic experience of having the baby hospitalized in the NICU that contributes the largest to the stress experienced. The meta-analysis also highlights that the stress tends to be higher for mothers compared to fathers and this finding could be explained by the different involvement in the parental role: while mothers tend to be involved as the primary caregiver, spending more time in NICUs, fathers often resume job engagement before the end of hospitalization, perceiving, therefore, less parental stress. In this sense, Schmoker et al. [27] explored the levels of stress in preterm infants' parents during the first postpartum year and found different patterns of symptoms between mothers and fathers (decrease across time in mothers, increase between 6 and 12 months in fathers), highlighting the need to deepen the distinction according to the parental role.

Another factor potentially contributing to a higher risk of depression in fathers might be the level of mothers' depressive symptomatology. In general, the literature focusing on perinatal depression in parents has frequently analyzed the relationship between maternal and paternal depressive symptoms, often finding a significant association in terms of correlational and predictive analyses [31,32]. According to Vismara et al. [33], the onset of depressive symptoms in first-time fathers and mothers was influenced by their own levels of anxiety and parenting stress as well as by the presence of depression in their partners. The study by Neri et al. [7] has further explored the characteristic of this mutual relationship in the context of preterm birth, highlighting the relevance of considering severity of prematurity. In fact, results showed that a reciprocal influence between partners was significant for VLBW infants' parents, specifically maternal depressive symptoms at 3 months contributed to paternal depressive ones at 9 months, but this did not happen for the ELBW group.

Based on all these premises, a longitudinal study was developed with the aim of better understanding the occurrence of depressive symptoms in fathers during the first postpartum year and the relationship between symptomatology, severity of prematurity, parenting stress, and mothers' depressive symptoms.

The first aim of the study was to investigate whether depressive symptoms in fathers differed according to categories of birth weight during the first postpartum year; based on the evidence of the literature, we expected to find higher levels of depressive symptoms in correspondence to a more severe preterm birth (ELBW).

A second aim was to investigate if the level of parenting stress in fathers was different according to the severity of prematurity during the first postpartum year; according to the previous literature, we expected a higher score in more severe preterm babies' fathers across time.

A third aim was to identify which variables could better predict fathers' perinatal depressive symptoms at 12 months after birth. We specifically aimed at exploring the role played by the severity of prematurity, depressive symptoms in fathers and mothers at 3 and 9 months after birth, and levels of paternal parenting stress.

2. Materials and Methods

2.1. Study Design and Participants

This study was part of wider longitudinal research aimed at assessing the parental affective states and infants' development from 3 to 12 months postpartum after preterm birth.

Families were recruited at the Neonatal Intensive Care Unit (NICU) of Bufalini Hospital (Cesena, Italy) during the period between April 2013 and December 2015; at the same time, the study was presented at the antenatal classes held at Health Services in the same town, in order to recruit a control group composed by parents of healthy FT infants. Eligible participants received complete information about all the aspects of the research from a member of the research team at the moment of NICU discharge or during antenatal classes. Exclusion criteria for all participants were: absence of fluency in Italian language, presence of previous or present psychiatric illness, presence of infants' chromosomal abnormalities, cerebral palsy, malformations, fetopathy, severe complications (leukomalacia, hydrocephalus, Intraventricular hemorrhage-grades III–IV). In case of twin birth, only the first-born one was included. Infants were monitored during the first year and in case of delays or severe complications they were excluded from the study.

At the end of the recruitment, the sample included 153 participants: 78 were fathers of FT infants, with a birth weight > 2500 g and gestational age > 36 weeks (FT group) and the remaining 75 were fathers of PT infants. According to infant birth weight, 42 fathers were included in VLBW group (birth weight between 1000 and 1500 g) and 33 in ELBW group (birth weight < 1000 g).

The study was approved by the Ethical Committee of the Department of Psychology (University of Bologna) before its start.

2.2. Procedure

The assessments took place at 3 months (T1), 9 months (T2), and 12 months (T3) postpartum (corrected age for PT infants) at Developmental Psychodynamic Laboratory (Department of Psychology, University of Bologna, Cesena). At first assessment, a psychologist, blind to infant birth weight, gave all parents a written informed consent to sign and asked them to complete an ad hoc questionnaire regarding socio-demographic and infant clinical information. In addition, during all steps of assessment (T1, T2, and T3) the same psychologist met parents and administer two self-report questionnaires to evaluate the presence of depressive symptomatology in both fathers and mothers and the levels of paternal parenting stress.

2.3. Measures

The Edinburgh Postnatal Depression Scale (EPDS) [34] is the most widely used self-report questionnaire for the screening of perinatal depressive symptomatology in both women and men [35]. It is composed of 10 items that investigate the presence of perinatal depressive symptoms in the previous 7 days. Items are scored from 0 to 3 points, and the total EPDS score ranges from 0 to 30, with higher total scores indicating higher levels of depressive symptomatology. A validated Italian version of EPDS questionnaire is available for the assessment of PND for both mothers [36] and fathers [37]. The internal consistency has been demonstrated to be good in both the maternal (Cronbach's alpha 0.78) and paternal (Cronbach's alpha 0.83) versions. A cut-off score of ≥ 10 for women and ≥ 13 for men has been suggested for the identification of clinically relevant symptoms of postpartum depression [36,37].

The Parenting Stress Index-Short Form (PSI-SF) [38] is a 36-item self-report questionnaire investigating stress specifically associated with parenting on a 5-point Likert scale. It provides a total score and 3 partial scores according to 3 subscales: parental distress (perception of difficulties in parental role related to feelings of being overwhelmed, trapped, and frustrated by parental responsibilities at the expense of other aspects of life); parent–child dysfunctional interaction (difficulties in the interaction with the child related to feelings of unsatisfaction, sensation of not being appreciated and sought by the infant); difficult child (difficulties tied to specific infant characteristics, perceived as irritable, moody, agitated, hyperactive, etc.). Scores of the 3 subscales range from 12 to 60 and the total score (the sum of 3 subscales) from 36 to 180, with higher scores associated with more severe stress symptoms. A Total PSI-SF score ≥ 90 (or above the 90th percentile) is considered to detect individuals with significant level of distress, as indicated by the Italian version validated by Guarino et al. [39]. The questionnaire has good overall psychometric proprieties, with an internal reliability coefficient (Cronbach's alpha) of 0.91 for the total score, and >0.80 for the 3 subscales.

2.4. Statistical Analysis

All statistical analyses were carried out using the IBM SPSS statistical package version 25.0 (IBM, Armonk, NY, USA).

Pearson's chi-square test and univariate ANOVA were run to verify the homogeneity regarding sociodemographic and clinical variables among ELBW, VLBW, and FT groups. In case of non-homogeneity, we considered the possibility to include those variables in subsequent analyses.

In line with our first aim, we ran repeated measures univariate analysis of variance to compare fathers' depressive symptoms as a function of birth weight (ELBW, VLBW, FT) and time of assessment (3, 9, and 12 months). Bonferroni's post hoc analyses were used for comparison within and between groups. Similarly, in line with our second aim, repeated measures multivariate analysis of variance was performed for exploring the impact of birth weight (ELBW, VLBW, FT) and time of assessment (3, 9, and 12 months) on total and 3 subscale scores of PSI-SF (parental distress, parent–child dysfunctional interaction and difficult child).

According to the third aim, a linear regression model was performed to identify possible predictors for fathers' EPDS scores at 12 months (dependent variable). Regression models were tested by backward method in order to reduce the risk of Type II error [40]. Selected predictors were: birth weight, fathers' and mothers' depressive symptoms (at 3 and 9 months), fathers' sources of parenting stress (at 3 and 9 months). Given that birth weight variable included more than two conditions, we split "birth weight" into 2 different categorical variables: birth weight 1 (FT vs. VLBW and ELBW fathers), and birth weight 2 (ELBW vs. VLBW and FT fathers).

3. Results

3.1. Sociodemographic and Clinical Characteristics

Descriptive analyses showed that the three birth weight groups were homogenous in relation to all sociodemographic and clinical variables, except for parity ($X^2_{(2)} = 38.85$; $p < 0.005$), and level of education ($X^2_{(2)} = 7.47$; $p = 0.024$). Specifically, FT fathers, compared to VLBW and ELBW ones, were nulliparous in a higher percentage, while FT and VLBW fathers had a higher level of education than ELBW ones (Table 1). Given the differences in the distribution of parity and level of education, and that their potential influence on paternal PND was recognized in previous studies [31,41–45], these variables were included in further analyses to control their possible influence.

Table 1. Sociodemographic and clinical characteristics of father–infant dyads.

	ELBW Group (n = 33)	VLBW Group (n = 42)	FT Group (n = 78)	F/X^2
Father characteristics				
Paternal age in years [a]	36.85 (5.2)	37.29 (5.3)	35.63 (5.5)	1.45
Level of education [b]				
Primary/secondary school	15 (45)	9 (21)	17 (22)	7.47 *
High school/university	18 (55)	33 (79)	61 (78)	
Marital status [b]				
Married/cohabit	33 (100)	39 (93)	70 (90)	3.66
Other	0 (0)	3 (7)	8 (10)	
Parity [b]				
Nulliparous	21 (70) [b]	16 (41)	69 (90)	30.85 **
Multiparous	9 (30)	23 (59)	8 (10)	
Infant characteristics				
Gender [b]				
Male	16 (49)	28 (67)	37 (47)	4.39
Female	17 (51)	14 (33)	41 (53)	
Gestational age in weeks [a]	27.55 (2.2)	29.87 (1.5)	40.33 (1.5)	937.63 **
Type of delivery [b]				
Spontaneous	9 (28)	10 (26)	65 (83)	48.41 **
Cesarean section	23 (72)	29 (74) [b]	13 (17)	

Table 1. Cont.

	ELBW Group (n = 33)	VLBW Group (n = 42)	FT Group (n = 78)	F/X²
Multiple birth [b]				
Yes	6 (18)	15 (36)	1 (1)	26.78 **
Not	27 (82)	27 (64)	77 (99)	

Note. ELBW = extremely low birth weight; VLBW = very low birth weight; FT = full-term. [a] Means (and standard deviations in parentheses) for interval data. [b] Number (and % in parentheses) for categorical data. * $p < 0.05$, ** $p < 0.005$.

Additionally, as expected, significant differences among the three groups emerged regarding type of delivery ($X^2_{(2)} = 48.41$; $p < 0.005$), multiple birth ($X^2_{(2)} = 26.78$; $p < 0.005$), and gestational age ($F_{(2, 150)} = 937.63$; $p < 0.005$). Specifically, in the FT group, cesarean section delivery and multiple births were less frequent compared to preterm groups, while a lower gestational age was found in preterm groups. Since these variables, along with the differences that emerged, were strictly linked to preterm status and are coherent with group belonging based on birth weight, they were not included in subsequent analyses.

3.2. Fathers' Depressive Symptoms

In line with our first aim, we compared fathers' EPDS scores among the three birth weight groups, controlling for confounding variables (parity and level of education).

Results showed no significant effect of birth weight on fathers' EPDS scores ($F_{(2, 143)} = 0.20$, $p = 0.817$), meaning that fathers, independently from the birth weight group, showed similar EPDS mean scores (Table 2).

When the interaction between birth weight and time of assessment was considered, a significant within effect emerged ($F_{(2, 143)} = 4.40$, $p = 0.014$) (Table 2): ELBW fathers' scores significantly decreased from 3 months to 9 and 12 months (Bonferroni post hoc $p = 0.037$; $p < 0.005$, respectively) (Figure 1); conversely, no significant differences emerged among EPDS scores of VLBW and FT fathers in the three times of assessment (Figure 1). Moreover, no between-group significant differences emerged at any time at Bonferroni post hoc.

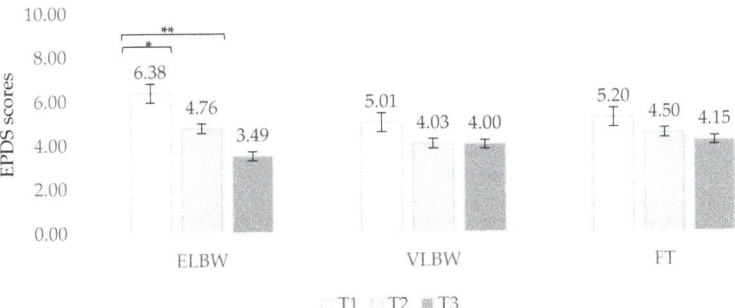

Figure 1. Fathers' EPDS mean scores related to birth weight and time of assessment. Note. ELBW = extremely low birth weight; VLBW = very low birth weight; FT = full-term; T1 = 3 months; T2 = 9 months; T3 = 12 months. * $p < 0.05$. ** $p < 0.005$.

Table 2. Fathers' mean scores for EPDS and PSI-SF to birth weight and time of assessment.

	Birth Weight			Birth Weight × Time of Assessment									F	
				ELBW			VLBW			FT				
	ELBW (n = 33)	VLBW (n = 42)	FT (n = 78)	T1	T2	T3	T1	T2	T3	T1	T2	T3	Birth Weight	Birth Weight × Time of Assessment
EPDS	4.62 ±0.49	4.88 ±0.61	4.35 ±0.56	6.38 ±0.77	4.76 ±0.69	3.49 ±0.62	5.01 ±0.70	4.03 ±0.63	4.00 ±0.57	5.20 ±0.62	4.50 ±0.56	4.15 ±0.50	0.20	4.40 *
Parental distress (PD)	22.34 ±1.10	21.00 ±0.99	22.62 ±0.88	25.01 ±1.27	20.96 ±1.24	21.04 ±1.33	20.70 ±1.15	21.82 ±1.12	20.48 ±1.20	22.30 ±1.02	23.68 ±1.00	21.89 ±1.06	0.81	3.39 *
Parent-child dysfunctional interaction (PCDI)	17.13 ±0.77	16.74 ±0.70	17.17 ±0.2	19.22 ±0.97	15.99 ±0.88	16.18 ±0.98	17.07 ±0.87	16.48 ±0.80	16.69 ±0.89	17.49 ±0.77	16.89 ±0.71	17.14 ±0.79	0.12	2.65
Difficult child (DC)	20.08 ±0.95	19.88 ±0.86	20.24 ±0.76	21.65 ±1.14	19.26 ±1.09	19.34 ±1.07	20.20 ±1.03	19.80 ±0.99	19.65 ±0.97	20.17 ±0.91	20.55 ±0.87	20.00 ±0.86	0.05	1.54
PSI total score	60.04 ±2.45	57.60 ±2.24	59.70 ±1.98	66.54 ±2.80	56.99 ±2.69	56.59 ±2.95	57.89 ±2.56	58.01 ±2.46	56.91 ±2.70	59.72 ±2.26	60.80 ±2.18	58.59 ±2.39	0.33	4.56 *

Note. ELBW = extremely low birth weight; VLBW = very low birth weight; FT = full-term; EPDS = Edinburgh Postnatal Depression Scale; T1 = 3 months; T2 = 9 months; T3 = 12 months. Values are means ± standard deviations. * $p < 0.05$.

3.3. Fathers' Parenting Stress

No significant differences according to birth weight emerged among the three groups in PSI total score [$F_{(2, 143)} = 0.33$; $p = 0.718$] nor in any of the PSI-SF subscales: Parental Distress [$F_{(2, 143)} = 0.81$, $p = 0.446$]; Parent–Child Dysfunctional Interaction [$F_{(2, 143)} = 0.12$, $p = 0.950$]; Difficult Child [$F_{(2, 143)} = 0.051$, $p = 0.950$] (Table 2).

Regarding the interaction between birth weight and time of assessment (Table 2), a significant within effect emerged for PSI total score [$F_{(2, 143)} = 4.56$; $p = 0.012$]: the level of distress in ELBW fathers significantly decreased from 3 months to 9 and 12 months (Bonferroni post hoc: $p < 0.005$; $p = 0.001$, respectively) (Figure 2), while no significant effects were found in case of VLBW and FT fathers (Figure 2). No differences among birth weight groups emerged at any time of assessment.

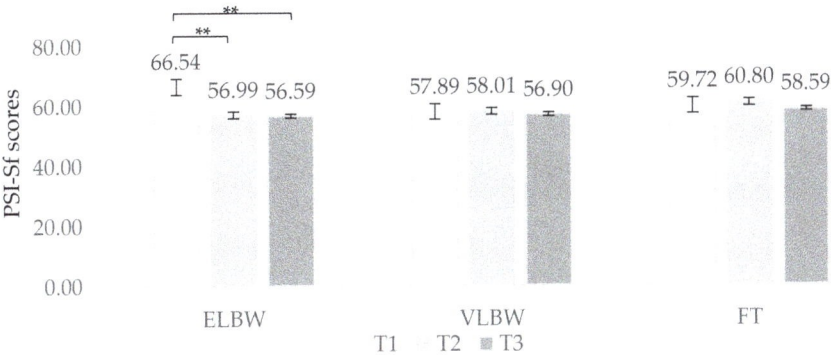

Figure 2. Fathers' PSI total score related to birth weight and time of assessment. Note. ELBW = extremely low birth weight; VLBW = very low birth weight; FT = full-term; T1 = 3 months; T2 = 9 months; T3 = 12 months. ** $p < 0.005$.

In the case of PSI subscales, the interaction between birth weight and time of assessment significantly influenced scores for the PD subscale [$F_{(2, 143)} = 3.29$; $p = 0.040$] (Table 2). According to Bonferroni post hoc analyses, at 3 months ELBW showed significantly higher scores than VLBW group ($p = 0.044$); moreover, ELBW fathers' scores significantly decreased from 3 to 9 and 12 months ($p = 0.001$; $p = 0.006$, respectively) (Figure 3).

No significant differences emerged when PCDI and DC subscales were considered (Figure 2).

3.4. Predictors of Fathers' Depressive Symptoms at 12 Months

At a preliminary level, to explore possible multicollinearity among variables, we ran correlation analyses considering if EPDS paternal scores at 12 months were associated with mothers' and fathers' EPDS and PSI at 3 and 9 months. Results showed that these variables were significantly but moderately correlated (all Pearson's $r \leq 0.70$).

Regression analysis showed a significant model [$F_{(5, 44)} = 45.523$, $p < 0.005$], with an R^2 Adjusted = 0.648. According to the model, fathers' EPDS scores at 12 months were significantly predicted by the following variables: birth weight condition (to be a father of a VLBW or FT infant); high fathers' EPDS scores at 3 and 9 months; high level of distress related to PCDI at 3 months and to DC at 9 months (Table 3). Among these, the predictors with higher β scores were paternal EPDS scores at 3 months, followed by fathers' EPDS and DC subscale scores, both related to 9 months.

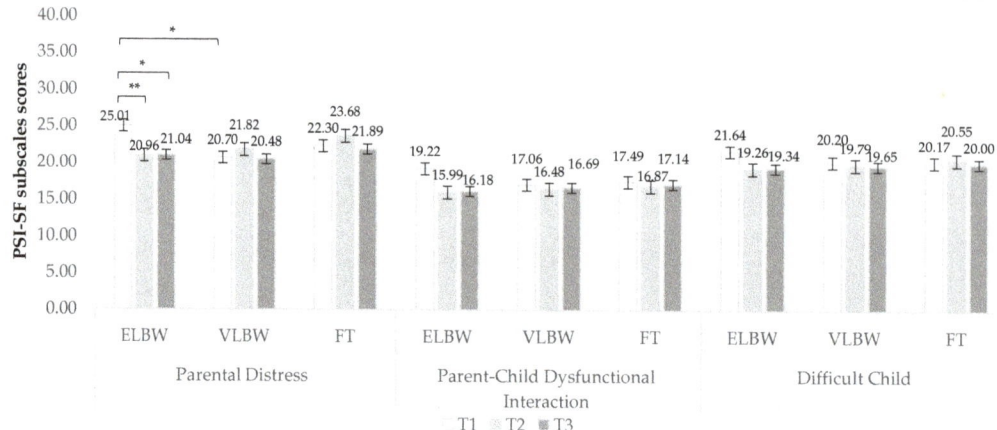

Figure 3. Fathers' PSI-subscales scores related to birth weight and time of assessment. Note. ELBW = extremely low birth weight; VLBW = very low birth weight; FT = full-term; T1 = 3 months; T2 = 9 months; T3 = 12 months. * $p < 0.05$. ** $p < 0.005$.

Table 3. Regression model identifying predictors of fathers' EPDS scores at 12 months.

	T	β	t	p
Constant	−3.470		−4.142	<0.001
Birth weight 2	1.314	0.160	3.118	0.002
Fathers' EPDS scores at 3 months	0.377	0.478	7.459	<0.001
Fathers' EPDS scores at 9 months	0.264	0.291	4.358	<0.001
Fathers' PCDI scores at 3 months	0.090	0.139	2.329	0.021
Fathers' DC scores at 9 months	0.164	0.280	4.398	<0.001

Note. Birth weight 2 = extremely low birth weight fathers vs other fathers (VLBW and FT); PD = Parental Distress subscale; PCDI = Parent–Child Dysfunctional Interaction subscale; DC = Difficult Child subscale.

Considering all the predictors included in the model, maternal EPDS scores and fathers' PD at any time of assessment did not significantly contribute to fathers' EPDS scores at 12 months, nor did parity or education.

4. Discussion

This study intended to explore the occurrence and characteristics of fathers' PND symptomatology across the first postpartum year, according to the severity of prematurity (ELBW, VLBW, and FT conditions). Additionally, it aimed to shed light on the predictive role of specific variables, at infant (birth weight), paternal (PND and parental distress), and maternal (PND symptoms) levels, on fathers' long-term depressive risk after preterm birth. This is one of the first research studies focused on the long-term emotional and psychological adaptation of fathers considering the severity of prematurity. Therefore, it will contribute to deepening the knowledge of fathers' postpartum well-being, given it is recognized as a potential risk or protective factor for child development, family, and parental functioning [46].

The first aim of this study was to investigate the impact of the severity of preterm birth on paternal PND symptomatology during the first postpartum year. A first result seemed to suggest that, as a function of birth weight, significant differences among ELBW, VLBW, and FT groups did not emerge. This result is in line with a recent study [20] reporting comparable levels of PND between VPT and FT fathers, but it is in contrast with our expected results and with a previous investigation [19], showing higher levels of depression in VPT fathers with respect to FT ones. The inconsistency of these findings might be explained by the different timeframe within whom the fathers were compared, and by the characteristics of the included samples. Differently from our study, in fact, the reported previous investigations were conducted within the first six months postpartum, and they included only one specific category of preterm population, without comparing the risk for PND connected to different degrees of prematurity.

Comparable levels of PND symptoms in ELBW, VLBW, and FT fathers at 3, 9, and 12 months postpartum emerged also when we considered the interaction between birth weight and time of assessment. Our results whereby at 3 months postpartum VLBW and FT fathers showed comparable depression levels are in line with previous investigations on PT and FT samples [12,15], but are in contrast with a study on VLBW fathers [17], indicating the need for better clarifying the relationship between severity of prematurity and risk for PND. The lack of significant differences could be explained by the influence of several factors: firstly, men tend to display depressive symptomatology more through externalizing behaviors (i.e., anger attacks, acting outs, addictions, etc.), rather than typically depressive-like responses and the use of screening tools originally developed for mothers (such as the EPDS) might not be appropriate [14,47]; secondly, they tend to see mental health difficulties as a sign of weakness, threatening masculinity, and they may feel it is culturally and socially unacceptable to express them [14,48]; thirdly, especially in cases of atypical and vulnerable conditions, they may suppress or minimize their depressive states for not compromising support offered to their partners [49]. All these factors could have made difficult an accurate identification of the depressive risk after preterm birth, especially if severe. For these reasons, and given the paucity of the literature, this issue needs to be further deepened.

However, in line with recent studies [7,11,19], an interesting trend did emerge that sees ELBW fathers showing high EPDS scores at 3 months, followed by a significant decrease at 9 months and by a stable trend till 12 months, while VLBW and FT fathers' symptoms remained quite constant across all the first postpartum year. These findings seem to suggest that the risk for PND is related to higher severity of prematurity (ELBW) and that the most challenging period for fathers' emotional and psychological adaptation is represented by the first months postpartum when the demands tied to the preterm birth are more relevant (infant hospitalization, medical complications, support to the partner, etc.). Additionally, the reduction in depressive symptoms observed in the following months seems to be in line with other studies [11,19,22], allowing prudent hope about the fact that the effects of severely preterm birth could be acute but not chronic.

The second aim of this study was to investigate the impact of the severity of prematurity on parental distress during the first year after birth. As a function of birth weight, we did not find differences (nor at global or subscale levels) among ELBW, VLBW, and FT groups. These results are partially in line with a recent study [20], which observed similar levels of perceived stress between VPT fathers and FT fathers, but more everyday problems related to parenting, spouse relationship, and physical and cognitive domains for VPT fathers in the first 6 months after birth. When we looked at the interaction between birth weight and time of assessment, we found that at 3 months postpartum only, ELBW fathers reported significantly higher mean scores on the PD subscale compared to VLBW ones (FT group reported a lower mean score too, but not significantly). On the contrary, the three groups did not differ at a global level or on PCDI and DC subscales. These findings seem to confirm that the consequences of preterm birth are related to its severity, with a greater psychological burden in terms of stress for fathers of severely preterm infants, particularly in the first months following birth, as evidenced by Ionio et al. [26] and Hames et al. [24]. In addition, they strengthen the empirical observation that the biggest source of stress is represented by parental role alteration, confirming previous studies [28–30]. Indeed, the traumatic and unexpected interruption of the process of the transition to parenthood catapults these "extremely preterm" fathers in their parental role, calling them to quickly adapt to the demands of the situation, while they must cope with feelings of fear, helplessness, and uncertainty related to the extreme vulnerability of their babies. These results add further support to the possibility that, given the stressful scenario in which the transition to parenthood happens, fathers of severely preterm babies might feel more overwhelmed by the demands of their parental role in the first postpartum months. Again, the results seem to confirm that, in the following months, "severely preterm" fathers gradually feel less stressed and more able to cope with their parental responsibilities, showing resilient behaviors and adaptability to the parental role.

However, it is noteworthy that the comparable levels of stress observed in our VLBW and FT fathers are not in line with previous longitudinal investigations where: for VPT infants' fathers an increase in stress levels was observed from 6 to 12 months postpartum [27]; in case of less severe preterm birth (moderately and late preterm infants), higher paternal distress levels were observed particularly at 6 and 12 months [50]. So far, as no previous studies on long-term adaptation to stress in fathers of severely preterm infants have been conducted to be compared to our findings, more research is needed for a better understanding of the course of fathers' parental distress across the first postpartum year.

For an accurate clinical interpretation of these findings, it is important to consider the specific characteristics of NICU care intervention [51]. Our preterm sample was recruited at the NICU of Bufalini hospital (Cesena), where treatment encompasses modern care principles (e.g., encouraging kangaroo care, early breastfeeding, parental participation in baby care, and unrestricted visiting) and care interventions were provided also after discharge, during follow-up meetings for monitoring infant growth, neurodevelopment, and psychological health. Therefore, these NICU peculiarities could partially explain the risk for PND similar between VLBW and FT fathers and the resilience shown by ELBW fathers (suggested by the reduction in depression and parental distress levels after the first trimester). The fact remains that these findings identify in fathers of severely preterm infants a potential "vulnerable" population, with distinct difficulties, needs, and resources.

The third aim of this study was to explore to what extent fathers' depressive symptoms at 12 months were predicted by birth weight, depressive symptoms in fathers and mothers, and paternal sources of parenting stress at 3 and at 9 months postpartum. First, birth weight condition significantly predicted higher levels of paternal depressive symptoms at 12 months postpartum in the case of the VLBW or FT condition, but not ELBW. This result is somehow unexpected but is coherent with our ANOVA results whereby the impact of severely preterm birth on fathers' emotional adaptation seems to be acute rather than chronic, configuring more a reaction of exogenous nature (to the trauma of early birth, to the experience of hospitalization, and to the infant's vulnerabilities), which tends to gradually go into remission across time, when the risks for infant's survival and health decrease and fathers are reassured by new developmental skills reached by their infants [52,53]. On the contrary, the EPDS scores of VLBW and FT infants' fathers seemed to be constant and did not regress as a result of an adaptation to fatherhood during the postpartum year. Given the role that different levels of prematurity might play in paternal depressive symptoms, the monitoring of paternal affective states across time is recommended.

Second, higher levels of paternal depressive symptoms at 3 and 9 months predicted higher EPDS scores at 12 months postpartum. This result is in line with the previous literature on both FT [33] and PT samples [7], highlighting that early depressive risk contributes to higher symptoms in subsequent months and the relevance, therefore, of monitoring the evolution of symptoms [11]. In fact, it is noteworthy that the EPDS score at 3 months resulted from the predictor which most significantly contributed to EPDS scores at 12 months.

Regarding the influence of maternal depressive symptoms at 3 and 9 months on fathers' depression at 12 months, our results did not show any significant contribution, and this is partially in line with a previous investigation by Neri et al. [7], where a significant role of mothers' depression was found only for VLBW condition, but not for FT and ELBW groups. Nevertheless, these authors aimed to assess only the reciprocal influence between maternal and paternal depressive symptomatology but did not consider the effects of other predictors such as sources of parenting distress. The inclusion of these variables in the present study led to a more complex model, where the role of each factor is weighted by the presence of the others. This complexity could help to reach a more accurate understanding of paternal experience. However, given the lack of this kind of study, future investigations are recommended.

Specific dimensions of parental distress, that is high PDCI scores at 3 months and high DC scores at 9 months, significantly contributed to fathers' depressive symptoms at 12 months postpartum. These findings are in line with cross-sectional studies on VLBW and FT fathers [54,55], where high levels of parenting stress tended to be associated with more severe postpartum depressive symptoms; also, they are coherent with the study by Vismara and colleagues [33], suggesting the predictive role of parental distress regarding PND in fathers. It is interesting to note that specific sources of stress predicted depressive symptoms at one year: at 3 months the source was represented by the stress related to the perception of a poor relationship, at 9 months greater stress was related to the infant's behavior and characteristics. Therefore, these findings open to the possibility that postpartum depressive symptoms might be differentially predicted by specific types of stressful experiences across the first 12 months and this interplay between parenting stress and depression needs to be further explored.

We must acknowledge some limitations of this study. First, the sample should be enlarged, and the three birth-weight groups should reach a similar size for further confirmation of the findings. Second, the EPDS, originally developed for screening in mothers, may not be fully appropriate for detecting gender-related differences in the expression of PND symptoms [56]. Additionally, the EPDS is a self-report tool and, given the well-known limitations of this kind of measure, it should be associated with a structured clinical interview. Third, the presence of anxious symptoms has not been assessed, despite them frequently occurring in comorbidity with depressive symptomatology [57]. Finally, we did not investigate the possible influence of both prenatal factors (such as the frequency of prenatal visits, length of hospitalization before the delivery, etc.), and of NICU care intervention on fathers' emotional postnatal adaptation.

5. Conclusions

To sum up, given the paucity of longitudinal studies on fathers' psychological adjustment after preterm birth, these results shed new light on this field of research, highlighting the relevance of paying particular attention to the situations where fathers may be more vulnerable to perinatal mental health problems, such as a highly severe preterm birth.

The findings of this study strengthen the clinical relevance of including routine screening programs for fathers in perinatal health services, for identifying those cases that, given a complex interplay between exogenous and endogenous risk factors, are at higher risk for a chronic course. This early identification would enable the implementation of targeted specialist interventions for fathers both for reducing the symptomatology and for supporting their parenting role [48,58]. The inclusion of fathers in assessment programs and interventions might also contribute to reducing a mother-centered bias in the practices of perinatal health services, emphasizing a systemic perspective where the whole family plays an essential role in sustaining infant development and health. Therefore, future studies following these points of reference are highly recommended.

Author Contributions: Conceptualization, F.A., E.N. and M.S.; methodology, F.A., E.N., F.G. and A.P.; software, E.N. and F.G.; formal analysis, E.N. and F.G.; investigation, F.A., E.N., A.B. and M.S.; resources, F.A., E.T., A.B. and M.S.; data curation, E.N. and F.G.; writing—original draft preparation, F.A., E.N., F.G. and A.P.; writing—review and editing, F.A., E.N., F.G., E.T. and A.P.; supervision, F.A., E.N., E.T., A.B. and M.S.; project administration, F.A., E.T., A.B. and M.S. All authors have read and agreed to the published version of the manuscript.

Funding: This research received no external funding.

Institutional Review Board Statement: The study was conducted according to the guidelines of the Declaration of Helsinki and approved by the Ethical Committee of the Department of Psychology (University of Bologna).

Informed Consent Statement: Informed consent was obtained from all subjects involved in the study.

Data Availability Statement: Data available on request due to privacy and ethical restrictions.

Acknowledgments: We wish to thank all the families who participated in the study and the medical staff who supported the realization of the research.

Conflicts of Interest: The authors declare no conflict of interest.

References

1. World Health Organization. *Born Too Soon: The Global Action Report on Preterm Birth*; World Health Organization: Geneva, Switzerland, 2012.
2. Lind, A.; Korkman, M.; Lehtonen, L.; Lapinleimu, H.; Parkkola, R.; Matomäki, J.; Haataja, L.; The Pipari Study Group. Cognitive and neuropsychological outcomes at 5 years of age in preterm children born in the 2000s. *Dev. Med. Child Neurol.* **2011**, *53*, 256–262. [CrossRef] [PubMed]
3. Biasini, A.; Neri, C.; China, M.C.; Monti, F.; Di Nicola, P.; Bertino, E. Higher protein intake strategies in human milk fortification for preterms infants feeding. Auxological and neurodevelopmental outcome. *J. Biol. Regul. Homeost. Agents* **2012**, *26*, 43–47.
4. Pisoni, C.; Spairani, S.; Manzoni, F.; Ariaudo, G.; Naboni, C.; Moncecchi, M.; Balottin, U.; Tinelli, C.; Gardella, B.; Tzialla, C.; et al. Depressive symptoms and maternal psychological distress during early infancy: A pilot study in preterm as compared with term mother–infant dyads. *J. Affect. Disord.* **2019**, *257*, 470–476. [CrossRef] [PubMed]
5. Bry, A.; Wigert, H. Psychosocial support for parents of extremely preterm infants in neonatal intensive care: A qualitative interview study. *BMC Psychol.* **2019**, *7*, 76. [CrossRef]
6. Neri, E.; Agostini, F.; Baldoni, F.; Facondini, E.; Biasini, A.; Monti, F. Preterm infant development, maternal distress and sensitivity: The influence of severity of birth weight. *Early Hum. Dev.* **2017**, *106–107*, 19–24. [CrossRef] [PubMed]
7. Neri, E.; Genova, F.; Monti, F.; Trombini, E.; Biasini, A.; Stella, M.; Agostini, F. Developmental Dimensions in Preterm Infants During the 1st Year of Life: The Influence of Severity of Prematurity and Maternal Generalized Anxiety. *Front. Psychol.* **2020**, *11*, 455. [CrossRef]
8. Murthy, S.; Haeusslein, L.; Bent, S.; Fitelson, E.; Franck, L.S.; Mangurian, C. Feasibility of universal screening for postpartum mood and anxiety disorders among caregivers of infants hospitalized in NICUs: A systematic review. *J. Perinatol.* **2021**, *41*, 1811–1824. [CrossRef]
9. Agostini, F.; Monti, F.; Neri, E.; Dellabartola, S.; de Pascalis, L.; Bozicevic, L. Parental anxiety and stress before pediatric anesthesia: A pilot study on the effectiveness of preoperative clown intervention. *J. Health Psychol.* **2014**, *19*, 587–601. [CrossRef]
10. Neri, E.; Agostini, F.; Salvatori, P.; Biasini, A.; Monti, F. Mother-preterm infant interactions at 3 months of corrected age: Influence of maternal depression, anxiety and neonatal birth weight. *Front. Psychol.* **2015**, *6*, 1234. [CrossRef]
11. Genova, F.; Neri, E.; Trombini, E.; Stella, M.; Agostini, F. Severity of preterm birth and perinatal depressive symptoms in mothers and fathers: Trajectories over the first postpartum year. *J. Affect. Disord.* **2022**, *298*, 182–189. [CrossRef]
12. Petersen, I.B.; Quinlivan, J.A. Fatherhood too soon. Anxiety, depression and quality of life in fathers of preterm and term babies: A longitudinal study. *J. Psychosom. Obstet. Gynecol.* **2021**, *42*, 162–167. [CrossRef] [PubMed]
13. de Paula Eduardo, J.A.F.; de Rezende, M.G.; Menezes, P.R.; Del-Ben, C.M. Preterm birth as a risk factor for postpartum depression: A systematic review and meta-analysis. *J. Affect. Disord.* **2019**, *259*, 392–403. [CrossRef] [PubMed]
14. Seidler, Z.E.; Dawes, A.J.; Rice, S.M.; Oliffe, J.L.; Dhillon, H.M. The role of masculinity in men's help-seeking for depression: A systematic review. *Clin. Psychol. Rev.* **2016**, *49*, 106–118. [CrossRef]
15. Cajiao-Nieto, J.; Torres-Giménez, A.; Merelles-Tormo, A.; Botet-Mussons, F. Paternal symptoms of anxiety and depression in the first month after childbirth: A comparison between fathers of full term and preterm infants. *J. Affect. Disord.* **2021**, *282*, 517–526. [CrossRef] [PubMed]
16. Candelori, C.; Trumello, C.; Babore, A.; Keren, M.; Romanelli, R. The experience of premature birth for fathers: The application of the Clinical Interview for Parents of High-Risk Infants (CLIP) to an Italian sample. *Front. Psychol.* **2015**, *6*, 1444. [CrossRef] [PubMed]
17. Helle, N.; Barkmann, C.; Bartz-Seel, J.; Diehl, T.; Ehrhardt, S.; Hendel, A.; Nestoriuc, Y.; Schulte-Markwort, M.; von der Wense, A.; Bindt, C. Very low birth-weight as a risk factor for postpartum depression four to six weeks postbirth in mothers and fathers: Cross-sectional results from a controlled multicentre cohort study. *J. Affect. Disord.* **2015**, *180*, 154–161. [CrossRef] [PubMed]
18. Winter, L.; Colditz, P.B.; Sanders, M.R.; Boyd, R.N.; Pritchard, M.; Gray, P.H.; Whittingham, K.; Forrest, K.; Leeks, R.; Webb, L.; et al. Depression, posttraumatic stress and relationship distress in parents of very preterm infants. *Arch. Women's Ment. Health* **2018**, *21*, 445–451. [CrossRef] [PubMed]
19. Pace, C.C.; Spittle, A.J.; Molesworth, C.M.-L.; Lee, K.J.; Northam, E.A.; Cheong, J.L.Y.; Davis, P.G.; Doyle, L.W.; Treyvaud, K.; Anderson, P.J. Evolution of Depression and Anxiety Symptoms in Parents of Very Preterm Infants during the Newborn Period. *JAMA Pediatr.* **2016**, *170*, 863–870. [CrossRef] [PubMed]

20. Ouwendijk-Andréa, M.; Bröring-Starre, T.; Molderink, A.C.; Laarman, C.A.; Oostrom, K.J.; van Dijk-Lokkart, E.M. Parental emotional distress after discharge from the neonatal intensive care unit: A pilot study. *Early Hum. Dev.* **2020**, *140*, 104892. [CrossRef]
21. McMahon, G.E.; Anderson, P.J.; Giallo, R.; Pace, C.C.; Cheong, J.L.; Doyle, L.W.; Spittle, A.J.; Spencer-Smith, M.M.; Treyvaud, K. Mental Health Trajectories of Fathers Following Very Preterm Birth: Associations with Parenting. *J. Pediatr. Psychol.* **2020**, *45*, 725–735. [CrossRef]
22. Vriend, E.; Leemhuis, A.; Flierman, M.; van Schie, P.; Nollet, F.; Jeukens-Visser, M. Mental health monitoring in parents after very preterm birth. *Acta Paediatr.* **2021**, *110*, 2984–2993. [CrossRef] [PubMed]
23. Cameron, E.E.; Sedov, I.D.; Tomfohr-Madsen, L.M. Prevalence of paternal depression in pregnancy and the postpartum: An updated meta-analysis. *J. Affect. Disord.* **2016**, *206*, 189–203. [CrossRef] [PubMed]
24. Hames, J.L.; Gasteiger, C.; McKenzie, M.R.; Rowley, S.; Serlachius, A.S.; Juth, V.; Petrie, K.J. Predictors of parental stress from admission to discharge in the neonatal special care unit. *Child Care Health Dev.* **2021**, *47*, 243–251. [CrossRef] [PubMed]
25. Carson, C.; Redshaw, M.; Gray, R.; Quigley, M.A. Risk of psychological distress in parents of preterm children in the first year: Evidence from the UK Millennium Cohort Study. *BMJ Open* **2015**, *5*, e007942. [CrossRef] [PubMed]
26. Ionio, C.; Mascheroni, E.; Colombo, C.; Castoldi, F.; Lista, G. Stress and feelings in mothers and fathers in NICU: Identifying risk factors for early interventions. *Prim. Health Care Res. Dev.* **2019**, *20*, 81. [CrossRef]
27. Schmöker, A.; Flacking, R.; Udo, C.; Eriksson, M.; Hellström-Westas, L.; Ericson, J. Longitudinal cohort study reveals different patterns of stress in parents of preterm infants during the first year after birth. *Acta Paediatr.* **2020**, *109*, 1778–1786. [CrossRef]
28. Prouhet, P.M.; Gregory, M.R.; Russell, C.L.; Yaeger, L. Fathers' Stress in the Neonatal Intensive Care Unit: A systematic review. *Adv. Neonatal Care* **2018**, *18*, 105–120. [CrossRef]
29. Baía, I.; Amorim, M.; Silva, S.; Kelly-Irving, M.; de Freitas, C.; Alves, E. Parenting very preterm infants and stress in Neonatal Intensive Care Units. *Early Hum. Dev.* **2016**, *101*, 3–9. [CrossRef]
30. Caporali, C.; Pisoni, C.; Gasparini, L.; Ballante, E.; Zecca, M.; Orcesi, S.; Provenzi, L. A global perspective on parental stress in the neonatal intensive care unit: A meta-analytic study. *J. Perinatol.* **2020**, *40*, 1739–1752. [CrossRef]
31. Canário, C.; Figueiredo, B. Anxiety and depressive symptoms in women and men from early pregnancy to 30 months postpartum. *J. Reprod. Infant Psychol.* **2017**, *35*, 431–449. [CrossRef]
32. Kiviruusu, O.; Pietikäinen, J.T.; Kylliäinen, A.; Pölkki, P.; Saarenpää-Heikkilä, O.; Marttunen, M.; Paunio, T.; Paavonen, E.J. Trajectories of mothers' and fathers' depressive symptoms from pregnancy to 24 months postpartum. *J. Affect. Disord.* **2020**, *260*, 629–637. [CrossRef] [PubMed]
33. Vismara, L.; Rollè, L.; Agostini, F.; Sechi, C.; Fenaroli, V.; Molgora, S.; Neri, E.; Prino, L.E.; Odorisio, F.; Trovato, A.; et al. Perinatal Parenting Stress, Anxiety, and Depression Outcomes in First-Time Mothers and Fathers: A 3- to 6-Months Postpartum Follow-Up Study. *Front. Psychol.* **2016**, *7*, 938. [CrossRef] [PubMed]
34. Cox, J.L.; Holden, J.M.; Sagovsky, R. Detection of Postnatal Depression: Development of the 10-item Edinburgh Postnatal Depression Scale. *Br. J. Psychiatry* **1987**, *150*, 782–786. [CrossRef] [PubMed]
35. Escribà-Agüir, V.; Artazcoz, L. Gender differences in postpartum depression: A longitudinal cohort study. *J. Epidemiol. Community Health* **2011**, *65*, 320–326. [CrossRef] [PubMed]
36. Benvenuti, P.; Ferrara, M.; Niccolai, C.; Valoriani, V.; Cox, J.L. The Edinburgh Postnatal Depression Scale: Validation for an Italian sample. *J. Affect. Disord.* **1999**, *53*, 137–141. [CrossRef]
37. Loscalzo, Y.; Giannini, M.; Contena, B.; Gori, A.; Benvenuti, P. The Edinburgh Postnatal Depression Scale for Fathers: A contribution to the validation for an Italian sample. *Gen. Hosp. Psychiatry* **2015**, *37*, 251–256. [CrossRef]
38. Abidin, R.R. *Parenting Stress Index: Professional Manual*, 3rd ed.; Psychological Assessment Resources, Inc.: Odessa, FL, USA, 1995.
39. Guarino, A.; Di Blasio, P.; D'Alessio, M.; Camisasca, E.; Serantoni, G. *Validazione Italiana del Parenting Stress Index Forma Breve per L'identificazione Precoce di Sistemi Relazionali Genitore-Bambino Stressanti*; Giunti O.S.: Firenze, Italia, 2008.
40. Field, A. *Exploring Statistics Using IBM SPSS*, 5th ed.; Sage: London, UK, 2017.
41. Bergström, M. Depressive Symptoms in New First-Time Fathers: Associations with Age, Sociodemographic Characteristics, and Antenatal Psychological Well-Being. *Birth* **2013**, *40*, 32–38. [CrossRef] [PubMed]
42. Carlberg, M.; Edhborg, M.; Lindberg, L. Paternal Perinatal Depression Assessed by the Edinburgh Postnatal Depression Scale and the Gotland Male Depression Scale: Prevalence and Possible Risk Factors. *Am. J. Mens Health* **2018**, *12*, 720–729. [CrossRef] [PubMed]
43. Deater-Deckard, K.; Pickering, K.; Dunn, J.F.; Golding, J. Family structure and depressive symptoms in men preceding and following the birth of a child. The Avon Longitudinal Study of Pregnancy and Childhood Study Team. *Am. J. Psychiatry* **2018**, *155*, 818–823. [CrossRef]
44. Figueiredo, B.; Conde, A. Anxiety and depression symptoms in women and men from early pregnancy to 3-months postpartum: Parity differences and effects. *J. Affect. Disord.* **2011**, *132*, 146–157. [CrossRef]
45. Ramchandani, P.G.; Stein, A.; O'Connor, T.G.; Heron, J.; Murray, L.; Evans, J. Depression in Men in the Postnatal Period and Later Child Psychopathology: A Population Cohort Study. *J. Am. Acad. Child Adolesc. Psychiatry* **2008**, *47*, 390–398. [CrossRef] [PubMed]
46. Letourneau, N.L.; Dennis, C.-L.; Benzies, K.; Duffett-Leger, L.; Stewart, M.; Tryphonopoulos, P.D.; Este, D.; Watson, W. Postpartum Depression is a Family Affair: Addressing the Impact on Mothers, Fathers, and Children. *Issues Ment. Health Nurs.* **2012**, *33*, 445–457. [CrossRef] [PubMed]

47. Matthey, S.; Agostini, F. Using the Edinburgh Postnatal Depression Scale for women and men—Some cautionary thoughts. *Arch. Women's Ment. Health* **2017**, *20*, 345–354. [CrossRef] [PubMed]
48. Darwin, Z.; Domoney, J.; Iles, J.; Bristow, F.; Siew, J.; Sethna, V. Assessing the Mental Health of Fathers, Other Co-parents, and Partners in the Perinatal Period: Mixed Methods Evidence Synthesis. *Front. Psychiatry* **2021**, *11*, 585479. [CrossRef]
49. Schuppan, K.M.; Roberts, R.; Powrie, R. Paternal Perinatal Mental Health: At-Risk Fathers' Perceptions of Help-Seeking and Screening. *J. Men's Stud.* **2019**, *27*, 307–328. [CrossRef]
50. Ravn, I.H.; Smith, L.; Lindemann, R.; Smeby, N.A.; Kyno, N.M.; Bunch, E.H.; Sandvik, L. Effect of early intervention on social interaction between mothers and preterm infants at 12 months of age: A randomized controlled trial. *Infant Behav. Dev.* **2011**, *34*, 215–225. [CrossRef]
51. Bergström, E.-B.; Wallin, L.; Thomson, G.; Flacking, R. Postpartum depression in mothers of infants cared for in a Neonatal Intensive Care Unit—Incidence and associated factors. *J. Neonatal Nurs.* **2012**, *18*, 143–151. [CrossRef]
52. Pignon, A. What happens after the NICU? Parents Experience of Caring for their Premature Infants at Home. *OCCUPATION* **2017**, *2*, 68–76.
53. Grunberg, V.A.; Geller, P.A.; Bonacquisti, A.; Patterson, C.A. NICU infant health severity and family outcomes: A systematic review of assessments and findings in psychosocial research. *J. Perinatol.* **2019**, *39*, 156–172. [CrossRef]
54. Huhtala, M.; Korja, R.; Lehtonen, L.; Haataja, L.; Lapinleimu, H.; Munck, P.; Rautava, P.; the PIPARI Study Group. Parental psychological well-being and cognitive development of very low birth weight infants at 2 years. *Acta Paediatr.* **2011**, *100*, 1555–1560. [CrossRef]
55. Rollè, L.; Prino, L.E.; Sechi, C.; Vismara, L.; Neri, E.; Polizzi, C.; Trovato, A.; Volpi, B.; Molgora, S.; Fenaroli, V.; et al. Parenting Stress, Mental Health, Dyadic Adjustment: A Structural Equation Model. *Front. Psychol.* **2017**, *8*, 839. [CrossRef] [PubMed]
56. Martin, L.A.; Neighbors, H.W.; Griffith, D.M. The Experience of Symptoms of Depression in Men vs Women: Analysis of the National Comorbidity Survey Replication. *JAMA Psychiatry* **2013**, *70*, 1100–1106. [CrossRef] [PubMed]
57. O'Hara, M.W.; Wisner, K.L. Perinatal mental illness: Definition, description and aetiology. *Best Pract. Res. Clin. Obstet. Gynaecol.* **2014**, *28*, 3–12. [CrossRef] [PubMed]
58. Sekhon, M.; Cartwright, M.; Francis, J.J. Acceptability of healthcare interventions: An overview of reviews and development of a theoretical framework. *BMC Health Serv. Res.* **2017**, *17*, 88. [CrossRef]

Article

Construct Validity and Responsiveness of Instruments Measuring Depression and Anxiety in Pregnancy: A Comparison of EPDS, HADS-A and CES-D

Hanna Margaretha Heller [1,2,*], Stasja Draisma [2,3] and Adriaan Honig [2,4]

1 Department of Psychiatry, Amsterdam UMC Location Vrije Universiteit Amsterdam, Boelelaan 1117, 1081 HV Amsterdam, The Netherlands
2 Amsterdam Public Health, Mental Health Program, 1007 MB Amsterdam, The Netherlands; sdraisma@trimbos.nl (S.D.); a.honig@olvg.nl (A.H.)
3 Department on Aging, Netherlands Institute of Health and Addiction (Trimbos Institute), Da Costakade 45, 3521 VS Utrecht, The Netherlands
4 Department of Psychiatry, OLVG Hospital, Jan Tooropstraat 164, 1061 AE Amsterdam, The Netherlands
* Correspondence: hm.heller@amsterdamumc.nl; Tel.: +31-204-440-196

Abstract: Depression and anxiety occur frequently in pregnancy and may have unfavourable consequences for mother and child. Therefore, adequate symptom measurement seems important. Commonly used instruments are the Center for Epidemiologic Studies Depression Scale (CES-D), the Edinburgh Postpartum Depression Scale (EPDS), and the Hospital Anxiety and Depression Scale, anxiety subscale (HADS-A). We compared the (1) structural and (2) longitudinal validity of these instruments. The data originated from a study on the effectiveness of an Internet intervention for pregnant women with affective symptoms. (1) A confirmatory factor analysis was used to estimate the construct validity. The theoretical factorial structure that was defined in earlier studies of the CES-D and the EPDS, but not the HADS-A, could be sufficiently replicated with acceptable CFI and RMSEA values. (2) Since there were two measurements in time, the hypotheses concerning plausible directions of the change scores of subscales that were (un)related to each other could be formulated and tested. In this way, longitudinal validity in the form of responsiveness was estimated. Ten of sixteen hypotheses were confirmed, corroborating the longitudinal validity of all constructs, except anhedonia, probably due to inconsistent conceptualization. The HADS-A seems less suitable to screen for anxiety in pregnancy. Anhedonia needs better conceptualisation to assess the change of symptoms over time with the CES-D and the EPDS.

Keywords: questionnaires; screening; structural validity; perinatal depression; perinatal anxiety; pregnancy; responsiveness

1. Introduction

Depression and anxiety symptoms are regularly found among women during the antenatal period. Recent reviews show prevalence rates between 12 and 17 percent for antenatal depression [1,2] and prevalence rates of 15–23 percent of antenatal anxiety varying from pregnancy-specific anxiety to general anxiety symptoms [3–5], with higher rates in middle-low income countries [6,7]. Both antenatal depression and anxiety have been associated with poor pregnancy outcomes [8], poor postpartum mental health [9–11], and negative influences on child development [4,12–15]. Hence, screening for antenatal depression and anxiety is of the utmost importance. However, the selection of suitable screening instruments with adequate psychometric quality to identify symptoms of anxiety and depression during pregnancy is complicated: first, because physical changes, such as altered sleep and eating patterns, occur among most pregnant women, while items in self-report instruments for depression and anxiety often cover such somatic symptoms.

This may inflate the estimated occurrence of anxiety and depression. Moreover, during pregnancy specific types of worries with respect to labour and the child often occur and are not addressed in commonly used self-report instruments. Therefore, they may be overlooked and underreported when assessed with these instruments [5].

For our study concerning the effectiveness of a guided Internet intervention [16] for pregnant women with depressive or anxiety symptoms, we chose three commonly used screening instruments that measure depressive and anxiety symptoms in pregnancy. These instruments were the Center for Epidemiologic Studies Depression Scale (CES-D) and the Edinburgh Postpartum Depression Scale (EPDS) for depressive symptoms, and the Hospital Anxiety and Depression Scale, anxiety subscale (HADS-A) for anxiety symptoms.

The CES-D is a self-rating scale meant for measuring depressive symptomatology in the general population, but it is also widely used in pregnancy [17,18]. The overview of Carleton et al. [19] of twenty-five studies investigating structural validity with factor analyses of this instrument found models with one to four factors. The authors proposed a new three factor structure, tested on five different samples.

The EPDS is the most common instrument that is used to assess depression, but it also includes a few anxiety items [20]. It was designed to assess postnatal depression, yet it has also been validated for antenatal depression [21]. However, its factor structure is not always well established or replicated, suggesting mostly three factors, including depression, anxiety, and anhedonia, but also two factors, including only depression and anxiety [22].

The HADS-A is part of the HADS, which consists of two reliable subscales, one for depression (HADS-D) and one for anxiety (HADS-A). These subscales can be used independently [23]. The HADS-A is a widely used anxiety screening scale, originally developed to assess anxiety in non-psychiatric hospital outpatients [24]. It does not contain questions about physical symptoms which makes it suitable for pregnant women [24,25] who experience physical changes that may relate to both anxiety as well as to pregnancy.

Various studies present psychometric properties of the CES-D, the EPDS and the HADS-A questionnaires [19,20,26–28], but few studies deal with the comparison of these psychometric properties in pregnancy [5,17,29,30]. To the best of our knowledge, only three studies were carried out in pregnancy and involved a comparison of the cross validity of the CES-D, the EPDS and the HADS-A based on single scores of these scales [17,30,31]. None assessed their longitudinal validity, which is defined by comparing their sensitivity to change. This is especially important in pregnancy due to the variability of depressive and anxiety scores [32,33] and for the assessment of treatment outcomes. Sensitivity to change is also referred to as the responsiveness of an instrument and can be defined as the ability of the instrument to detect clinically important change over time [34].

The first aim of our study is to assess the (structural) construct validity of the CES-D, the EPDS and the HADS-A in a population of pregnant Dutch women by using a confirmatory factor analysis (CFA) cross-sectionally with baseline data. Most studies about the structure of these three instruments only applied an exploratory factor analysis. However, a confirmatory factor analysis is more appropriate to replicate earlier found factor structures as part of the validation of an instrument.

Secondly, validity is explored in a longitudinal way by formulating and testing hypotheses about relations between the change scores for different subscales. We do this to estimate the responsiveness of instruments over time in pregnancy to explore their sensitivity in measuring changes of symptoms. The hypotheses concern the subthemes: depression, anxiety and anhedonia, and are presented in the methods section.

2. Methods

2.1. Design and Participants

A secondary data analysis was performed with data that were collected in a randomized controlled trial (RCT) concerning the effectiveness of a guided Internet intervention (MamaKits) for pregnant women with moderate to severe symptoms of anxiety or depression, or both. The MamaKits study is described in more detail elsewhere [16]. In short, the study included self-referred pregnant women expressing interest in an Internet intervention to treat their depressive or anxiety symptoms. The inclusion criteria were being aged above 18 years, less than 30 weeks pregnant, having depressive symptoms above threshold (i.e., CES-D > 16) or anxiety symptoms above threshold (i.e., HADS-A > 8), or both. The single exclusion criterion was being suicidal. All participants signed their informed consent. The participants were randomly allocated to receive either a guided Internet intervention or care as usual. The EPDS was used as an additional measurement instrument. Further information was collected using one question of the Web Screening Questionnaire (WSQ) to asses suicidality [35], the Trimbos/institute for Medical Technology Assessment, Erasmus University Rotterdam questionnaire for costs associated with Psychiatric Illness for additional information about mental health [36], de Client Satisfaction Questionnaire (CSQ-8) to measure satisfaction about the intervention [37] and data on perinatal child outcome through self-report. Eligible women were recruited throughout the Netherlands via general media and flyers in prenatal care waiting rooms or via obstetricians and midwives. A total of 349 women expressed interest in the study, of which 91 withdrew their participation for several reasons, such as feeling better already. A further 99 were excluded because they did not fulfil the inclusion criteria, such as not reaching the symptom threshold. A total of 159 women completed one measurement at inclusion (T0) and met the inclusion criteria. About 10 weeks after randomization 119 of them also filled out the second measurement (T1). Due to inclusion in different stages of pregnancy T0 and T1 were taken at different moments in pregnancy. The study received approval from the Medical Ethics Committee of the VU University Medical Center (2013.275) and was registered in the Netherlands Trial Register (NL4162). All data were collected by Internet.

2.2. Measures

2.2.1. CES-D

The Center for Epidemiologic Studies Depression Scale (CES-D) [18] is a widely used instrument for screening depressive symptoms, also used in pregnancy, with 20 items concerning the last seven days. Symptoms are scored on a Likert-type scale from 0 to 3 ("rarely or none of the time" to "most or all of the time"), with a total score range from 0 (no depressive symptoms) to 60 (high number of depressive symptoms). The standard cut-off score is ≥ 16 for possible depression. The validity of the CES-D has been investigated in different populations, including pregnant women [30,38,39], on paper and online [40]. The scale has a sensitivity of 95.1% and a specificity of 85.0% [39] and the internal consistency (Cronbach's alpha) of the online version in the population at large is 0.89–0.93 [40]. The factor structure varies but the most frequently used consists of the following three or four factors: Somatic symptoms (6 items: item 1, 2, 5, 7, 11 and 20); negative affect (depressed) (4 items: item 3, 6, 14 and 18); positive affect (anhedonia) (4 items: item 4, 8, 12 and 16); and interpersonal affect if four factors were used (two items: item 15 and 19) (Carleton 2013). However, in other studies, a two, or another three or four factor model was found [40–42]. Anxiety is not included as a factor, but the instrument as a whole contains one item about anxiety (item 10, "I felt fearful").

2.2.2. EPDS

The EPDS is a 10-item depression scale, primarily developed to detect depression in the postpartum period, but it is also validated and widely used during pregnancy [21]. It is also used to measure anxiety [5,22,43] and its items address depressive and anxiety symptoms concerning the past seven days. Depending on the trimester, the cut-off score varies worldwide from 6.5 to 14.5, and in the Netherlands, it varies from 10 to 11 [21]. The item response options are 0 to 3 [21] and the total score range is 0 to 30 [21]. The internal consistency (Cronbach's alpha) was 0.87–0.90 in an online version [40,44]. Several factor models are investigated, but in most studies a three-factor model seems to fit best to the data [20,45]. The three factors most frequently found are: anhedonia (2 items: 1 and 2), anxiety (4 items: 3, 4, 5 and 6) and depression (4 items: 7, 8, 9 and 10) [5,20,45–47].

2.2.3. HADS-A

The Hospital Anxiety and Depression Scale, anxiety subscale (HADS-A) [24,27,48] is a screener for anxiety with item responses on a 0 to 3 scale, concerning the last week. Internal consistency as calculated with Cronbach's alpha varies but is 0.89 in the paper version [48] and 0.80 in the Internet version [49]. The HADS-A consists of 7 items (item 1, 3, 5, 7, 9, 11, 13) and has an optimal cut-off ≥ 8 to predict an anxiety disorder, with a sensitivity of 0.89 and a specificity of 0.75 [24,25,48]. The total score range is 0 to 21. The HADS-A is also used to measure anxiety in pregnancy [25,32] and it consists of one factor.

2.3. Data Analysis

2.3.1. Construct Validity

A confirmatory factor analysis (CFA) is commonly used to evaluate the latent factor structure of instrument items, to find support for an assumed grouping of items into subscales. For conceptualization of the factors of the three instruments that were involved, the factor structure was restricted a priori, according to the subscales that were found in recent studies. According to the study of Carleton [19], which consisted of five medium to large samples of people with different backgrounds, ages, gender, with and without medical and psychiatric problems, a three factor structure was found for the CES-D, consisting of the factors somatic symptoms, negative affect and anhedonia. The three-factor structure that was evaluated for the EPDS consisted of anhedonia, anxiety and depression [20,45–47]. The original HADS contains two factors, HADS-A- anxiety- and HADS-D –depression [26]. Since the MamaKits study only applied the HADS-A part of the instrument, only this factor, anxiety, was calculated and evaluated.

The LAVAAN package in R was used to assess whether the factors that were identified in the literature could be reproduced. Data of 159 included women from the baseline assessment were used. As measures for model fit, RMSEA (root mean square error of approximation) and CFI (comparative fit index) were used. RMSEA was assumed to be close to good when it was between 0.05 and 0.08, worse when >0.08 [50], TLI cut-off value close to 0.95 and SRMR cut-off value to 0.8. The CFI was acceptable when ≥ 0.90 and good when ≥ 0.95 [51].

2.3.2. Responsiveness

We studied the responsiveness of the three instruments by formulating hypotheses about expected differences and similarities in the change scores between T0 and T1. The hypotheses were based on theoretical contrasts between the different factors. An example is that the change scores between anxiety factors of different instruments are presumed to correlate more with each other than a change score of an anxiety factor with a depression factor. A hypothesis was corroborated when the expected difference in correlations of the change scores was at least 0.1 [52]. We used the criteria of de Boer [53] to assess responsiveness. This states that responsiveness is high if less than 25% of the hypotheses are refuted, moderate if 25 to 50% are refuted and low if more than 50% are refuted. The factors that we studied were 'negative or depressive affect', 'anxiety' and 'anhedonia'. We did not use the 'somatic symptoms' factor of the CES-D because this factor does not feature in any of the other instruments. The factor 'negative or depressive affect' refers to depressed mood (criterion A1 DSM-5 depressive disorder) [54]. The second factor, 'anhedonia' (criterion A2 DSM-5 depressive disorder) refers to the absence of almost all positive feelings and the inability to enjoy most or all aspects of life. The third factor 'anxiety' forms the main criterion of all anxiety disorders, as well as an additional feature to the classification of DSM-5 depressive disorder.

We formulated the following hypotheses:

<u>Negative (depressive) affect</u> We expected that the change scores in different subscales measuring depressive (negative) affect would be more strongly correlated to each other than to anxiety subscales (hypothesis 1 and 2) because depressive affect subscales contain no items measuring anxiety. Second, we hypothesized that the change scores of CES-D

negative affect would correlate more with the change scores in EPDS depression than with the EPDS anhedonia change scores (hypothesis 3), because negative/depressive affect scales refer to gloominess or a black mood, whereas anhedonia reflects the in ability to enjoy life.

Anhedonia We expected that EPDS and CES-D scales measuring change in anhedonia scores would correlate more with each other than with the EPDS depression, the CES-D negative affect and the HADS-A anxiety scales (hypotheses 4, 5, 6) since they measure the same construct expressing the absence of the ability to enjoy life, which is conceptually different from anxiety and negative/depressive affect.

Anxiety First, we expected the CES-D change in item 10 anxiety to be more strongly correlated with the HADS-A total scale change, since they indicate the same construct, whereas the CES-D negative affect, the EPDS depression, the CES-D anhedonia and the EPDS anhedonia represent other factors (hypotheses 7, 8, 9 and 10). Second, we hypothesized that the change score of the HADS-A and the change score of the anxiety scale of the EPDS correlate more with each other than with those of the CES-D negative affect, the EPDS depression, the EPDS anhedonia and the CES-D anhedonia (hypotheses 11, 12, 13 and 14). Finally, we hypothesized that the HADS-A change score is equally correlated to the EPDS anxiety score as to the CES-D anxiety score (hypothesis 15).

Comparison of questionnaires We expected a stronger correlation of changes between the CES-D and the EPDS total scales than each instrument with the HADS-A (hypothesis 16) since the EPDS and the CES-D consist of almost the same factors, while the HADS-A contains only one common (anxiety) factor.

3. Results

3.1. General Results

A total of 159 women who completed T0 and met the inclusion criteria were enrolled, of which 74.8% (n = 119) completed T1. Their median CES-D scores at the two time points (T0, T1) were 28 and 17 (interquartile range were 9–48 and 2–55, respectively); the median EPDS scores were 14 and 8 (interquartile range, respectively, 3–28 and 0–26); and the median HADS-A scores were 12 and 8 (interquartile range, respectively, 4–20 and 1–19). A more extensive description of the results is described elsewhere [16]. Table 1 contains the description of the sample.

3.2. Cross-Sectional Results

Cronbach's α's for the total scales of the three instruments were: CESD 0.84, EPDS 0.80 and HADS-A 0.72, denoting the sufficient reliability of the scales. Results of the CFA (Table 2) indicated that the theoretical factorial structure of both EPDS [20] and CESD [19] could be replicated sufficiently with acceptable CFI's and cut-off values of RMSEA's that were close to 0.08. However, the one factor model for the HADS-A was not replicated adequately; RMSEA was higher than the cut-off of 0.08 and CFI was too small. The SRMR values were close to 0.07. The acceptable range for the SRMR index is between 0 and 0.08 [51], therefore these values are adequate. The TLI values are all rather low, lower than the required 0.95. These values indicate poor model fit, maybe due to low inter-item correlations. A notable finding in Table 3 is that two items about restlessness did not load on the same factors as in the previous research, neither in the factor somatic symptoms of the CES-D (item 11) [19], nor in the factor anxiety of the HADS (item 11) [26]. Both items correlated weakly with other items of the same factor.

Table 1. Sociodemographic and clinical characteristics at baseline for intervention group and control group.

Variables	
Demographic factors ($n = 159$)	
Maternal age, years (mean ± SD)	32.01 (4.71)
Background (Dutch)	134 (84.3%)
Education [a]	
low	4 (2.5%)
middle	35 (22.0%)
high	120 (75.5%)
Marital status	
Relationship, yes	152 (95.6%)
Living together	144 (90.6%)
Employed, yes	111 (69.8%)
Pregnancy ($n = 159$)	
Duration by study entrance	
<12 weeks	16 (10.1%)
>12 and <26 weeks	92 (57.9%)
>26 weeks	51 (32.1%)
Previous mental health [b] ($n = 159$)	
Depressive disorder	53 (33.3%)
Anxiety disorder	45 (28.3%)
Other mental problems	11 (6.9%)
No diagnosis	61 (38.4%)
Affective symptoms (mean ± SD)	
T0 ($n = 159$)	
CES-D	28.38 (8.31)
EPDS	14.11 (4.91)
HADS-A	11.67 (3.43)
T1 ($n = 119$)	
CES-D	19.02 (9.74)
EPDS	9.17 (5.52)
HADS-A	8.52 (3.91)

[a] Dutch Standard Classification of Education: Standaard Onderwijsindeling 2006—Editie 2016/'2017, StatLine, the electronic database of Statistics Netherlands. [b] note that women can be both in the category 'depressive disorder' and in the category 'anxiety disorder'.

Table 2. Fit measures of confirmatory factor analysis of the three instruments ($n = 159$).

	Chi Square (*p* Value)	CFI	TLI	RMSEA (CI)	SRMR
CESD (3 factors somatic, neg. affect/depression, anhedonia)	118.848 (df = 74, $p = 0.001$)	0.923	0.906	0.062 (0.040–0.082)	0.070
EPDS (3 factors, anxiety, depression, anhedonia)	62.55 (df = 32, $p = 0.001$)	0.929	0.899	0.077 (0.048–0.106)	0.069
HADS (1 factor anxiety)	51.996 (df = 14, $p = 0.000$)	0.831	0.747	0.131 (0.093–0.171)	0.075

Table 3. Factor loadings for items of the CESD, HADS-A and EPDS (n = 159).

Factor	Item Content	Symptoms		
	CES-D	Somatic	Depression	Anhedonia
Somatic	1. I was bothered by things that usually don't bother me.	0.297		
	2. I did not feel like eating; my appetite was poor.	0.356		
	5. I had trouble keeping my mind on what I was doing.	0.300		
	7. I felt that everything I did was an effort.	0.583		
	11. My sleep was restless.	0.048		
Depressed	3. I felt that I could not shake off the blues.		0.581	
	6. I felt depressed.		0.669	
	14. I felt lonely.		0.476	
	18. I felt sad.		0.598	
	20. I could not get "going"		0.557	
Anhedonia	4. I felt that I was just as good as other people.			0.368
	8. I felt hopeful about the future.			0.298
	12. I was happy.			0.533
	16. I enjoyed life.			0.593
	EPDS	Anhedonia	Anxiety	Depression
Anhedonia	1. I have been able to laugh and see the funny side of things.	0.509		
	2. I have looked forward with enjoyment to things.	0.766		
Anxiety	3. I have blamed myself unnecessarily when things went wrong.		0.392	
	4. I have been anxious or worried for no good reason.		0.521	
	5 I have felt scared or panicky for no very good reason.		0.553	
	6. Things have been getting on top of me.		0.385	
Depression	7. I have been so unhappy that I have had difficulty sleeping.			0.505
	8. I have felt sad or miserable.			0.606
	9. I have been so unhappy that I have been crying.			0.641
	10. The thought of harming myself has occurred to me.			0.437
	HADS-A	Anxiety		
Anxiety	1. I feel tense or wound up.	0.384		
	3. I get a sort of frightened feeling as if something awful is about to happen.	0.648		
	5. Worrying thoughts go through my mind.	0.511		
	7. I can sit at ease and feel relaxed.	0.376		
	9. I get a sort of frightened feeling like 'butterflies' in the stomach.	0.432		
	11. I feel restless as if I have to be on the move.	0.140		
	13. I get sudden feelings of panic.	0.413		

3.3. Responsiveness Results

The majority of hypotheses–10 out of 16–concerning change could be confirmed, 37.5% were rejected, which indicates moderate responsiveness (Table 4).

More specifically, the change scores in CES-D and EPDS measuring depressive (negative) affect were more correlated to each other than to the changes scores in anxiety, but unexpectedly, they were also correlated to the EPDS factor anhedonia (difference 0.064).

Change scores of the factors measuring anhedonia were even less correlated to each other than to the factors measuring negative affect/depression and almost equally to the HADS-A.

The change scores of the anxiety items of all instruments were equally strongly correlated. However, the correlation of the change scores between the anxiety item (s) of the CES-D and the HADS-A was almost equal to the correlation with the EPDS anhedonia change (difference 0.04). This also applied to the correlation of change between the anxiety items of EPDS and the HADS-A with the CES-D anhedonia change (difference 0.08).

Concerning the measurement instruments as a whole, the change scores of the EPDS correlated more strongly with the CES-D change scores than with the HADS-A change scores, as was expected.

Table 4. Outcome of hypotheses for responsiveness of constructs of CES-D, HADS-A and EPDS.

Hypothesis:	Correlations *	Confirmed
CES-D negative affect change is more strongly correlated to EPDS depression change		
1 than to HADS-A (anxiety) change	0.694 vs. 0.313	Yes
2 than to EPDS anxiety change	0.694 vs. 0.248	Yes
3 than to EPDS anhedonia change	0.694 vs. 0.630	No < 0.1
CES-D anhedonia change is more strongly correlated to EPDS anhedonia change		
4 than to EPDS depression change	0.486 vs. 0.543	No
5 than to CES-D negative affect change	0.486 vs. 0.510	No
6 than to HADS-A change	0.486 vs. 0.462	No < 0.1
CES-D anxiety change (1 item) is more strongly correlated to HADS-A change		
7 than to CES-D negative affect change	0.458 vs. 0.286	Yes
8 than to EPDS depression change	0.458 vs. 0.355	Yes
9 than to CES-D anhedonia change	0.458 vs. 0.345	Yes
10 than to EPDS anhedonia change	0.458 vs. 0.418	No < 0.1
HADS-A (anxiety) change is more strongly correlated to EPDS anxiety change		
11 than to CES-D negative affect change	0.554 vs. 0.313	Yes
12 than to EPDS depression change	0.554 vs. 0.418	Yes
13 than to EPDS anhedonia change	0.554 vs. 0.295	Yes
14 than to CES-D anhedonia change	0.554 vs. 0.462	No < 0.1
HADS-A anxiety change is equally correlated to EPDS anxiety change		
15 than to CES-D anxiety (1 item) change	0.554 vs. 0.458	Yes
CES-D total scale change score is more strongly correlated to EPDS total scale change score		
16 than to HADS-A change score	0.732 vs. 0.485	Yes

* Correlations are calculated between change scores (T0–T1) of two subscales. Resulting correlations of two sets are compared, differences > 1 are considered significant.

4. Discussion

Our evaluation of cross-sectional construct validity as assessed by CFA of the three instruments for measuring depression and anxiety in pregnancy, delivered predominantly adequate results, apart from those of HADS-A.

For the CES-D, the three-factor structure ('somatic symptoms', 'negative affect' and 'anxiety' [19]) was replicated sufficiently. The EPDS three-factor structure of anhedonia, anxiety and depression [20] was also found to be adequate. The factor structure of the HADS-A turned out relatively weak according to low fit measures. One possible explanation for the poor outcomes of the total HADS-A subscale in our study is that only HADS-A anxiety items were used, whereas in a meta-CFA it was found that the HADS mainly measures distress, without a distinction between depression and anxiety [26,28]. Furthermore, the HADS-A seems to be sensitive to biological changes, assessing anxiety as autonomic arousal [28,55]. Since biology during pregnancy changes considerably, this could negatively impact the validity of the instrument. Unlike the HADS-A, the EPDS item formulations for anxiety contain more cognitive-emotional expressions (such as, 'feeling scared for no good reason', 'being anxious or worried for no good reason') which may explain our replication of the proposed latent structure of the EPDS. However, since this scale was especially designed for use in the perinatal period, items that could be influenced by physical symptoms were avoided [56]. A third reason for the poor outcome of the HADS could be that the anxiety in pregnancy is different from other anxiety disorders and specific for the prenatal period [57].

In our study we added a new approach by exploring construct validity in a longitudinal way. We did this by formulating and testing hypotheses to assess the responsiveness of instruments over time and their difference in measuring changes of symptoms. As the majority of hypotheses concerning change scores could be confirmed, six of eight hypotheses considering anhedonia (hypotheses 3, 4, 5, 6, 10 and 14) had to be refuted. The most remarkable finding was that the correlation of change scores of the EPDS construct anhedonia was even less strongly correlated to the change score of the CES-D construct anhedonia than to the change scores of the constructs of CES-D negative affect and EPDS depression. It was about equally strongly correlated to the HADS anxiety scale. An explanation for this finding is the inconsistent conceptualization of the concept anhedonia. In the DSM-5, anhedonia is defined as the absence of the ability to have interest and/or enjoy activities that were previously considered pleasurable [54]. However, in the description of the factors of the CES-D, for example by Carleton [19] anhedonia is defined as the absence of positive affect. Considering the EPDS validation studies [20,46] the factor anhedonia is sometimes defined as inability to feel pleasure from normally pleasurable experiences and in other studies as having low positive affect.

So, although the CES-D and the EPDS both contain a factor anhedonia, the items loading on the factors differ substantially, which make them not comparable.

5. Limitations

The instruments were used in different stages of pregnancy, reducing comparability and hence, validity. Second, including the HADS-D instrument for depression could have resulted in better outcomes for the factor analysis of the HADS. Third, to deliver more robust results of the CFA of the instruments, we probably needed to include a larger sample of women. This is especially applicable to the TLI and the RMSEA [51]. Fourth, the fact that the women in our sample were relatively highly educated may have influenced the results of the cross sectional, as well as the longitudinal analyses.

6. Conclusions

Based on their high construct validity, CES-D and the EPDS, but not the HADS-A, seem to be reliable instruments to assess depression and anxiety in pregnancy.

The reason that HADS-A is probably less useful as an instrument to measure prenatal anxiety is its sensitivity to biological changes which occur frequently in pregnancy. Secondly, prenatal anxiety seems to be a distinct kind of anxiety which requires a specific type of questionnaire.

The responsiveness of the three instruments was moderate, probably due to the change scores of the anhedonia constructs which need more theoretical and empirical substantiation.

More research is needed to develop a sensitive questionnaire to measure anxiety in pregnancy and to investigate how to improve the responsiveness of instruments. Existing questionnaires measuring pregnancy-specific anxiety, such as the Pregnancy Related Anxiety Questionnaire and the Pregnancy-Related Anxiety scale need more extensive validation.

Furthermore, we recommend testing of the instruments in larger samples of women at the same stage of pregnancy, but with a more diverse background, such as a varying level of education.

Author Contributions: Conceptualization, S.D. and A.H.; Formal analysis, H.M.H. and S.D.; Funding acquisition, H.M.H. and A.H.; Investigation, H.M.H.; Methodology, S.D.; Project administration, A.H.; Supervision, A.H.; Writing–original draft, H.M.H.; Writing–review and editing, H.M.H., S.D. and A.H. All authors have read and agreed to the published version of the manuscript.

Funding: The authors disclosed receipt of the following financial support: the randomized controlled trial MamaKits was supported by the Stichting tot Steun VCVGZ. The funding number is 197.

Institutional Review Board Statement: The original MamaKits study was conducted in accordance with the Declaration of Helsinki and approved by the Institutional Ethics Committee of VU University Medical Center (protocol code 2013.275; date of approval 27 November 2013).

Informed Consent Statement: Informed consent was obtained from all subjects involved in the study.

Data Availability Statement: Data sharing is not applicable to this article. No new data were created or analysed in this study.

Acknowledgments: We thank Liesbeth Ribbink for her contribution to the editing.

Conflicts of Interest: The authors declare no conflict of interest. The funders had no role in the design of the study; in the collection, analyses, or interpretation of data; in the writing of the manuscript, or in the decision to publish the results.

References

1. Underwood, L.; Waldie, K.; D'Souza, S.; Peterson, E.R.; Morton, S. A review of longitudinal studies on antenatal and postnatal depression. *Arch. Women's Ment. Health* **2016**, *19*, 711–720. [CrossRef] [PubMed]
2. Woody, C.A.; Ferrari, A.J.; Siskind, D.J.; Whiteford, H.A.; Harris, M.G. A systematic review and meta-regression of the prevalence and incidence of perinatal depression. *J. Affect. Disord.* **2017**, *219*, 86–92. [CrossRef] [PubMed]
3. Dennis, C.L.; Falah-Hassani, K.; Shiri, R. Prevalence of antenatal and postnatal anxiety: Systematic review and meta-analysis. *Br. J. Psychiatry J. Ment. Sci.* **2017**, *210*, 315–323. [CrossRef]
4. Grigoriadis, S.; Graves, L.; Peer, M.; Mamisashvili, L.; Tomlinson, G.; Vigod, S.N.; Dennis, C.L.; Steiner, M.; Brown, C.; Cheung, A.; et al. Maternal Anxiety During Pregnancy and the Association With Adverse Perinatal Outcomes: Systematic Review and Meta-Analysis. *J. Clin. Psychiatry* **2018**, *79*, 813. [CrossRef]
5. Sinesi, A.; Maxwell, M.; O'Carroll, R.; Cheyne, H. Anxiety scales used in pregnancy: Systematic review. *BJPsych Open* **2019**, *5*, e5. [CrossRef]
6. Biaggi, A.; Conroy, S.; Pawlby, S.; Pariante, C.M. Identifying the women at risk of antenatal anxiety and depression: A systematic review. *J. Affect. Disord.* **2016**, *191*, 62–77. [CrossRef]
7. Fellmeth, G.; Fazel, M.; Plugge, E. Migration and perinatal mental health in women from low- and middle-income countries: A systematic review and meta-analysis. *BJOG Int. J. Obstet. Gynaecol.* **2017**, *124*, 742–752. [CrossRef] [PubMed]
8. Jarde, A.; Morais, M.; Kingston, D.; Giallo, R.; MacQueen, G.M.; Giglia, L.; Beyene, J.; Wang, Y.; McDonald, S.D. Neonatal Outcomes in Women With Untreated Antenatal Depression Compared With Women Without Depression: A Systematic Review and Meta-analysis. *JAMA Psychiatry* **2016**, *73*, 826–837. [CrossRef] [PubMed]
9. Gelaye, B.; Rondon, M.B.; Araya, R.; Williams, M.A. Epidemiology of maternal depression, risk factors, and child outcomes in low-income and middle-income countries. *Lancet Psychiatry* **2016**, *3*, 973–982. [CrossRef]
10. Meltzer-Brody, S. Heterogeneity of postpartum depression: A latent class analysis. *Lancet Psychiatry* **2015**, *2*, 59–67. [CrossRef]
11. Robertson, E.; Grace, S.; Wallington, T.; Stewart, D.E. Antenatal risk factors for postpartum depression: A synthesis of recent literature. *Gen. Hosp. Psychiatry* **2004**, *26*, 289–295. [CrossRef] [PubMed]
12. Barker, E.D.; Jaffee, S.R.; Uher, R.; Maughan, B. The contribution of prenatal and postnatal maternal anxiety and depression to child maladjustment. *Depress. Anxiety* **2011**, *28*, 696–702. [CrossRef] [PubMed]
13. Goodman, J.H. Women's attitudes, preferences, and perceived barriers to treatment for perinatal depression. *Birth* **2009**, *36*, 60–69. [CrossRef]
14. Grigoriadis, S.; VonderPorten, E.H.; Mamisashvili, L.; Tomlinson, G.; Dennis, C.L.; Koren, G.; Steiner, M.; Mousmanis, P.; Cheung, A.; Radford, K.; et al. The impact of maternal depression during pregnancy on perinatal outcomes: A systematic review and meta-analysis. *J. Clin. Psychiatry* **2013**, *74*, e321–e341. [CrossRef] [PubMed]
15. Verbeek, T.; Bockting, C.L.; van Pampus, M.G.; Ormel, J.; Meijer, J.L.; Hartman, C.A.; Burger, H. Postpartum depression predicts offspring mental health problems in adolescence independently of parental lifetime psychopathology. *J. Affect. Disord.* **2012**, *136*, 948–954. [CrossRef] [PubMed]
16. Heller, H.M.; Hoogendoorn, A.W.; Honig, A.; Broekman, B.F.P.; van Straten, A. The Effectiveness of a Guided Internet-Based Tool for the Treatment of Depression and Anxiety in Pregnancy (MamaKits Online): Randomized Controlled Trial. *J. Med. Internet Res.* **2020**, *22*, e15172. [CrossRef] [PubMed]
17. Mosack, V.; Shore, E.R. Screening for depression among pregnant and postpartum women. *J. Community Health Nurs.* **2006**, *23*, 37–47. [CrossRef]
18. Radloff, L.S. The CES-D Scale: A Self-Report Depression Scale for Research in the General Population. *Appl. Psychol. Meas.* **1977**, *1*, 385–401. [CrossRef]
19. Carleton, R.N.; Thibodeau, M.A.; Teale, M.J.; Welch, P.G.; Abrams, M.P.; Robinson, T.; Asmundson, G.J. The center for epidemiologic studies depression scale: A review with a theoretical and empirical examination of item content and factor structure. *PLoS ONE* **2013**, *8*, e58067. [CrossRef]
20. Coates, R.; Ayers, S.; de Visser, R. Factor structure of the Edinburgh Postnatal Depression Scale in a population-based sample. *Psychol. Assess.* **2017**, *29*, 1016–1027. [CrossRef]

21. Bergink, V.; Kooistra, L.; Lambregtse-van den Berg, M.P.; Wijnen, H.; Bunevicius, R.; van Baar, A.; Pop, V. Validation of the Edinburgh Depression Scale during pregnancy. *J. Psychosom. Res.* **2011**, *70*, 385–389. [CrossRef]
22. Brouwers, E.P.; van Baar, A.L.; Pop, V.J. Does the Edinburgh Postnatal Depression Scale measure anxiety? *J. Psychosom. Res.* **2001**, *51*, 659–663. [CrossRef]
23. Herrmann, C. International experiences with the Hospital Anxiety and Depression Scale–a review of validation data and clinical results. *J. Psychosom. Res.* **1997**, *42*, 17–41. [CrossRef]
24. Zigmond, A.S.; Snaith, R.P. The hospital anxiety and depression scale. *Acta Psychiatr. Scand.* **1983**, *67*, 361–370. [CrossRef]
25. Rubertsson, C.; Hellström, J.; Cross, M.; Sydsjö, G. Anxiety in early pregnancy: Prevalence and contributing factors. *Arch. Women's Ment. Health* **2014**, *17*, 221–228. [CrossRef] [PubMed]
26. Norton, S.; Cosco, T.; Doyle, F.; Done, J.; Sacker, A. The Hospital Anxiety and Depression Scale: A meta confirmatory factor analysis. *J. Psychosom. Res.* **2013**, *74*, 74–81. [CrossRef] [PubMed]
27. Bjelland, I.; Dahl, A.A.; Haug, T.T.; Neckelmann, D. The validity of the Hospital Anxiety and Depression Scale. An updated literature review. *J. Psychosom. Res.* **2002**, *52*, 69–77. [CrossRef]
28. Karimova, G.; Martin, C. A psychometric evaluation of the Hospital Anxiety and Depression Scale during pregnancy. *Psychol. Health Med.* **2003**, *8*, 89–103. [CrossRef]
29. Chorwe-Sungani, G.; Chipps, J. A systematic review of screening instruments for depression for use in antenatal services in low resource settings. *BMC Psychiatry* **2017**, *17*, 112. [CrossRef]
30. Tandon, S.D.; Cluxton-Keller, F.; Leis, J.; Le, H.N.; Perry, D.F. A comparison of three screening tools to identify perinatal depression among low-income African American women. *J. Affect. Disord.* **2012**, *136*, 155–162. [CrossRef]
31. Evans, K.; Spiby, H.; Morrell, C.J. A psychometric systematic review of self-report instruments to identify anxiety in pregnancy. *J. Adv. Nurs.* **2015**, *71*, 1986–2001. [CrossRef]
32. Matthey, S.; Ross-Hamid, C. Repeat testing on the Edinburgh Depression Scale and the HADS-A in pregnancy: Differentiating between transient and enduring distress. *J. Affect. Disord.* **2012**, *141*, 213–221. [CrossRef]
33. Banti, S.; Mauri, M.; Oppo, A.; Borri, C.; Rambelli, C.; Ramacciotti, D.; Montagnani, M.S.; Camilleri, V.; Cortopassi, S.; Rucci, P.; et al. From the third month of pregnancy to 1 year postpartum. Prevalence, incidence, recurrence, and new on-set of depression. Results from the perinatal depression-research & screening unit study. *Compr. Psychiatry* **2011**, *52*, 343–351. [CrossRef]
34. Terwee, C.B.; Bot, S.D.; de Boer, M.R.; van der Windt, D.A.; Knol, D.L.; Dekker, J.; Bouter, L.M.; de Vet, H.C. Quality criteria were proposed for measurement properties of health status questionnaires. *J. Clin. Epidemiol.* **2007**, *60*, 34–42. [CrossRef]
35. Donker, T.; van Straten, A.; Marks, I.; Cuijpers, P. A brief Web-based screening questionnaire for common mental disorders: Development and validation. *J. Med. Internet Res.* **2009**, *11*, e19. [CrossRef] [PubMed]
36. Bouwmans, C.; Hakkaart-van Roijen, L. *Manual Trimbos/iMTA Questionnaire for Costs Associated with Psychiatric Illness (in Dutch)*; Institute for Medical Technology Assessment: Rotterdam, The Netherlands, 2013.
37. De Brey, H. A cross-national validation of the client satisfaction questionnaire: The Dutch experience. *Eval. Program Plan.* **1983**, *6*, 395–400. [CrossRef]
38. Beekman, A.T.; Deeg, D.J.; Van Limbeek, J.; Braam, A.W.; De Vries, M.Z.; Van Tilburg, W. Criterion validity of the Center for Epidemiologic Studies Depression scale (CES-D): Results from a community-based sample of older subjects in The Netherlands. *Psychol. Med.* **1997**, *27*, 231–235. [CrossRef] [PubMed]
39. Wada, K.; Tanaka, K.; Theriault, G.; Satoh, T.; Mimura, M.; Miyaoka, H.; Aizawa, Y. Validity of the Center for Epidemiologic Studies Depression Scale as a screening instrument of major depressive disorder among Japanese workers. *Am. J. Ind. Med.* **2007**, *50*, 8–12. [CrossRef] [PubMed]
40. van Ballegooijen, W.; Riper, H.; Cuijpers, P.; van Oppen, P.; Smit, J.H. Validation of online psychometric instruments for common mental health disorders: A systematic review. *BMC Psychiatry* **2016**, *16*, 45. [CrossRef]
41. Leykin, Y.; Torres, L.D.; Aguilera, A.; Muñoz, R.F. Factor structure of the CES-D in a sample of Spanish- and English-speaking smokers on the Internet. *Psychiatry Res.* **2011**, *185*, 269–274. [CrossRef]
42. Thombs, B.D.; Hudson, M.; Schieir, O.; Taillefer, S.S.; Baron, M. Reliability and validity of the center for epidemiologic studies depression scale in patients with systemic sclerosis. *Arthritis Rheum.* **2008**, *59*, 438–443. [CrossRef] [PubMed]
43. Loyal, D.; Sutter, A.L.; Rascle, N. Screening Beyond Postpartum Depression: Occluded Anxiety Component in the EPDS (EPDS-3A) in French Mothers. *Matern. Child Health J.* **2020**, *24*, 369–377. [CrossRef]
44. Spek, V.; Nyklícek, I.; Cuijpers, P.; Pop, V. Internet administration of the Edinburgh Depression Scale. *J. Affect. Disord.* **2008**, *106*, 301–305. [CrossRef]
45. Long, M.M.; Cramer, R.J.; Bennington, L.; Morgan, F.G., Jr.; Wilkes, C.A.; Fontanares, A.J.; Sadr, N.; Bertolino, S.M.; Paulson, J.F. Psychometric assessment of the Edinburgh Postnatal Depression Scale in an obstetric population. *Psychiatry Res.* **2020**, *291*, 113161. [CrossRef]
46. Kozinszky, Z.; Töreki, A.; Hompoth, E.A.; Dudas, R.B.; Németh, G. A more rational, theory-driven approach to analysing the factor structure of the Edinburgh Postnatal Depression Scale. *Psychiatry Res.* **2017**, *250*, 234–243. [CrossRef]
47. Tuohy, A.; McVey, C. Subscales measuring symptoms of non-specific depression, anhedonia, and anxiety in the Edinburgh Postnatal Depression Scale. *Br. J. Clin. Psychol.* **2008**, *47*, 153–169. [CrossRef]

48. Olssøn, I.; Mykletun, A.; Dahl, A.A. The Hospital Anxiety and Depression Rating Scale: A cross-sectional study of psychometrics and case finding abilities in general practice. *BMC Psychiatry* **2005**, *5*, 46. [CrossRef]
49. Whitehead, L. Methodological issues in Internet-mediated research: A randomized comparison of internet versus mailed questionnaires. *J. Med. Internet Res.* **2011**, *13*, e109. [CrossRef] [PubMed]
50. Cangur, S.; Ercan, I. Comparison of Model Fit Indices Used in Structural Equation Modeling Under Multivariate Normality. *J. Mod. Appl. Stat. Methods* **2015**, *14*, 152–167. [CrossRef]
51. Hu, L.t.; Bentler, P.M. Cutoff criteria for fit indexes in covariance structure analysis: Conventional criteria versus new alternatives. *Struct. Equ. Model. A Multidiscip. J.* **1999**, *6*, 1–55. [CrossRef]
52. De Boer, M.R.; Terwee, C.B.; de Vet, H.C.; Moll, A.C.; Völker-Dieben, H.J.; van Rens, G.H. Evaluation of cross-sectional and longitudinal construct validity of two vision-related quality of life questionnaires: The LVQOL and VCM1. *Qual. Life Res. Int. J. Qual. Life Asp. Treat. Care Rehabil.* **2006**, *15*, 233–248. [CrossRef]
53. De Boer, M.R.; Moll, A.C.; de Vet, H.C.; Terwee, C.B.; Völker-Dieben, H.J.; van Rens, G.H. Psychometric properties of vision-related quality of life questionnaires: A systematic review. *Ophthalmic Physiol. Opt. J. Br. Coll. Ophthalmic Opt.* **2004**, *24*, 257–273. [CrossRef] [PubMed]
54. American Psychiatric Association. *Diagnostic and Statistical Manual of Mental Disorders*, 5th ed.; American Psychiatric Association: Washington, DC, USA, 2013.
55. Jomeen, J.; Martin, C.R. Is the hospital anxiety and depression scale (HADS) a reliable screening tool in early pregnancy? *Psychol. Health* **2004**, *19*, 787–800. [CrossRef]
56. Cox, J.L.; Holden, J.M.; Sagovsky, R. Detection of postnatal depression. Development of the 10-item Edinburgh Postnatal Depression Scale. *Br. J. Psychiatry J. Ment. Sci.* **1987**, *150*, 782–786. [CrossRef] [PubMed]
57. Brunton, R.J.; Dryer, R.; Saliba, A.; Kohlhoff, J. Pregnancy anxiety: A systematic review of current scales. *J. Affect. Disord.* **2015**, *176*, 24–34. [CrossRef] [PubMed]

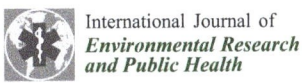

Article

A Comparison of Three Measures to Identify Postnatal Anxiety: Analysis of the 2020 National Maternity Survey in England

Gracia Fellmeth [1,*], Siân Harrison [1], Maria A. Quigley [1] and Fiona Alderdice [1,2]

[1] NHIR Policy Research Unit in Maternal and Neonatal Health and Care, National Perinatal Epidemiology Unit, Nuffield Department of Population Health, University of Oxford, Oxford OX3 7LF, UK; sian.harrison@npeu.ox.ac.uk (S.H.); maria.quigley@npeu.ox.ac.uk (M.A.Q.); fiona.alderdice@npeu.ox.ac.uk (F.A.)

[2] School of Nursing and Midwifery, Queen's University Belfast, Belfast BT7 1NN, UK

* Correspondence: gracia.fellmeth@ndph.ox.ac.uk

Abstract: Perinatal anxiety affects an estimated 15% of women globally and is associated with poor maternal and infant outcomes. Identifying women with anxiety is essential to prevent these adverse associations, but there are a number of challenges around measurement. We used data from England's 2020 National Maternity Survey to compare the prevalence of anxiety symptoms at six months postpartum using three different measures: the two-item Generalised Anxiety Disorders Scale (GAD-2), the anxiety subscales of the Edinburgh Postnatal Depression Scale (EPDS-3A) and a direct question. The concordance between each pair of measures was calculated using two-by-two tables. Survey weights were applied to increase the representativeness of the sample and reduce the risk of non-response bias. The prevalence of postnatal anxiety among a total of 4611 women was 15.0% on the GAD-2, 28.8% on the EPDS-3A and 17.1% on the direct question. Concordance between measures ranged between 78.6% (95% CI 77.4–79.8; Kappa 0.40) and 85.2% (95% CI 84.1–86.2; Kappa 0.44). Antenatal anxiety was the strongest predictor of postnatal anxiety across all three measures. Women of Black, Asian or other minority ethnicity were less likely to report self-identified anxiety compared with women of White ethnicity (adjusted odds ratio 0.44; 95% CI 0.30–0.64). Despite some overlap, different anxiety measures identify different groups of women. Certain population characteristics such as women's ethnicity may determine which type of measure is most likely to identify women experiencing anxiety.

Keywords: postnatal; anxiety; identifying; screening; GAD; EPDS

Citation: Fellmeth, G.; Harrison, S.; Quigley, M.A.; Alderdice, F. A Comparison of Three Measures to Identify Postnatal Anxiety: Analysis of the 2020 National Maternity Survey in England. *IJERPH* **2022**, *19*, 6578. https://doi.org/10.3390/ijerph19116578

Academic Editor: Francesca Agostini

Received: 9 May 2022
Accepted: 27 May 2022
Published: 28 May 2022

Publisher's Note: MDPI stays neutral with regard to jurisdictional claims in published maps and institutional affiliations.

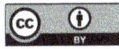

Copyright: © 2022 by the authors. Licensee MDPI, Basel, Switzerland. This article is an open access article distributed under the terms and conditions of the Creative Commons Attribution (CC BY) license (https://creativecommons.org/licenses/by/4.0/).

1. Introduction

Anxiety disorders are common during the perinatal period [1]. Anxiety disorders are characterised by core symptoms of anxiety, including cognitive distortions, physiological arousal and behavioural avoidance [2]. Globally, an estimated 15% of women experience anxiety symptoms postnatally, with significantly higher rates in low- and middle-income countries (LMIC) [3–5]. Figures from the UK are slightly lower, with one review estimating prevalence to be 12–15% during pregnancy and 8% postnatally [6]. Exposure to the physiological and psychosocial impacts of anxiety during this critical period has been associated with poor maternal, infant and child outcomes, including delayed cognitive and behavioural development [7–9]. Timely identification and treatment of perinatal anxiety are therefore essential to prevent adverse outcomes for women and their children.

A number of challenges exist around measuring perinatal anxiety [2]. Although several self-report measures have been validated to facilitate the recognition of anxiety, uncertainty remains around which instrument is most suitable for perinatal women and best able to identify women who need support [10]. The number of items included on a measure and the time required for completion have been highlighted as barriers to their administration. Shortened measures have been suggested as a solution to this. In the UK, the National Institute for Health and Care Excellence (NICE) recommends administering the two-item version of the Generalised Anxiety Scale (GAD-2) to all women at their first antenatal appointment and in the early postnatal period [11,12]. However, there remains uncertainty around the psychometric properties of the GAD-2 in perinatal populations, and direct comparisons of how the GAD-2 performs against other self-report measures are lacking.

An alternative method of identifying women with anxiety is to ask women directly whether they self-identify as having anxiety. This measure of 'self-identified anxiety' may offer advantages in certain contexts. For instance, it may help to identify women who have anxiety but whose symptoms differ from those captured by self-report measures. Self-identified anxiety may also help to identify women with anxiety who do not meet the severity threshold of standardised measures. A direct question may be preferable in communities less familiar with the culture of 'test-taking' [10,13,14]. In a previous study of postnatal women in the UK, almost half (42%) of women who self-identified as having anxiety scored below the threshold on the anxiety subscale of the Edinburgh Postnatal Depression Scale (EPDS-3A) [15]. Results suggested that eliciting women's own views of their psychological wellbeing through a direct question may help to ensure that more women experiencing symptoms of anxiety are identified and offered appropriate support.

In this analysis, we compared the prevalence of anxiety symptoms identified using the GAD-2—the currently recommended measure for postnatal women in the UK [11]—with the prevalence of anxiety symptoms identified using the EPDS-3A and using a direct question. We use data from England's 2020 National Maternity Survey (NMS), which captures the experiences of women who gave birth during the first wave of the COVID-19 pandemic in May 2020 [16]. We built upon existing work by assessing symptoms of anxiety at six months postpartum, where previous analyses focused on earlier postnatal periods. By directly comparing the GAD-2 with another standardised measure as well as with a direct question, we built on previous studies that were limited to comparing self-identified anxiety against a single standardised measure. Our aims were to determine the prevalence of anxiety symptoms identified by the GAD-2, EPDS-3A and a direct question; to assess the extent of concordance between the three measures; and to compare the characteristics of women with anxiety on each of the three measures.

2. Materials and Methods

2.1. Study Setting and Participants

We conducted an analysis of data from the 2020 NMS in England. The survey methods have been described in detail elsewhere [16]. In summary, a random population-based sample of 16,050 women aged 16 years or older who were living in England and had given birth during a two-week period in May 2020 was identified by the Office for National Statistics (ONS) using birth registration records. Women were sent questionnaires six months after they had given birth. The survey included questions on care during pregnancy, labour and birth, and the postnatal period and included mental health outcomes. Women had a choice of completing questionnaires on paper, online or over the telephone with an interpreter if required. Reminder packs were sent to non-respondents using a tailored reminder system [17].

2.2. Anxiety Measures

Self-identified anxiety was assessed using a single, direct question asking women whether they had experienced anxiety in the postpartum period, worded as follows: 'Did you experience any of the following after the birth of your baby?'. Anxiety was listed as one of the conditions. Women were asked to indicate if they had experienced anxiety at one month, three months and/or six months after the baby's birth. Responses were coded as either 'yes' or 'no' (binary) for each time point. Because surveys were sent to women at approximately six months postpartum, women's responses about experiencing anxiety at one and three months postpartum relied on their recall. In order to minimise the risk of recall bias, we used women's responses about anxiety at six months postpartum as our measure of self-identified anxiety. This also maximised comparability with the two standardised measures, which were also administered at six months postpartum. For the purpose of our analyses, therefore, women who responded 'yes' to having anxiety at six months postpartum were defined as having self-identified anxiety.

We used two standardised self-report measures of anxiety: the GAD-2 and the EPDS-3A. The GAD-2 is a shortened version of the original seven-item Generalised Anxiety Disorder scale (GAD) [18]. The GAD is used to identify symptoms of anxiety and is designed for use in the general (non-perinatal) population. The GAD-2 asks respondents to rate the frequency with which they have experienced the following two symptoms of anxiety over the previous two weeks: *feeling nervous, anxious, or on edge* and *not being able to stop or control worrying*. Each item is scored on a four-point Likert scale from 0 (not at all) to 3 (nearly every day), with the total score ranging from 0 to 6. A score of ≥ 3 on the GAD-2 was identified as an acceptable cut-off for identifying clinically significant anxiety symptoms in the general population, with sensitivity and specificity of 86% and 83%, respectively [19]. In our analysis, GAD-2 scores ≥ 3 were considered to suggest possible clinically significant anxiety.

The Edinburgh Postnatal Depression Scale (EPDS) is one of the most widely used screening instruments for depression during the perinatal period [20]. The original scale consists of ten items that ask women to rate the intensity of depressive symptoms they have experienced within the previous seven days. Each item is scored 0–3 with a maximum total score of 30 and higher scores representing greater symptom severity. Items 3, 4 and 5 of the EPDS assessed symptoms of anxiety and were administered as a stand-alone anxiety subscale (EPDS-3A) [21,22]. The three items of the EPDS-3A are as follows: *I have blamed myself unnecessarily when things went wrong*; *I have been anxious or worried for no good reason*; and *I have felt scared or panicky for no very good reason*. Each item was scored on a four-point Likert scale from 0 (never or not at all) to 3 (very often or most of the time). Scores range from 0 to 9, with a threshold of ≥ 6 considered to indicate possible anxiety [23]. In our analysis, EPDS-3A scores ≥ 6 were considered indicative of possible clinically significant anxiety. EPDS-3A and GAD-2 items, along with their scoring criteria, are summarised in Supplementary Table S1. The three measures of anxiety were presented in the following order in the questionnaire: first the self-identified measure, followed by the EPDS-3A and finally the GAD-2.

2.3. Sociodemographic, Clinical and Psychological Variables

We selected socio-demographic, clinical and psychological variables, which are known to be associated with perinatal anxiety. Socio-demographic variables were age (under 25 years; 25–34 years; 35 years and over); education (under 16 years; 17–18 years; 19 years and over); ethnicity (White; Black or minority ethnic (BME)); country of birth (UK; outside of UK); index of multiple deprivation (IMD) based on the area of residence (from most (1) to least (5) deprived); whether the pregnancy was planned (yes; no); and women's reaction to the pregnancy (pleased or happy; no particular feelings or unhappy). The IMD ranks small geographic areas in England by the level of deprivation, assessed according to the following seven domains: income, employment, education and skills, health and disability, crime, barriers to housing and services and the quality of the local living environment [24]. Clinical variables were multiple births (singleton; multiple), the presence of any chronic health conditions complicating pregnancy or pregnancy-related problems (yes; no) and whether children of participating women required admission to the neonatal intensive care unit (NICU) (yes; no). The psychological variable was antenatal anxiety, assessed using a single direct question as follows: 'Did you have any mental health problems during your pregnancy?'. Women who selected 'Yes—anxiety' were classified as having had antenatal anxiety.

2.4. Statistical Analysis

Descriptive characteristics of participants were summarised. Because respondents differed from non-respondents on key socio-demographic characteristics, we calculated non-response weights to adjust the sample in order to increase representativeness and reduce the risk of non-response bias [16]. The weighted prevalence of anxiety symptoms according to each measure was determined along with the proportion of women who reported symptoms on more than one measure. Weighted mean EPDS-3A and GAD-2 scores were calculated for women with and without self-identified anxiety to assess differences in scores between these two groups. The distribution of GAD-2 and EPDS-3A scores and the percentage who scored 0, 1 and 2 on individual items of the scales were plotted. Cronbach's alpha was calculated for the GAD-2 and EPDS-3A to assess their reliability. Agreement between the measures was assessed by calculating the proportion and 95% confidence intervals (CI) of women with concordance on each pair of measures by summing the diagonal in a two-by-two table. Cohen's kappa coefficient was used to quantify the statistical agreement between each pair of measures, taking into account the possibility of the agreement occurring by chance [25]. Kappa coefficients were interpreted using the following cut-offs: 0.00–0.20 'no agreement', 0.21–0.39 'minimal agreement', 0.40–0.59 'weak agreement', 0.60–0.79 'moderate agreement', 0.80–0.90 'strong agreement' and >0.90 'almost perfect agreement' [25].

Associations between socio-demographic (age, education, ethnicity, country of birth, IMD, planned pregnancy, reaction to pregnancy), clinical (multiple births, health condition, NICU admission) and psychological (antenatal anxiety) factors and postnatal anxiety were explored in univariable and multivariable logistic regression analyses. Unadjusted and adjusted odds ratios (OR) of associations between these variables and postnatal anxiety were calculated for each of the three anxiety measures. Variables that remained statistically significant at the $p < 0.05$ level in the final adjusted model were considered to be significantly associated with anxiety. Full case analysis was used throughout. Analyses were conducted using STATA version 15 (StataCorp LLC, College Station, TX, USA). All means, proportions and odds ratios were survey-weighted using the *svy* command in STATA.

3. Results

Completed questionnaires were returned by 4611 women, giving a valid response rate of 28.9% when excluding those returned as undeliverable [16]. Baseline characteristics of the sample are reported in detail elsewhere [16]. After applying survey weights, a third of women who participated in the survey were aged 30–34 years (33.7%), 69.1% were born in the UK, just under half (47.5%) were living in areas in the two most deprived quintiles on the IMD and 44.3% were primiparous [16]. Anxiety measures were complete for 4508 (97.8%) women; subsequent analyses are based on these complete cases.

3.1. Prevalence of Anxiety Symptoms

The weighted prevalence of anxiety symptoms on each measure is summarised in Table 1. At six months postpartum, 17.1% of women had self-identified anxiety, 15.0% had elevated GAD-2 scores and 28.8% had elevated EPDS-3A scores. One-third (36.0%) of women reported anxiety symptoms on at least one measure, and 7.3% reported symptoms on all three measures. Weighted mean GAD-2 scores were 3.04 and 0.83 among women with and without self-identified anxiety, respectively. Weighted mean EPDS-3A scores were 6.27 and 3.49 among women with and without persistent self-identified anxiety, respectively. Among those with self-identified anxiety, these mean scores fall above the cut-off for the GAD-2 and EPDS-3A. Figure 1 shows the distribution of total GAD-2 and EPDS-3A scores, and Figure 2 shows the distribution of responses to individual question items on the GAD-2 and EPDS-3A. Lower total scores were seen on the GAD-2, with the majority of women scoring zero and few scoring above the threshold of 3. Higher total scores were seen on the EPDS-3A, with fewer women scoring zero. When comparing the individual items, EPDS item 5 (*I feel scared or panicky for no good reason*) showed a similar response pattern to GAD-2 items 1 and 2, with more women scoring 0 on this item. Cronbach alpha was 0.88 for the GAD-2 and 0.76 for the EPDS-3A.

Table 1. Prevalence of postnatal anxiety symptoms on different measures (n = 4508).

Measure	n	%
Single measure		
Self-identified anxiety	786	17.1
GAD-2 score ≥3	645	15.0
EPDS-3A score ≥6	1295	28.8
Anxiety on at least one measure	1609	36.0
Multiple measures	382	8.5
Self-identified anxiety and GAD-2 score ≥3	382	8.5
Self-identified anxiety and EPDS-3A score ≥6	558	12.1
GAD-2 score ≥3 and EPDS-3A score ≥6	511	11.6
Anxiety on all three measures	334	7.3
No anxiety on any measure	2971	65.9

Note: Prevalence estimates (%) are weighted; counts (n) are unweighted.

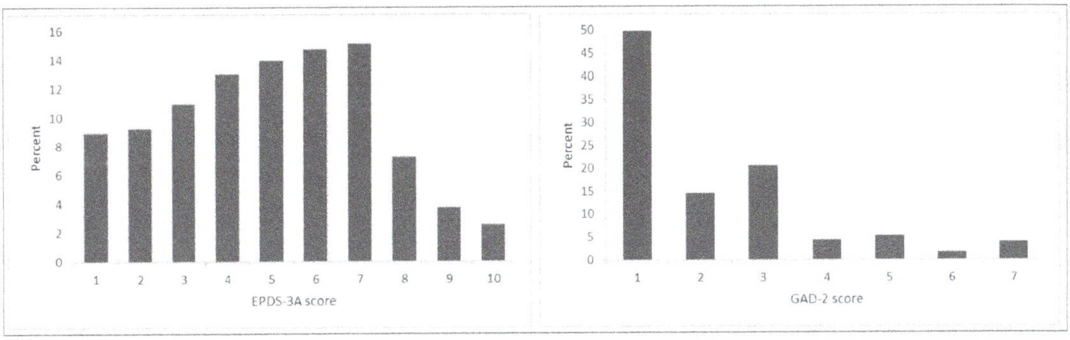

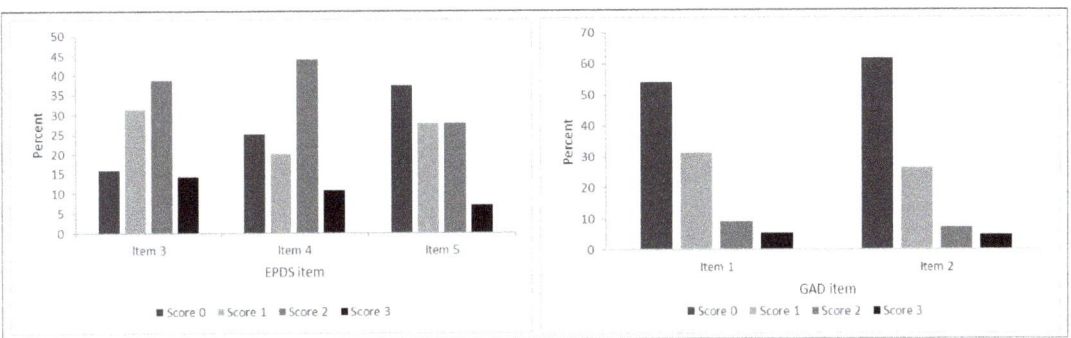

Figure 1. Distribution of total GAD-2 and EPDS-3A scores.

Figure 2. Distribution of scores on individual items of the GAD-2 and EPDS-3A.

3.2. Agreement between Anxiety Measures

Tables 2–4 show the concordance between each pair of anxiety measures. The concordance between self-identified anxiety and the GAD-2 was 85.2% (95% CI 84.1–86.2; Kappa

0.439). Concordance between self-identified anxiety and the EPDS-3A was 78.6% (95% CI 77.4–79.8; Kappa 0.399). Concordance between the GAD-2 and EPDS-3A was 79.6% (95% CI 78.4–80.1; Kappa 0.415). The Kappa coefficient for all three measures was 0.414. The Kappa coefficients suggest a 'weak level of agreement' between measures. Figure 3 shows the overlap between the three measures.

Table 2. Concordance and kappa values for self-identified anxiety and GAD-2 (n = 4508).

		GAD-2		Concordance % (95% CI) [Kappa]
		Anxiety	No Anxiety	
Self-identified	Anxiety	8.5% (382)	8.6% (404)	85.2% (84.1–86.2) [0.439]
	No anxiety	6.5% (263)	76.4% (3459)	

Note: Proportions and Kappa values are weighted; counts are unweighted.

Table 3. Concordance and kappa values for self-identified anxiety and EPDS-3A (n = 4508).

		EPDS-3A		Concordance % (95% CI) [Kappa]
		Anxiety	No Anxiety	
Self-identified	Anxiety	12.1% (558)	5.0% (228)	78.6% (77.4–79.8) [0.399]
	No anxiety	16.7% (737)	66.2% (2985)	

Note: Proportions and Kappa values are weighted; counts are unweighted.

Table 4. Concordance and kappa values for GAD-2 and EPDS-3A (n = 4508).

		EPDS-3A		Concordance % (95% CI) [Kappa]
		Anxiety	No Anxiety	
GAD-2	Anxiety	11.6% (511)	3.4% (134)	79.6% (78.4–80.1) [0.415]
	No anxiety	17.2% (784)	67.8% (3079)	

Note: Proportions and Kappa values are weighted; counts are unweighted.

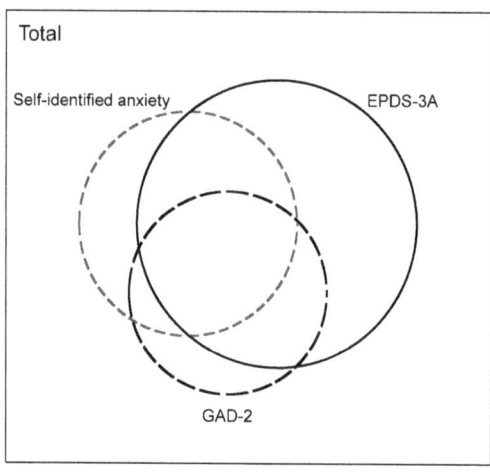

Figure 3. Venn diagram illustrating proportional overlap between self-identified anxiety, GAD-2 and EPDS-3A.

3.3. Characteristics of Women with Anxiety

Table 5 summarises the characteristics of women with anxiety. After controlling for all other variables in the multivariable model, antenatal anxiety was the strongest predictor of postnatal anxiety across all three measures. Antenatal anxiety was associated with an increased likelihood of self-identified anxiety (aOR 5.35; 95% CI 4.37–6.55), elevated EPDS-3A scores (aOR 3.64; 95% CI 3.03–4.36) and elevated GAD-2 scores (aOR 4.16; 95% CI 3.35–5.15). Women of Black, Asian or other minority ethnicity were less likely to report self-identified anxiety compared with women of White ethnicity (aOR 0.44; 95% CI 0.30–0.64), while women born outside of the UK were less likely than women born in the UK to have elevated GAD-2 scores (aOR 0.66; 95% CI 0.49–0.89). Women aged over 35 years were less likely than those aged 25–34 years to have elevated EPDS-3A scores (aOR 0.80; 95% CI 0.67–0.96). Women who were unhappy with or had mixed feelings about their pregnancy were more likely to have elevated GAD-2 scores compared with women who felt pleased about pregnancy (aOR 1.71; 95% CI 1.30–2.25) compared with those who were pleased about their pregnancy. Women with a health condition were more likely than those without to have elevated EPDS-3A scores (aOR 1.49; 95% CI 1.16–1.93).

Table 5. Unadjusted and adjusted odds ratios of associations between participant characteristics and anxiety according to different measures.

	Self-Identified Anxiety (6 m)			EPDS-3A			GAD-2		
	n (%)	uOR (95% CI)	aOR (95% CI)	n (%)	uOR (95% CI)	aOR (95% CI)	n (%)	uOR (95% CI)	aOR (95% CI)
Age									
Under 25 years	78 (23.5)	1.52 (1.12–2.07)	1.29 (0.91–1.84)	123 (39.4)	1.63 (1.24–2.14)	1.32 (0.96–1.82)	75 (22.5)	1.71 (1.25–2.34)	1.23 (0.85–1.79)
25–34 years	478 (16.8)	Ref	Ref	800 (28.6)	Ref	Ref	380 (14.5)	Ref	Ref
35 years and over	226 (15.1)	0.89 (0.73–1.07)	0.89 (0.72–1.09)	363 (24.9)	0.83 (0.70–0.98)	0.80 (0.67–0.96)	183 (12.7)	0.85 (0.69–1.05)	0.88 (0.70–1.10)
Education									
Under 16 years	94 (19.4)	1.26 (0.95–1.67)	0.83 (0.61–1.15)	164 (33.2)	1.41 (1.11–1.79)	1.05 (0.80–1.37)	94 (19.1)	1.57 (1.18–2.09)	1.06 (0.76–0.47)
17–18 years	213 (18.1)	1.16 (0.94–1.42)	0.86 (0.68–1.09)	370 (32.2)	1.34 (1.13–1.59)	1.07 (0.88–1.30)	188 (16.7)	1.33 (1.07–1.66)	0.99 (0.76–1.28)
19 years and over	473 (16.1)	Ref	Ref	748 (26.2)	Ref	Ref	354 (13.1)	Ref	Ref
Ethnicity									
White	726 (19.3)	Ref	Ref	1130 (30.1)	Ref	Ref	577 (16.0)	Ref	Ref
Black or minority ethnic	54 (8.0)	0.36 (0.26–0.51)	0.44 (0.30–0.64)	148 (23.4)	0.71 (0.56–0.90)	0.93 (0.71–1.21)	60 (10.8)	0.64 (0.46–0.88)	0.86 (0.59–1.25)
Country of birth									
UK	681 (20.0)	Ref	Ref	1097 (31.7)	Ref	Ref	557 (17.4)	Ref	Ref
Outside of UK	102 (10.7)	0.48 (0.37–0.62)	0.79 (0.59–1.04)	191 (22.5)	0.62 (0.51–0.76)	0.81 (0.64–1.01)	83 (9.6)	0.50 (0.38–0.66)	0.66 (0.49–0.89)
IMD									
1 (most deprived)	120 (17.2)	1.05 (0.79–1.40)	1.06 (0.77–1.46)	209 (30.9)	1.14 (0.90–1.45)	1.05 (0.81–1.36)	123 (18.2)	1.45 (1.08–1.95)	1.34 (0.97–1.87)
2	152 (17.4)	1.06 (0.82–1.38)	1.20 (0.91–1.60)	239 (28.7)	1.03 (0.82–1.29)	1.00 (0.78–1.29)	131 (15.6)	1.21 (0.91–1.60)	1.22 (0.90–1.66)
3	166 (17.2)	1.05 (0.81–1.36)	1.04 (0.79–1.36)	266 (27.6)	0.98 (0.79–1.21)	0.94 (0.75–1.18)	137 (14.1)	1.08 (0.82–1.43)	1.05 (0.78–1.41)
4	184 (17.0)	1.04 (0.81–1.33)	1.04 (0.79–1.35)	301 (28.2)	1.01 (0.82–1.23)	1.00 (0.80–1.25)	125 (12.4)	0.93 (0.70–1.23)	0.91 (0.68–1.23)
5 (least deprived)	164 (16.5)	Ref	Ref	280 (28.1)	Ref	Ref	129 (13.2)	Ref	Ref

Table 5. Cont.

	Self-Identified Anxiety (6 m)			EPDS-3A			GAD-2		
	n (%)	uOR (95% CI)	aOR (95% CI)	n (%)	uOR (95% CI)	aOR (95% CI)	n (%)	uOR (95% CI)	aOR (95% CI)
Planned pregnancy									
Planned	608 (16.1)	Ref	Ref	987 (26.7)	Ref	Ref	471 (13.2)	Ref	Ref
Unplanned	175 (20.4)	1.33 (1.08–1.66)	1.05 (0.79–1.40)	299 (35.1)	1.49 (1.24–1.79)	1.12 (0.89–1.41)	168 (20.1)	1.65 (1.32–2.06)	1.01 (0.76–1.36)
Reaction to pregnancy									
Pleased or happy	610 (16.0)	Ref	Ref	993 (26.9)	Ref	Ref	461 (12.7)	Ref	Ref
Mixed or unhappy	164 (22.0)	1.48 (1.18–1.85)	1.13 (0.85–1.50)	275 (36.3)	1.55 (1.28–1.88)	1.22 (0.96–1.55)	173 (23.6)	2.12 (1.69–2.65)	1.71 (1.30–2.25)
Multiple birth									
Singleton	780 (17.3)	Ref	Ref	1273 (28.8)	Ref	Ref	638 (15.1)	Ref	Ref
Twin	6 (9.3)	0.49 (0.18–1.35)	0.56 (0.18–1.78)	15 (26.2)	0.88 (0.41–1.85)	0.89 (0.39–2.01)	5 (9.1)	0.56 (0.19–1.68)	0.40 (0.10–1.62)
Antenatal anxiety									
No	386 (10.4)	Ref	Ref	770 (22.0)	Ref	Ref	316 (9.5)	Ref	Ref
Yes	398 (40.9)	5.93 (4.89–7.18)	5.35 (4.37–6.55)	517 (53.2)	4.03 (3.39–4.80)	3.64 (3.03–4.36)	327 (34.5)	5.00 (4.08–6.13)	4.16 (3.35–5.15)
Chronic health conditions									
No	677 (16.3)	Ref	Ref	1097 (27.2)	Ref	Ref	544 (14.1)	Ref	Ref
Yes	107 (23.3)	1.56 (1.19–2.05)	1.16 (0.85–1.59)	189 (41.0)	1.87 (1.48–2.35)	1.49 (1.16–1.93)	99 (22.1)	1.73 (1.31–2.27)	1.21 (0.89–1.65)
NICU admission									
No	688 (18.7)	Ref	Ref	1148 (28.7)	Ref	Ref	577 (15.2)	Ref	Ref
Yes	95 (16.9)	1.13 (0.85–1.51)	1.01 (0.74–1.39)	141 (29.6)	1.05 (0.81–1.36)	0.94 (0.71–1.26)	67 (15.0)	1.01 (0.72–1.41)	0.86 (0.61–1.20)

Notes: Bold denotes statistical significance at $p < 0.05$ level. **Abbreviations:** aOR adjusted odds ratio; CI confidence interval; EPDS-3A Edinburgh Postnatal Depression Scale anxiety subscale; GAD-2 two-item Generalised Anxiety Disorder scale; IMD index of multiple deprivation; m months; NICU neonatal intensive care unit; Ref reference category; uOR unadjusted odds rat.

4. Discussion

We compared the prevalence of anxiety symptoms at six months postpartum on two standardised self-report measures and one direct question on self-identified anxiety. We found wide variation in the prevalence depending on the measure used. Prevalence was highest using the EPDS-3A, which yielded an estimate of 28.7%, while prevalence using the GAD-2 was almost half of this at 15.0%. The prevalence of self-identified anxiety was at the lower end of this range, with 17.1% of women reporting anxiety on the direct question. Previous estimates of postnatal anxiety from meta-analyses have reported a prevalence of 15% in high-income settings [3]. These pooled estimates pre-date the COVID-19 pandemic. Our data were collected during the first wave of the COVID-19 pandemic in the UK when higher levels of anxiety might be expected. It is possible that the higher rates seen on the EPDS-3A may reflect this trend, although there is no evidence to suggest that only EPDS-3A scores and not GAD-2 scores or self-identified anxiety would be affected. Alternatively, the high prevalence of symptoms accoding to the EPDS-3A may suggest that this measure is overly inclusive when used with the recommended threshold of ≥ 6. In the absence of a clinical interview—the 'gold standard' for the diagnosis of mental disorders—we cannot conclude whether this is the case or whether, in fact, the GAD-2 is over-excluding women with anxiety. Both overly inclusive and overly exclusive measures are problematic: while the former can result in women being incorrectly identified as having anxiety, creating unnecessary strains on mental health services, the latter risks women with anxiety being missed and left unsupported.

The wording and scoring of EPDS-3A and GAD-2 items may have contributed to the difference in prevalence observed. On both measures, a score of zero denotes 'never' or 'not at all' experiencing that particular symptom. However, a score of one represents significantly different levels of symptoms on each measure. A score of one on the EPDS-3A is defined as experiencing the symptom 'not very often' or 'hardly ever', while a score of one on the GAD-2 is defined as experiencing the symptom on 'several days' (Supplementary Table S1). This may pose a difficulty for women with occasional symptoms of anxiety: these women can select the category of 'not very often' or 'hardly ever' on the EPDS (a score of one), but on the GAD, they must select between either 'no symptoms' (a score of zero) or having symptoms on 'several days' (a score of one). It is possible that this larger conceptual gap between a score of zero and one on the GAD-2 may be pushing women with mild anxiety towards selecting zero, thereby underestimating the true prevalence of symptoms.

Although there was overlap between the three measures, the Kappa values were relatively low, corresponding to a weak level of agreement between them. The GAD-2, EPDS-3A and direct questions on anxiety each identified different groups of women. Although the prevalence estimates were similar for the GAD-2 and self-identified anxiety, the overlap between these measures shows that they are not identifying all the same women. Perhaps of greatest concern are the women with self-identified anxiety who are not being identified by either of the standardised measures. Women who report anxiety on a direct question are likely to benefit from support, even without scoring above the EPDS-3A or GAD-2 thresholds. Hence it may be appropriate for women to be asked about self-identify anxiety alongside completing standardised measures in order to avoid missing those who may need follow-up.

When we compared the characteristics of women with anxiety on each of the three measures, the factor most strongly associated with postnatal anxiety across all measures was antenatal anxiety. Antenatal anxiety was associated with an approximately four-fold increase in the likelihood of experiencing postpartum anxiety. The strongest association was between antenatal anxiety and self-identified postnatal anxiety. In part, this might be explained by the fact that antenatal anxiety was also self-identified: women who self-identified as having postnatal anxiety may be most likely to also self-identify as having had antenatal anxiety. The association between antenatal and postnatal anxiety also has important clinical implications, as it suggests a trend of anxiety symptoms that persist throughout the perinatal period. Ideally, women with anxiety should be identified during pregnancy and offered timely support to address symptoms [26]. Routinely asking all women about anxiety symptoms during antenatal appointments, as recommended by NICE, can help to ensure that women with anxiety are identified and supported from an early stage and prevent symptoms from continuing into the postnatal period.

Women from ethnic minority backgrounds were less likely than women of White ethnicity to report self-identified anxiety, while women born outside the UK were less likely to have elevated EPDS-3A and GAD-2 scores compared to women born in the UK. These results suggest that different groups of women may have different preferences for the type of measures used. Our findings are of particular importance given that women from minority groups—including migrant populations and those from low- and middle-income countries of origin—are at greater risk of perinatal mental disorders [5,27–29]. Women from minority ethnic backgrounds may be less likely to respond to a direct question on anxiety due to cultural sensitivities, social desirability or stigmatising attitudes around mental disorders [30]. Among some groups, there may also be a lower awareness of what constitutes anxiety, resulting in women who experience symptoms of anxiety not ascribing their symptoms to anxiety. Standardised self-report measures offer an alternative means of bringing to light problematic symptoms without needing to label these as 'anxiety'. Conversely, standardised measures may fail to identify culturally diverse manifestations of anxiety, which could be contributing to the lower likelihood of women from minority ethnic groups having anxiety on the GAD-2 and EPDS-3A [30]. Future research should examine in more depth the acceptability of different screening measures among populations of diverse ethnicities [26].

Age was also significantly associated with anxiety. Compared with women aged 25–34 years, those aged over 34 years were less likely to have anxiety on the EPDS-3A. Although results for self-identified anxiety according to age did not reach statistical significance, the trend suggests that younger women may feel more at ease in discussing anxiety. Finally, the method of administration may play a role: while some women may prefer the less personal means of disclosure offered by a self-report measure that they complete independently, others may welcome the opportunity for a more personal discussion as offered by a direct question from a health professional [31]. Importantly, a direct question can be nuanced to assess anxiety symptoms over a longer time period and therefore provide a marker of chronicity and severity, while standardised measures provide only a snapshot in time [2]. The impact of mode of administration upon disclosure of anxiety symptoms warrants further research.

5. Strengths and Limitations

Our data stem from a large, population-based survey of women across England. To our knowledge, this is the first comparison of two standardised measures—including one that is recommended for routine use in the perinatal period—with a direct question on self-identified anxiety. There are also a number of limitations. One of the main limitations is the low survey response rate of 28.9%. Response rates to the NMS and to surveys generally have been declining over recent decades [32]. There are many possible reasons for this, including increasing demands on people's time, survey fatigue and concerns around access to and use of personal information [33]. We used evidence-based recommendations to optimise response rates, including offering incentives and sending reminders [34]. Women who were younger, multiparous, not married at the time of registering the birth of their baby and those born outside of the UK were under-represented in the survey. In order to address the under-representation of these groups, survey weights were applied to analyses of prevalence to reduce the effect of non-response bias. The fact that self-identified anxiety was based on a single question while the GAD-2 and EPDS-3A were based on two and three questions, respectively, may have introduced bias and made the self-identified measure less sensitive. Furthermore, the order in which anxiety measures were presented may have introduced a bias, with women possibly being more inclined to report symptoms on the later questions, having been 'primed' to think about their mental health. The absence of a diagnostic clinical interview meant we were unable to conclude which of the three measures most accurately identifies women with anxiety. Finally, our self-reported measure of anxiety did not assess the level of impairment resulting from anxiety symptoms. Eliciting the level of distress and impairment associated with symptoms could provide an additional indicator of when further psychological intervention might be called for, and future research would benefit from including such assessments.

6. Conclusions

A comparison of three measures of postnatal anxiety suggests that, despite some overlap, different measures identify different groups of women. Certain population characteristics such as women's ethnicity and age may determine which type of measure is most likely to identify women experiencing anxiety. Our findings suggest that using a direct question alongside a self-report measure such as the GAD-2 may improve the identification of women who need support and highlight the importance of being attentive to what women say rather than relying solely on standardised measures.

Supplementary Materials: The following supporting information can be downloaded at: https://www.mdpi.com/article/10.3390/ijerph19116578/s1. Table S1: Response categories on the EPDS-3A and GAD-2.

Author Contributions: Conceptualisation, G.F., S.H., M.A.Q. and F.A.; Methodology, G.F., S.H., M.A.Q. and F.A.; Data Curation, S.H., M.A.Q. and F.A.; Analysis, G.F. and S.H.; Writing—Original Draft Preparation, G.F.; Writing—Review and Editing, G.F., S.H., M.A.Q. and F.A. All authors have read and agreed to the published version of the manuscript.

Funding: This research was funded by the National Institute for Health Research (NIHR) Policy Research Programme, conducted through the Policy Research Unit in Maternal and Neonatal Health and Care, PR-PRU-1217-21202. The views expressed are those of the authors and not necessarily those of the NIHR or the Department of Health and Social Care. GF is funded by a Nuffield Department of Population Health Clinical Research Fellowship. The funders had no role in the study design, data collection, data analysis, data interpretation or writing of the report.

Institutional Review Board Statement: The authors assert that all procedures contributing to this work comply with the ethical standards of the relevant national and institutional committees on human experimentation and with the Helsinki Declaration of 1975, as revised in 2008. All procedures involving human subjects/patients were approved by London Bloomsbury NRES Committee (reference: 18/LO/0271).

Informed Consent Statement: Return of the questionnaire was taken as implicit consent from all participants.

Data Availability Statement: Data are archived by the NPEU at the University of Oxford. Requests for any data access can be made to the Director of the NPEU. Any requests will be considered by the NPEU data access committee following the NPEU data sharing policy and will be subject to further regulatory approval should access be required for any purposes other than those outlined in the NMS study protocol.

Acknowledgments: Most thanks are due to the many women who responded and participated in the survey. Staff at the Office for National Statistics drew the sample and managed the mailings but bear no responsibility for the analysis or interpretation of the data. Ciconi Ltd. printed and prepared the survey packs, set up and managed the online survey and was responsible for the data entry.

Conflicts of Interest: The authors declare no conflict of interest.

References

1. Howard, L.M.; Molyneaux, E.; Dennis, C.L.; Rochat, T.; Stein, A.; Milgrom, J. Non-psychotic mental disorders in the perinatal period. *Lancet* **2014**, *384*, 1775–1788. [CrossRef]
2. Harrison, S.; Alderdice, F. Challenges of defining and measuring perinatal anxiety. *J. Reprod. Infant. Psychol.* **2020**, *38*, 1–2. [CrossRef] [PubMed]

3. Dennis, C.-L.; Falah-Hassani, K.; Shiri, R. Prevalence of antenatal and postnatal anxiety: Systematic review and meta-analysis. *Br. J. Psychiatry* **2017**, *210*, 315–323. [CrossRef] [PubMed]
4. Fawcett, E.J.; Fairbrother, N.; Cox, M.L.; White, I.R.; Fawcett, J.M. The Prevalence of Anxiety Disorders During Pregnancy and the Postpartum Period: A Multivariate Bayesian Meta-Analysis. *J. Clin. Psychiatry* **2019**, *80*, 1181. [CrossRef]
5. Nielsen-Scott, M.; Fellmeth, G.; Opondo, C.; Alderdice, F. Prevalence of perinatal anxiety in low- and middle-income countries: A systematic review and meta-analysis. *J. Affect. Disord.* **2022**, *306*, 71–79. [CrossRef]
6. Centre for Mental Health and London School of Economics. *The Costs of Perinatal Mental Health Problems*; Centre for Mental Health: London, UK, 2014. Available online: http://eprints.lse.ac.uk/59885/1/__lse.ac.uk_storage_LIBRARY_Secondary_libfile_shared_repository_Content_Bauer%2C%20M_Bauer_Costs_perinatal_%20mental_2014_Bauer_Costs_perinatal_mental_2014_author.pdf (accessed on 27 May 2022).
7. Gelaye, B.; Rondon, M.B.; Araya, R.; Williams, M.A. Epidemiology of maternal depression, risk factors, and child outcomes in low-income and middle-income countries. *Lancet Psychiatry* **2016**, *3*, 973–982. [CrossRef]
8. Abel, K.M.; Hope, H.; Swift, E.; Parisi, R.; Ashcroft, D.; Kosidou, K.; Osam, C.S.; Dalman, C.; Pierce, M. Prevalence of maternal mental illness among children and adolescents in the UK between 2005 and 2017: A national retrospective cohort analysis. *Lancet Public Health* **2019**, *4*, e291–e300. [CrossRef]
9. O'Hara, M.W.; Wisner, K. Perinatal mental illness: Definition, description and aetiology. *Best Pr. Res. Clin. Obstet. Gynaecol.* **2013**, *28*, 3–12. [CrossRef]
10. Smith, M.S.; Cairns, L.; Pullen, L.S.W.; Opondo, C.; Fellmeth, G.; Alderdice, F. Validated tools to identify common mental disorders in the perinatal period: A systematic review of systematic reviews. *J. Affect. Disord.* **2021**, *298*, 634–643. [CrossRef]
11. NICE (National Institute for Health and Care Excellence). *Antenatal and postnatal mental health: Clinical management and service guidance (CG192)*; NICE: London, UK, 2014.
12. Silverwood, V.; Nash, A.; Chew-Graham, C.A.; Walsh-House, J.; Sumathipala, A.; Bartlam, B.; Kingstone, T. Healthcare professionals' perspectives on identifying and managing perinatal anxiety: A qualitative study. *Br. J. Gen. Pract.* **2019**, *69*, e768–e776. [CrossRef]
13. Downe, S.M.; Butler, E.; Hinder, S. Screening tools for depressed mood after childbirth in UK-based South Asian women: A systematic review. *J. Adv. Nurs.* **2007**, *57*, 565–583. [CrossRef] [PubMed]
14. Brealey, S.D.; Hewitt, C.; Green, J.M.; Morrell, J.; Gilbody, S. Screening for postnatal depression—Is it acceptable to women and healthcare professionals? A systematic review and meta-synthesis. *J. Reprod. Infant Psychol.* **2010**, *28*, 328–344. [CrossRef]
15. Fellmeth, G.; Harrison, S.; McNeill, J.; Lynn, F.; Redshaw, M.; Alderdice, F. Identifying postnatal anxiety: Comparison of self-identified and self-reported anxiety using the Edinburgh Postnatal Depression Scale. *BMC Pregnancy Childbirth* **2022**, *22*, 180. [CrossRef] [PubMed]
16. Harrison, S.; Alderdice, F.; McLeish, J.; Quigley, M.A. You and Your Baby: A national survey of health and care during the 2020 Covid-19 pandemic. In *National Perinatal Epidemiology Unit*; University of Oxford: Oxford, UK, 2021.
17. Dillman, D.A. Mail and internet surveys. In *the Tailored Design Method*, 2nd ed.; John Wiley & Sons: Hoboken, NJ, USA, 2007.
18. Spitzer, R.L.; Kroenke, K.; Williams, J.B.; Löwe, B. A brief measure for assessing generalized anxiety disorder: The GAD-7. *Arch Intern. Med.* **2006**, *166*, 1092–1097. [CrossRef] [PubMed]
19. Kroenke, K.; Spitzer, R.L.; Williams, J.B.; Monahan, P.O.; Löwe, B. Anxiety disorders in primary care: Prevalence, impairment, comorbidity, and detection. *Ann Intern. Med.* **2007**, *146*, 317–325. [CrossRef] [PubMed]
20. Cox, J.L.; Holden, J.M.; Sagovsky, R. Detection of postnatal depression. Development of the 10-item Edinburgh Postnatal Depression Scale. *Br. J. Psychiatry* **1987**, *150*, 782–786. [CrossRef]
21. Swalm, D.; Brooks, J.; Doherty, D.; Nathan, E.; Jacques, A. Using the Edinburgh postnatal depression scale to screen for perinatal anxiety. *Arch. Women's Ment. Health* **2010**, *13*, 515–522. [CrossRef]
22. Matthey, S.; Fisher, J.; Rowe, H. Using the Edinburgh postnatal depression scale to screen for anxiety disorders: Conceptual and methodological considerations. *J. Affect. Disord.* **2013**, *146*, 224–230. [CrossRef]
23. Bowen, A.; Bowen, R.; Maslany, G.; Muhajarine, N. Anxiety in a Socially High-Risk Sample of Pregnant Women in Canada. *Can. J. Psychiatry* **2008**, *53*, 435–440. [CrossRef]
24. Department for Communities and Local Government. *The English Index of Multiple Deprivation (IMD) 2015–Guidance*; Department for Communities and Local Government: London, UK, 2015. Available online: https://assets.publishing.service.gov.uk/government/uploads/system/uploads/attachment_data/file/464430/English_Index_of_Multiple_Deprivation_2015_-_Guidance.pdf (accessed on 27 May 2022).
25. McHugh, M.L. Interrater reliability: The kappa statistic. *Biochem. Med.* **2012**, *22*, 276–282. [CrossRef]
26. Bhat, A.; Nanda, A.; Murphy, L.; Ball, A.L.; Fortney, J.; Katon, J. A systematic review of screening for perinatal depression and anxiety in community-based settings. *Arch. Women's Ment. Health* **2021**, *25*, 33–49. [CrossRef] [PubMed]
27. Fellmeth, G.; Fazel, M.; Plugge, E. Migration and perinatal mental health in women from low- and middle-income countries: A systematic review and meta-analysis. *Bjog* **2017**, *124*, 742–752. [CrossRef]
28. Gennaro, S.; O'Connor, C.; McKay, E.A.; Gibeau, A.; Aviles, M.; Hoying, J.; Melnyk, B.M. Perinatal Anxiety and Depression in Minority Women. *MCN: Am. J. Matern. Nurs.* **2020**, *45*, 138–144. [CrossRef] [PubMed]

29. Sidebottom, A.; Vacquier, M.; LaRusso, E.; Erickson, D.; Hardeman, R. Perinatal depression screening practices in a large health system: Identifying current state and assessing opportunities to provide more equitable care. *Arch. Women's Ment. Health* **2020**, *24*, 133–144. [CrossRef]
30. Watson, H.; Harrop, D.; Walton, E.; Young, A.; Soltani, H. A systematic review of ethnic minority women's experiences of perinatal mental health conditions and services in Europe. *PLoS ONE* **2019**, *14*, e0210587. [CrossRef]
31. Button, S.; Thornton, A.; Lee, S.; Shakespeare, J.; Ayers, S. Seeking help for perinatal psychological distress: A meta-synthesis of women's experiences. *Br. J. Gen. Pract.* **2017**, *67*, e692–e699. [CrossRef]
32. Harrison, S.; Alderdice, F.; Henderson, J.; Redshaw, M.; Quigley, M.A. Trends in response rates and respondent characteristics in five National Maternity Surveys in England during 1995–2018. *Arch. Public Health* **2020**, *78*, 46. [CrossRef]
33. Galea, S.; Tracy, M. Participation rates in epidemiologic studies. *Ann. Epidemiol.* **2007**, *17*, 643–653. [CrossRef]
34. Harrison, S.; Henderson, J.; Alderdice, F.; Quigley, M.A. Methods to increase response rates to a population-based maternity survey: A comparison of two pilot studies. *BMC Med Res. Methodol.* **2019**, *19*, 65. [CrossRef]

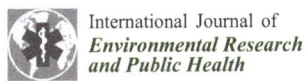

Article

Factor Structure of the Edinburgh Postnatal Depression Scale in a Sample of Postpartum Slovak Women

Zuzana Škodová [1], Ľubica Bánovčinová [1], Eva Urbanová [1], Marián Grendár [2] and Martina Bašková [1,*]

[1] Department of Midwifery, Jessenius Faculty of Medicine, Comenius University, 03601 Martin, Slovakia; zuzana.skodova@uniba.sk (Z.Š.); lubica.banovcinova@uniba.sk (Ľ.B.); eva.urbanova@uniba.sk (E.U.)
[2] Bioinformatic Unit, Biomedical Center Martin, Jessenius Faculty of Medicine, Comenius University, 03601 Martin, Slovakia; Marian.Grendar@uniba.sk
* Correspondence: martina.baskova@uniba.sk

Abstract: Background: Postpartum depression has a negative impact on quality of life. The aim of this study was to examine the factor structure and psychometric properties of the Slovak version of the Edinburgh Postnatal Depression Scale (EPDS). Methods: A paper and pencil version of the 10-item EPDS questionnaire was administered personally to 577 women at baseline during their stay in hospital on the second to fourth day postpartum (age, 30.6 ± 4.9 years; 73.5% vaginal births vs. 26.5% operative births; 59.4% primiparas). A total of 198 women participated in the online follow-up 6–8 weeks postpartum (questionnaire sent via e-mail). Results: The Slovak version of the EPDS had Cronbach's coefficients of 0.84 and 0.88 at baseline (T1) and follow-up, respectively. The three-dimensional model of the scale offered good fit for both the baseline ($\chi^2_{(df=28)}$ = 1339.38, $p < 0.001$; CFI = 0.99, RMSEA = 0.02, and TLI = 0.99) and follow-up ($\chi^2_{(df=45)}$ = 908.06, $p < 0.001$, CFI = 0.93, RMSEA = 0.09, and TL = 0.90). A risk of major depression (EPDS score ≥ 13) was identified in 6.1% in T1 and 11.6% in the follow-up. Elevated levels of depression symptoms (EPDS score ≥ 10) were identified in 16.7% and 22.7% of the respondents at baseline and follow-up, respectively. Conclusions: The Slovak translation of the EPDS showed good consistency, convergent validity, and model characteristics. The routine use of EPDS can contribute to improving the quality of postnatal health care.

Keywords: Edinburgh Postnatal Depression Scale (EPDS); Slovakia; validity; postpartum depression

1. Introduction

Significant geographical and socio-demographical differences in the estimates of the prevalence of postpartum depression have been reported by several studies. In a systematic review by Shorey et al. [1], the average prevalence of depression was 17% among healthy mothers without a prior history of depression, with significant differences between geographical regions, with the Middle East having the highest prevalence (26%) and Europe having the lowest (8%). In a large-sample multinational study by Lupattelli et al. [2], significant differences in the prevalence of postpartum depression between European regions were found as well, with Eastern European countries having a significantly higher prevalence of postpartum depression. Similarly, differences in prevalence in high-income countries (9.5%) and low/middle-income countries (18.7%) were found in a systematic review by Woody et al. [3]; the overall pooled prevalence in this study was 11.9% among women during the perinatal period. The prevalence of depressive symptoms in a longitudinal ELSPAC study was 10–11% in a representative sample of postpartum women in the Czech Republic [4]. Only a few studies have estimated the postpartum depression occurrence in the Slovak Republic. A prevalence of 18% was reported in a small sample of Slovak postpartum women by Izakova [5]; similarly, 25% prevalence was reported by Banovcinova et al. [6].

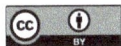

In the etiopathogenesis of postnatal depression, genetic predisposition, together with anamnestic risk factors and the accumulation of psychosocial stressors, seems to play an important role. According to a systematic review by Hutchens and Kearney [7], the risk factors for postnatal depression are high life stress, lack of social support, current or past abuse, prenatal depression, marital or partner dissatisfaction, and prenatal depression. There is evidence that depressive symptoms that begin during the antenatal period tend to persist into the postnatal period. Up to one-third of women with postnatal depression have a diagnosis of depression or anxiety disorder in their medical history. Furthermore, as many as half of postpartum women with depression experienced depressive symptoms during pregnancy [8]. Depression or anxiety disorder in medical anamnesis prior to pregnancy is also a major risk factor for postpartum depression. However, a significant proportion of women experience depressive symptoms only during the postpartum period and have no increased risk of depression without a relationship to pregnancy or birth. A specific sensitivity of the mood-regulation system influencing pregnancy-related hormones might play a role in this case [9].

The association between the mode of delivery and postpartum depression remains unclear. Whereas some studies reported elevated levels of postpartum depressive symptoms amongst women who underwent operative birth or had perinatal factors such as significant blood loss or longer duration of stage II or III of labor [10]; other studies, including systematic reviews, found no significant association [11,12]. However, subjective perception of the birth experience and level of birth satisfaction might be more important risk factors of postpartum depression than the objective mode of delivery. Women's negative perception of their birth experience, including factors such as lack of respect, privacy, support, inclusion in decision making, and feeling nurtured, may contribute to postnatal depression [12].

The Edinburgh Postnatal Depression Scale (EPDS) is a widely used measuring instrument for postpartum depression screening, providing a quick and simple administration and scoring system. The EPDS has been translated into over 60 languages and validated both as an antenatal and postpartum screen for minor or major depression in several countries [13]. High heterogeneity has been found regarding the sensitivity and specificity of the cut-off scores in different studies, possibly due to differences in study methodology, language, and diagnostic criteria used. Therefore, the validity of the EPDS as a screening instrument for postpartum depression may vary across different settings [14].

The EPDS was originally designed as a unidimensional measure. However, as shown in a comprehensive overview of the EPDS validation studies [15], most of the researchers confirmed the multidimensionality of the scale. In some studies, a two-factor structure has been found [16,17]; others have identified three factors of the EPDS: anxiety, anhedonia, and depression [18,19]. A theoretically driven four-factor model of the EPDS performed well in a Hungarian sample of postpartum women [20].

According to available information, the Slovak version of the EPDS has not yet been validated. The adaptation of the Slovak version of the Edinburgh Scale of Postnatal Depression and the examination of its psychometric properties and factor structure in a research sample of postpartum women in Slovakia were the main research aims in this study.

2. Materials and Methods

2.1. Data Collection and Sample

A longitudinal follow-up design was used in this study, with data collection at two time points: T1 (paper and pencil questionnaire completed 2–4 days after birth) and T2 (electronic data collection 6–8 weeks postpartum). A convenient sampling method was used in the process of the data collection.

T1 data, baseline: The inclusion criteria at T1 were 2–4 days postpartum and informed consent. The exclusion criteria in T1 point were actual perinatal loss or stillbirth (previous perinatal loss in the anamnesis was not an exclusion criterium) and a history of severe psychiatric disorder in the anamnesis (psychotic disorder). Data for the T1 point were collected in 2 hospital birth centers in Slovakia: Bratislava (located in the capital city) and Martin (located in the central part of the country). Both centers are large university hospital facilities providing complex perinatal care, including specialized perinatological care for high-risk pregnancies and pathological births. Each participant filled out a paper and pencil questionnaire during their second to fourth day postpartum hospital stay (4 days is the standard length of hospital stay after a physiological birth in Slovakia). Data were collected by midwives working in the birth center between September 2018 and April 2020. Each participant in T1 data collection was personally approached by a midwife and invited to participate in the research. A total of 577 postpartum women participated in T1 data collection; the response rate for T1 was 82.3%.

T2 data, follow-up: All women who participated in the T1 data collection received an e-mail 6–8 weeks postpartum with the invitation to participate in the follow-up and an electronic version of the questionnaire (the e-mail addresses were provided when signing the informed consent letter). Altogether, 198 women participated in the follow-up (response rate of 34.9%).

Most of the validation studies of the EPDS include women 6–8 weeks postpartum, or later. However, validation studies in Serbia, and Greece have also included women immediately after the birth [18,21]. Some of the authors [22–24] reported that the use of the EPDS in early postpartum is valid, and have argued that using the EPDS shortly after birth might have clinical value, especially in detecting the symptoms of anxiety or atypical depression, and in identifying women eligible for depression screening later during postpartum. Zanardo et al. [25] have found a strong association between high maternity blues scores and EPDS scores, and suggested that women who experienced strong symptoms of maternity blues may represent a distinct subgroup of postpartum women with a significantly increased risk of developing postpartum depression. Using the EPDS shortly after the birth also has significant practical advantages, as administering the questionnaire during the stay in the hospital allows approaching a larger proportion of postpartum women compared to online or telephone contact a few weeks of month postpartum.

Given the high attrition rate in T2 follow-up, differences between respondents and nonrespondents in the T2 follow-up were examined with chi-square statistics. The results of the nonresponse bias analysis showed significant differences regarding education ($p \leq 0.001$) and type of birth ($p \leq 0.05$). Among women who responded in the T2 follow-up, higher rates of participants with high education were found compared with the nonresponse group (68% vs. 53%). Women after physiological birth were also more likely to respond in T2 (79% in the response group compared with 72% in the nonresponse group). No significant differences between respondents and nonrespondents were found regarding age, parity, preterm birth, perinatal loss in anamnesis, complications in pregnancy, support person during birth, positive psychiatric anamnesis reported in T1, or positive depression symptoms (<13 points in EPDS) in T1. Total EPDS scores in response and nonresponse groups were compared using Student independent samples t-test, and no significant differences were found (t = 1.90, $p > 0.05$).

2.2. Measuring Instruments

The Edinburgh Postnatal Depression Scale (EPDS) was used for both T1 and T2 of the data collection. The EPDS was developed by Cox et al. [26]. The EPDS is a 10-item self-rated questionnaire; each item asks about a common depressive symptom. Due to the specifics of the postpartum period, the EPDS does not contain items asking about somatic symptoms (as distinguishing somatic symptoms caused by physiological postpartum changes from those associated with depression is problematic). The scale also does not include items focused on assessing a mother–child relationship. Each EPDS item contains 4 response choices per statement (rated on a Likert scale). Items 3, 5, 6, 7, 8, 9, and 10 are reversely scored. The possible total score of the scale ranges from 0–30 points, with a higher score indicating a higher level of depression symptoms.

Different cut-off points of the EPDS have been used. According to the EPDS manual, second edition [15], a cut-off point of 10 or higher is recommended for research use, indicating elevated levels of depressive symptoms. For clinical use, a cut-off score of 12.5 has been shown to detect women at risk of major depression. As the EPDS is a screening measure, not a diagnostic tool, a woman who meets this threshold should be further assessed by a mental health professional for diagnosis.

Permission to use the EPDS for this study was obtained from the Royal College of Psychiatrists (U.K.). The back-translation process of the EPDS was performed with an additional assessment of the accuracy of the translation. Strong emphasis was placed on possible ambiguous questions and culturally sensitive items.

In a longitudinal follow-up (T2), the Zung self-rated depression scale was used along with the EPDS as a measure of the convergent validity of the EPDS. The Zung self-rated depression scale [27] is a self-reported 20-item scale measuring the symptoms of depression. The items' responses are ranked from 1 to 4, with higher scores corresponding to elevated depressive symptoms. Ten positively worded items (2, 5, 11, 12, 14, 16, 17, 18, and 20) are scored reversely. The total score on the Zung depression scale indicates the level of depressive symptoms rather than a clinical diagnosis of major depression. The maximum total score is 80, and four categories can be identified based on the total score of the scale: 1, total score < 50 = no signs of depressive symptoms; 2, total score 50–60 = minimal signs of depression; 3, total score 60–69 = moderately to notably expressed signs of depression; and 4, total score > 70 = severe symptoms of depression. The Zung SDS is an established measure and in Slovakia, it is frequently used as a screening measure for depression. The Zung SDS has shown good psychometric properties and validity in the general population [28], in a population with depression [18], and in women of reproductive age [29].

At T1 baseline data collection, a sociodemographic and anamnestic questionnaire was used in the study together with the EPDS. The anamnestic questionnaire contained questions on basic sociodemographic variables (age and education) and perinatal data (type of birth, parity, support person during birth, preterm birth, perinatal loss in the anamnesis, and complications in pregnancy). Previous or actual onset of psychiatric disorders of the participants was measured by self-reported questions focused on a history of depression or other psychiatric illness before or during pregnancy.

2.3. Statistical Procedures

Statistical analysis was performed using IBM SPSS Statistics for Windows, version 25.0, and statistical software R, version 3.5.0 (2018). Student's *t*-test for independent samples and ANOVA with Sheffe's post hoc tests were used when testing differences in the mean EPDS sores in the different groups of respondents according to basic demographic and perinatal characteristics. For the analysis of the reliability of the EPDS, Cronbach's α and the Spearman–Brown coefficient were employed. Chi-square tests were used for testing differences between respondents and nonrespondents in T2. The convergent validity of the EPDS was tested based on the correlation coefficients between the total EPDS score and the total Zung self-rated depression inventory score only in the T2 sample (6–8 weeks postpartum). Interclass correlation coefficients between the EPDS and Zung SDS were calculated as well; average measures value greater than 0.6 were considered acceptable.

Exploratory factor analysis (EFA) was employed to test the factor structure in both T1 and T2 samples. Multiple factor solutions (direct oblimin rotation) were run. Eigenvalues, scree plots, and the amount of variance explained were examined to determine the number of factors in each model. Factors with eigenvalues greater than one were retained, with a meaningful factor solution explaining at least 50% of the variance. An item loading significantly on a factor was determined by a loading of ≥ 0.3.

In the next step, confirmatory factor analysis (CFA) was performed in both the T1 and T2 samples with the goal of evaluating the EFA-based models' fit to the data. The structural equation modeling (SEM) approach was employed to perform the CFA, using the statistical software R, version 3.5.0 [30], including the lavaan [31] and semPlot statistical packages [32]. A maximum likelihood (ML) approach to model estimation was adopted. Multiple goodness-of-fit tests were used to evaluate the models, including the chi-square statistic, comparative fit index (CFI), toot mean square error of approximation (RMSEA), and the Tucker–Lewis index (TLI). A CFI greater than 0.90 was employed as an indicator of an acceptable fit to the data, and a CFI equal to or greater than 0.95 indicated a good fit to the data. An RMSEA less than 0.08 was a threshold for an acceptable fit to the data; values of less than 0.05 indicated a good fit to the data. TLI values greater than 0.9 were considered the threshold for a good model fit [33,34].

2.4. Ethical Issues

All the participants were thoroughly informed about the project aims and ethical issues (anonymity, personal data protection, and voluntary participation). An informed consent letter was signed by each participant prior to their participation. Ethical approval was obtained from the Ethical committee of the Jessenius Faculty of Medicine in Martin, Slovakia, no. EK 36/2018.

3. Results

3.1. Distribution of the EPDS Scores

The basic demographic and anamnestic characteristics of the respondents who participated at both T1 and T2 are provided in Table 1, along with the mean EPDS scores in the different groups of participants. The T1 sample included 577 postpartum women with a mean age of 30.6 ± 4.9 years. Altogether, 375 (65%) participants were from Martin university hospital and 202 (35%) from Bratislava university hospital. Most of the respondents had higher education (57.9%), and 59.4% were primiparas. The majority of women in the research sample (73.5%) had a vaginal birth.

There were 198 postpartum women participants at T2, with a mean age of 30.9 ± 4.8 years; most of them had higher education (68.2%). Altogether, 58.1% of women were primiparas, and 79% had a vaginal birth. More detailed information on the study participants at T1 and T2 is provided in Table 1. In the T1 sample, statistically significant differences in EPDS scores were found regarding parity (primiparas scored significantly higher in the EPDS than multiparas), type of birth (women after operative birth scored significantly higher in EPDS than women after spontaneous birth). In both T1 and T2 samples, significant differences regarding the history of psychiatric disorders were found: women with a history of psychiatric disorders scored significantly higher than those without a history of psychiatric illness).

The mean EPDS score T1 at (2–4 days postpartum) was 5.24 (SD = 4.35), and 6.21 (SD = 4.93) at T2 (6–8 weeks postpartum); the difference in the EPDS scores between samples was statistically significant ($t = -2.61$, $p \leq 0.009$).

A risk of major depression (EPDS score ≥ 13) was identified in 6.1% of women at T1 and 11.6% women at T2. An elevated level of depression symptoms (EPDS score ≥ 10) was reported by 16.7% and 22.7% of the respondents at T1 and T2, respectively. According to the results of the Zung self-rated depression scale, 17.7% of women reported having mild signs of depression, and 5.1% as having moderate signs of depression (results only from T2 sample).

The mean EPDS score at T1 (2–4 days postpartum) was 5.24 (SD = 4.35), and 5.71 (SD = 4.42) at T2 (6–8 weeks postpartum); the difference in the EPDS scores between samples was not statistically significant ($t = 1.288$, $p \leq 0.19$).

The risk of major depression (EPDS score ≥ 13) was identified in 6.1% of women at T1 and 8.4% women at T2. An elevated level of depression symptoms (EPDS score ≥ 10) was recorded in 16.7% and 19.5% of respondents at T1 and T2, respectively. According to the results of the Zung self-rated depression scale, 16.8% of women were identified as having mild signs of depression and 2.6%, as having moderate signs of depression (results only from the T2 sample).

Table 1. Characteristics of the study participants.

Variable		T1 Total Sample n = 584	EPDS Score (SD)	p Value	T2 Total Sample n = 204	EPDS Score (SD)	p-Value
Age (years)	Mean (SD) Range	30.6 (±4.9) 16–44	-	-	30.9 (±4.8) 20–44	-	-
Education	Primary	13 (2.3%)	4.0 (±3.1)	0.41	1 (0.5%)	4.0 (-)	0.90
	Secondary	229 (39.7%)	5.1 (±4.2)		62 (31.3%)	6.3 (±5.3)	
	Tertiary	334 (57.9%)	5.4 (±4.5)		135 (68.2%)	6.2 (±4.8)	
	Missing	1 (0.2%)					
Parity	Primipara	343 (59.4%)	5.6 (±4.6)	0.05	115 (58.1%)	6.4 (±4.9)	0.44
	Multipara	229 (39.7%)	4.7 (±3.8)		81 (40.9%)	5.8 (±4.9)	
	Missing	5 (0.9%)			2 (1%)		
Preterm birth	Yes	119 (20.6%)	5.8 (±4.1)	0.14	40 (20.2%)	5.8 (±4.6)	0.50
	No	457 (79.2%)	5.1 (±4.4)		158 (79.8%)	6.3 (±5.0)	
	Missing	1 (0.2%)					
Type of birth	Vaginal	424 (73.5%)	4.8 (±4.2)	0.001	157 (79.3%)	6.2 (±4.8)	0.68
	Operative	153 (26.5%)	6.5 (±4.4)		41 (20.7%)	6.5 (±4.5)	
Chronic health conditions in anamnesis	Yes	52 (9.0%)	5.9 (±5.9)	0.27	19 (9.6%)	6.4 (±4.9)	0.88
	No	522 (90.5%)	5.2 (±4.2)		179 (90.4%)	6.2 (±5.0)	
	Missing	3 (0.5%)					
Perinatal loss in anamnesis	Yes	127 (22.0%)	5.2 (±3.8)	0.85	41 (20.7%)	6.1 (±4.9)	0.90
	No	448 (77.6%)	5.3 (±4.5)		157 (79.3%)	6.2 (±4.7)	
	Missing	2 (0.3%)					
Support person during labor	Yes	402 (69.7%)	5.2 (±4.3)	0.86	145 (73.2%)	6.3 (±4.6)	0.77
	No	174 (30.2%)	5.3 (±4.6)		53 (26.8%)	6.0 (±5.8)	
	Missing	1 (0.2%)					
History of psychiatric disorder	Yes	27 (4.7%)	8.8 (±6.1)	0.001	7 (3.5%)	11.3 (±4.6)	0.05
	No	550 (95.3%)	5.1 (±4.2)		191 (96.5%)	6.0 (±4.8)	
Risk of major depression	EPDS score ≥ 13	35 (6.1%)	-	-	23 (11.6%)	-	-
	EPDS score < 13	542 (93.9%)			175 (88.4%)		
Elevated depressive symptoms	EPDS score ≥ 10	96 (16.7%)	-	-	45 (22.7%)	-	-
	EPDS score < 10	481 (83.4%)			153 (77.3%)		
Zung self-rated depression scale		No signs of depression			153 (77.3%)	-	-
		Minimal signs of depression			35 (17.6%)		
		Moderate signs of depression			10 (5.1%)		
		Severe signs of depression			-		

3.2. Convergent Validity

The total score of the Slovak version of the EPDS was statistically significantly correlated with the Zung self-rated depression scale scores (Pearson's r = 0.718, $p \leq 0.001$) in the sample of 204 postpartum women (T2, 6–8 weeks postpartum). According to Cohen's interpretation of Pearson correlation coefficients, this represents a strong correlation between variables. The interclass correlation coefficients calculation showed an average measure value of 0.798 (95% CI: 0.73, 0.85). These results showed that the construct validity of the Slovak version of the EPDS is satisfactory.

3.3. Reliability of the EPDS Scores

Table 2 shows the internal consistency of the individual as well as total EPDS scores. The EPDS showed good reliability (Cronbach's α 0.84 at T1 and 0.88 at T2). The α coefficients for individual EPDS items were above 0.80, indicating good homogeneity. The Spearman–Brown coefficient was 0.80 at T1 and 0.87 at T2, indicating the good split-half reliability of the scale.

Table 2. Cronbach's α values for the EPDS items.

Item No.	EPDS Cronbach's α without the Item at T1	EPDS Cronbach's α without the Item at T2
1. I have been able to laugh and see the funny side of things	0.83	0.87
2. I have looked forward with enjoyment to things	0.83	0.87
3. I have blamed myself unnecessarily when things went wrong	0.83	0.88
4. I have been anxious and worried for no good reason	0.81	0.86
5. I have felt scared or panicky for no very good reason	0.81	0.87
6. Things have been getting on top of me	0.82	0.87
7. I have been so unhappy that I have had difficulty sleeping	0.83	0.88
8. I have felt sad or miserable	0.81	0.86
9. I have been so unhappy that I have been crying	0.82	0.87
10. The thought of harming myself has occurred to me	0.84	0.88
EPDS scale: Cronbach's α	0.84	0.88
EPDS scale: Spearman Brown coefficient	0.80	0.87

3.4. Exploratory Factor Analysis (EFA) of the Data from the T1 Sample

The Kaiser–Meyer–Olkin measure of sampling adequacy for T1 data was 0.82, and the result of the Bartlett's test of sphericity was significant (p-value < 0.001), which indicated that the collected data were suitable for factor analysis.

The results of the EFA revealed two components with eigenvalues greater than one: the first was 5.605, and represented a factor consisting of items 3–10; the second was 1.333 and contained items 1 and 2. However, there were items that loaded significantly on both factors: item 6 loaded almost similarly on factors 1 and 2, and item 8 loaded higher on factor 1 and lower but significantly on factor 2 (Table 3). The combination of the two factors explained 57.5% of the variance, and the correlation between factors was 0.43. the internal reliability of the first factor was 0.90, and 0.86 for the second factor.

Table 3. Factor matrix for the EPDS in the T1 Slovak sample (exploratory factor analysis with oblimin rotation).

Item No.	Two-Factor Solution		Three-Factor Solution		
	Factor 1	Factor 2	Factor 1	Factor 2	Factor 3
Item 1		0.819		0.755	
Item 2		0.974		0.923	
Item 3	0.520				0.336
Item 4	0.333				0.570
Item 5	0.742				0.997
Item 6	0.420	0.420		0.341	
Item 7	0.641		0.719		
Item 8	0.616	0.363	0.840		
Item 9	0.547		0.754		
Item 10	0.975		0.574		0.473

The three-factor solution was suggested by parallel analysis. This solution contained a first factor (items 7–10); a second factor, which comprised items 1 and 2; and a third factor with items 3–5. Item 6 loaded significantly on both factors 1 and 2, with higher loading on factor 2. Item 10 loaded significantly on all three factors, with the highest loading on factor 1. The combination of the three factors explained 58.7% of the variance, and the correlation between factors varied from 0.30 to 0.64. the internal reliability of the first, second, and third factors was 0.87, 0.86, and 0.84, respectively.

3.5. EFA of the Data from the T2 Sample

The Kaiser–Meyer–Olkin measure of sampling adequacy for T2 was 0.82, and the p-value for Bartlett's test of sphericity was less than 0.001.

The results of the EFA revealed only one component with an eigenvalue greater than one (eigenvalue = 6.52). The factor loadings for each item ranged from 0.66 to 0.88 (Table 4), and this single factor explained 61.6% of the variance. Cronbach's α of the factor was 0.94.

Table 4. Factor matrix for the EPDS in the T2 Slovak sample (exploratory factor analysis with oblimin rotation).

Item No.	One-Factor Solution	Two-Factor Solution		Three-Factor Solution		
	Factor 1	Factor 1	Factor 2	Factor 1	Factor 2	Factor 3
Item 1	0.888	0.742		0.453	0.372	
Item 2	0.826	0.732			0.901	
Item 3	0.667	0.364	0.368			0.333
Item 4	0.832		0.720			0.634
Item 5	0.690		0.907			0.936
Item 6	0.793	0.439	0.431		0.584	0.369
Item 7	0.662	0.626		0.801		
Item 8	0.832	0.799		0.432	0.440	
Item 9	0.826	1.017		0.827		
Item 10	0.796	0.733		0.752		

The two-factor solution was suggested by parallel analysis. This solution contained a first factor (items 1–2, 6, and 7–10) and a second factor that comprised items 3–5. Items 3 and 6 loaded significantly on both factors 1 and 2. The combination of the two factors explained 58.4% of the variance, and the correlation between factors was 0.76. The internal reliability of the first and second factors was 0.93 and 0.87, respectively.

The three-factor solution for the T2 data was examined as well. This solution contained a first factor (items 1 and 7–10); a second factor, which comprised items 2 and 6; and a third factor containing items 3–5. Item 1 loaded significantly on both factors 1 and 2, with a higher loading on factor 1, and item 6 loaded significantly on the second and third factors, with a higher loading on factor 2. Item 8 also loaded significantly on factors 1 and 2, with a slightly higher loading on factor 1 (Table 4). The combination of the three factors explained 56.1% of the variance, and the correlation between factors was 0.95–0.97. This three-factor model differs from the three-factor model identified by EFA using T1 data in one feature: in the T2 EFA model, item 1 loaded significantly on the first factor together with items 7–10; in the T1 EFA model, item 1 loaded on the second factor together with items 2 and 6.

3.6. Confirmatory Factor Analysis (CFA)

The first step in the CFA was the evaluation of the two multidimensional structural models (two-factor and three-factor solutions) as well as the unidimensional model on data from the T1 baseline sample. As shown in Figure 1, the structure of the three-factor model of the Slovak version of the EPDS was found to have a good fit with the baseline data ($\chi^2_{(df=32)}$ = 159.84, $p < 0.001$; CFI = 0.94, RMSEA = 0.08, and TLI = 0.91). The two-factor solution was found to poorly fit the baseline data; the CFA and RMSEA values did not meet the threshold for an acceptable fit to the data ($\chi^2_{(df=45)}$ = 1982.96, $p < 0.001$; CFI = 0.87, RMSEA = 0.114, TLI = 0.82). Similar results were found for the unidimensional model of the EPDS ($\chi^2_{(df=45)}$ = 1982.78, $p < 0.001$; CFI = 0.80, RMSEA = 0.138, TLI = 0.74).

As the second step in CFA, both multidimensional structural models (two-factor and three-factor solutions) and the unidimensional model on data from the T2 sample were evaluated. A single-factor model of the Slovak version of the EPDS was found to poorly fit the data ($\chi^2_{(df=45)}$ = 908.06, $p < 0.001$, CFI = 0.88, RMSEA = 0.12, TLI = 0.84). The two-factor model showed an acceptable fit to the T2 data ($\chi^2_{(df=45)}$ = 908.06, $p < 0.001$, CFI = 0.93, RMSEA = 0.09 and TLI = 0.90), as did the three-factor EPDs model ($\chi^2_{(df=45)}$ = 908.06, $p < 0.001$, CFI = 0.93, RMSEA = 0.09 and TLI = 0.90).

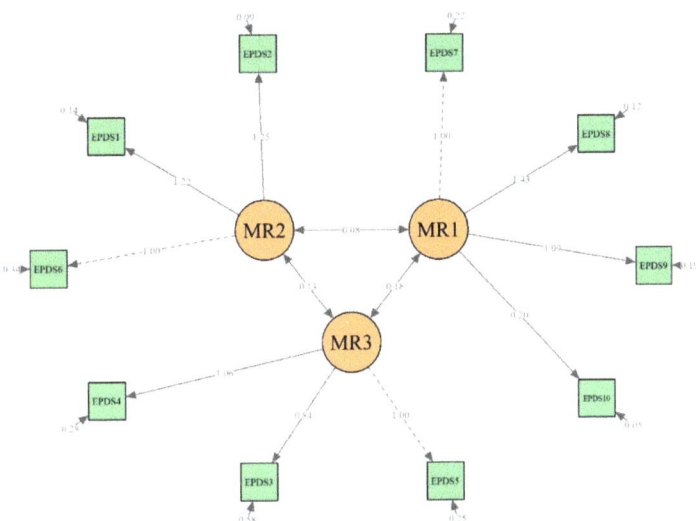

Figure 1. Confirmatory factor analysis of T1 data, 3-factor model (3–4 days postpartum).

An additional confirmatory factor analysis of the T2 data was performed as well using the three-factor model identified on T1 data. This step of the CFA revealed similar results: an acceptable fit of this model to the T2 data ($\chi^2_{(df=45)}$ = 908.05, $p < 0.001$, CFI = 0.94, RMSEA = 0.09, and TL =0.91) (Figure 2).

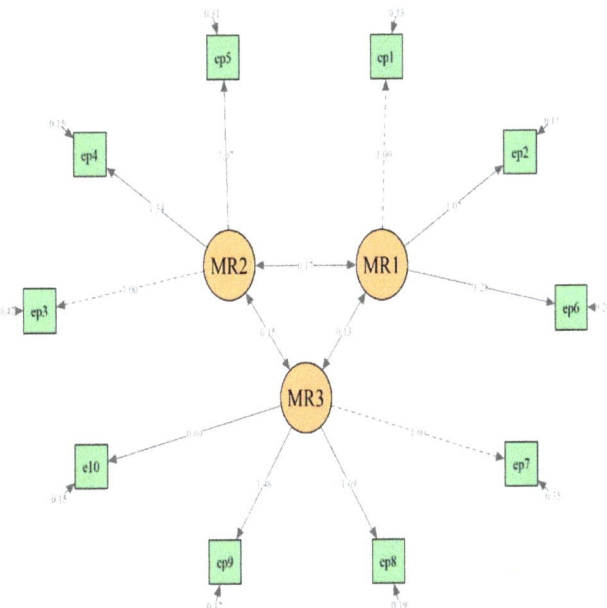

Figure 2. Confirmatory factor analysis of T2 data, 3-factor model (6–8 weeks postpartum).

4. Discussion

To the best of our knowledge, this is the first study examining the factor structure and psychometric properties of the Edinburgh Postnatal Depression Scale in Slovakia. The Slovak translation of the EPDS showed good consistency, convergent validity, and acceptable model characteristics among postpartum women. The three-factor model best fit the Slovak data for both the baseline data (2–4 days postpartum) and the follow-up data (6 weeks postpartum). The three dimensions identified by factor analysis in our study might be seen as representing three factors: (1) depression (items 7–10 with/without item 1), (2) anxiety (items 3, 4, and 5), and (3) anhedonia (items 2 and 6, with/without item 1). Despite the authors of the EPDS presuming its single-dimensional character [26], many studies have reported the multidimensional nature of the EPDS, as shown in a study by Kozinszkyi et al. [20]. Our study findings agree with previous validation studies of the EPDS and confirm the multidimensionality of the scale. The three-factor model in the present study is similar to those found by Coates et al. [19] on a large representative U.K. sample and Odalovic et al. [18] on a smaller Serbian sample. The two-factor model was identified as an alternative model with an acceptable fit for the follow-up data (6 weeks postpartum) in our sample: (1) items 1, 2, and 7–10; (2) items 3, 4, and 5. This two-factor model is identical to the two-factor model proposed by Gollan et al. [17] in a study on a large representative USA sample. However, the two-factor model performed unsatisfactorily for our T1 data, which led us to the conclusion that the three-factor model best fit the Slovak data.

Both exploratory and confirmatory factor analysis revealed differences in the models for the T1 and T2 samples in our study. A possible explanation for these discrepancies might be the differences between the T1 and T2 samples in our study. The high attrition rate in the T2 sample, which resulted in a low number of participants at T2, might have contributed to the differences in the results of the EPDS factor analysis of the T1 and T2 samples. Another factor potentially influencing the different results of EFA and CFA in the T2 sample is the nonresponse bias according to lower education and operative birth in our sample. Moreover, the validity of using the EPDS shortly after birth might be problematic. Although the use of the EPDS early postpartum was found to be valid by some studies [24], a critical point against the EPDS validity 1–2 weeks postpartum was recently raised [35]. Petrozzi et al. [22] argued that symptoms measured by the EPDS in a short time postpartum are symptoms of anxiety rather than depressive symptoms, and they propose more focus on differentiating the EPDS anxiety and depression subscales. Dennis et al. [24] showed that the 1-week EPDS accurately classified approximately half of women at 16 weeks postpartum with elevated EPDS scores. Thus, it seems that using the EPDS shortly after the birth needs to reflect the heterogeneity in the EPDS results at different time points, and the relevance of using the EPDS in early postpartum needs to be examined closer.

In our sample, the risk of major depression (EPDS score higher than or equal to 13 points) was identified among 6.1% of women at T1 and 11.6% at the 6–8 weeks follow-up. When using the EPDS cut-off point of 10 points or higher, the prevalence of depressive symptoms was 16.7% at T1 and 22.7% at T2. Lupattelli et al. [2] reported a 30% prevalence of mild to moderate depressive symptoms (EPDS scores 10–16), and a 5–6% prevalence of moderate to severe symptoms (EPDS scores > 17) in Eastern European countries, which is higher than in our study. Similarly, higher prevalence compared with our study (24.8%) was found among Serbian postpartum women using the 13-point criterion [18]. One of the possible reasons for this might be that data were collected over a longer timespan after birth (1 year) in both of these studies. However, depressive syndrome prevalence in our study was similar to the findings of an ELSPAC study in a large representative sample of Czech women 6 weeks postpartum, where the prevalence of 21.9% was found (using the 10-point criterion), and 11.8% when the stricter cut-off point was used [4]. Similar to our study, 10,1% prevalence of 6–8 weeks postpartum was found in a study by Coates et al. [19] in a large UK sample; and 10.8% prevalence of 3–24 weeks postpartum was found by Nagy et al. [36]

in Hungarian sample. In both studies, a 13-point cut-off of the EPDS criterion was used. In a review by Lyubenova et al. [37], the pooled prevalence of postpartum depression ranged from 27.8% when a cut-off of nine points was used to 9.0% when a 14-points cut-off was employed. Comparison of depressive symptoms prevalence across different studies is complicated using different cut-off points and data collection time spans; however, it seems that the prevalence of depressive symptoms found in our study is similar to that of other studies, and depressive symptoms occurrence might have an increasing tendency with time during the postpartum period. The prevalence of depressive symptoms among postpartum women across research studies highlights the importance of the detection of depression as a part of postpartum screening programs. According to Cox [38], in some countries, the EPDS is included in the national screening programs for perinatal women (for instance, in the USA, Sweden, and Australia), and in the U.K., its use is recommended).

Some of the methodological limitations of this study need to be mentioned. When comparing our sample with birthing women in Slovakia based on national statistical reports [39], some of the sociodemographic and perinatal characteristics in our sample differed significantly from the population of Slovak women giving birth. The respondents in our sample were more often highly educated (58.2%) compared with the population of birthing women in Slovakia (34.7%) and more often primiparas (59.9% vs. 45.9% in the whole population). The type of birth in our sample was vaginal in 73.8%, whereas it was 67.8% in the whole population of women giving birth in Slovakia. These differences influence the possibility of generalizing our results to the whole population of Slovak women. The second limitation of the study is the high attrition rate at T2, which may have occurred due to the differences in the data collection process: women were approached personally during baseline T1 data collection, which contributed to the higher response rate compared with online data collection via e-mail for the T2 follow-up. The analysis of response bias showed that women with lower education and after operative birth were less likely to respond at T2. As both these characteristics might be seen as risk factors for developing postpartum depression, these differences might have influenced the results of our analysis. Using the Zung depression scale in the process of validation is also a possible methodological limitation of our study, as well as convergent validity only being assessed for the T2 sample. Although the Zung SDS has been established as a widely used screening measure and has been validated in the general population [28], a population with depression [40], and women of reproductive age [29], the appropriateness of its use among perinatal women has not been sufficiently explored. No history of depression diagnosis (other than one self-report question) is also a methodological weakness in our research. Another limitation in our study is that we did not analyze the possible impact of ethnicity on our results. The largest ethnic minority in Slovakia, Roma, accounts for approximately 8–9% of the population. A significant proportion of this ethnic minority lives in socially excluded communities with severely disadvantaged socioeconomic conditions, which can significantly impact postpartum depression prevalence in this group. Finally, we have considered only cut-off values validated in different countries in our study, and we did not establish the exact cut-off values appropriate and sensitive for use in the Slovak population, as we did not consider a formal diagnosis of postnatal depression in our research. This issue needs to be addressed in future studies, which should focus on establishing the cut-off scores sensitive to the characteristics of the Slovak population of postpartum women, using, for instance, ROC curves.

5. Conclusions

The Slovak translation of the EPDS showed good consistency, convergent validity, and good model characteristics in a sample of postpartum Slovak women. Postpartum depression remains undiagnosed and untreated in a high percentage of cases in Slovakia. Multidisciplinary cooperation of experts, particularly in the fields of psychiatry, clinical psychology, gynecology, and midwifery, is required to improve postpartum depression screening and treatment. Routine screening for postpartum depression may significantly help to identify women with an increased risk of developing depression, thereby contributing to improving disease prevention and effective treatment. The administration and scoring of the Edinburgh Postnatal Depression Scale are quick and simple, and its use in routine screening programs in postpartum care may contribute to improved quality of health care with increased emphasis on mental health in Slovakia. Further studies should focus on establishing the sensitivity and specificity of the Slovak version of the EPDS on a larger and more representative sample using a psychiatric diagnostics interview as the acknowledged standard in the EPDS validation.

Author Contributions: Conceptualization, Z.Š., Ľ.B., E.U., and M.B.; methodology, Z.Š. and Ľ.B.; software, M.G.; validation, Z.Š.; formal analysis, M.G.; investigation, E.U.; resources, M.B.; data curation, Z.Š. and Ľ.B.; writing—original draft preparation, Z.Š.; writing—review and editing, Z.Š. and M.B.; visualization, M.G.; supervision, M.B.; project administration, Z.Š. and Ľ.B.; funding acquisition, Z.Š. All authors have read and agreed to the published version of the manuscript.

Funding: This work was financially supported by the VEGA (research grant agency of the Ministry of Education, Science, Research and Sport of the Slovak Republic) under contract no. VEGA-1/0211/19.

Institutional Review Board Statement: The study was conducted according to the guidelines of the Declaration of Helsinki and approved by the Ethics Committee of Jessenius Faculty of Medicine in Martin, Slovakia, no. EK 36/2018.

Informed Consent Statement: Informed consent was obtained from all subjects involved in the study.

Data Availability Statement: The data presented in this study are available on request from the corresponding author. The data are not publicly available due to ethical and privacy restrictions.

Conflicts of Interest: The authors declare no conflict of interest.

References

1. Shorey, S.; Chee, C.Y.I.; Ng, E.D.; Chan, Y.H.; Tam, W.W.S.; Chong, Y.S. Prevalence and incidence of postpartum depression among healthy mothers: A systematic review and meta-analysis. *J. Psychiatr. Res.* **2018**, *104*, 235–248. [CrossRef] [PubMed]
2. Lupattelli, A.; Twigg, M.J.; Zagorodnikova, K.; Moretti, M.E.; Drozd, M.; Panchaud, A.; Rieutord, A.; Juraski, R.G.; Odalovic, M.; Kennedy, D.; et al. Self-reported perinatal depressive symptoms and postnatal symptom severity after treatment with antidepressants in pregnancy: A cross-sectional study across 12 European countries using the Edinburgh Postnatal Depression Scale. *Clin. Epidemiol.* **2018**, *10*, 655–669. [CrossRef] [PubMed]
3. Woody, C.A.; Ferrari, A.J.; Siskind, D.J.; Whiteford, H.A.; Harris, M.G. A systematic review and meta-regression of the prevalence and incidence of perinatal depression. *J. Affect. Disord.* **2017**, *219*, 86–92. [CrossRef] [PubMed]
4. Fiala, A.; Švancara, J.; Klánová, J.; Kašpárek, T. Sociodemographic and delivery risk factors for developing postpartum depression in a sample of 3233 mothers from the Czech ELSPAC study. *BMC Psychiatry* **2017**, *17*, 104. [CrossRef]
5. Izáková, Ľ. Incidence of depressive symptoms in the postpartum period. *Psychiatr. Praxi* **2013**, *14*, 26–29.
6. Banovcinova, L.; Skodova, Z.; Jakubcikova, K. Predictors of increased depressive symptoms in the postpartum period. *Kontakt* **2018**, *21*, 32–38. [CrossRef]
7. Hutchens, B.F.; Kearney, J.J. Risk Factors for Postpartum Depression: An Umbrella Review. *J. Midwifery Womens Health* **2020**, *65*, 96–108. [CrossRef]
8. Underwood, L.; Waldie, K.; D'Souza, S.; Peterson, E.R.; Morton, S. A review of longitudinal studies on antenatal and postnatal depression. *Arch. Women's Ment. Health* **2016**, *19*, 711–720. [CrossRef]
9. Brummelte, S.; Galea, L.A. Postpartum depression: Etiology, treatment and consequences for maternal care. *Horm. Behav.* **2016**, *77*, 153–166. [CrossRef]
10. Zaręba, K.; Banasiewicz, J.; Rozenek, H.; Wójtowicz, S.; Jakiel, G. Peripartum Predictors of the Risk of Postpartum Depressive Disorder: Results of a Case-Control Study. *Int. J. Environ. Res. Public Health* **2020**, *17*, 8726. [CrossRef]
11. Clout, D.; Brown, R. Sociodemographic, pregnancy, obstetric, and postnatal predictors of postpartum stress, anxiety and depression in new mothers. *J. Affect. Disord.* **2015**, *188*, 60–67. [CrossRef]
12. Bell, A.F.; Andersson, E. The birth experience and women's postnatal depression A systematic review. *Midwifery* **2016**, *39*, 112–123. [CrossRef]
13. Cox, J. Use and misuse of the Edinburgh Postnatal Depression Scale (EPDS): A ten point 'survival analysis'. *Arch. Womens Ment. Health* **2017**, *20*, 789–790. [CrossRef]
14. Cox, J.L.; Holden, J.M.; Henshaw, C. *Perinatal Mental Health. The Edinburgh Postanatal Depression Scale (EPDS) Manual*, 2nd ed.; The Royal College of Psychiatrists: London, UK, 2014.
15. Gibson, J.; McKenzie-McHarg, K.; Shakespeare, J.; Price, J.; Gray, R. A systematic review of studies validating the Edinburgh Postnatal Depression Scale in antepartum and postpartum women. *Acta Psychiatr. Scandidavica* **2009**, *119*, 350–364. [CrossRef]

16. Toreki, A.; Andó, B.; Dudas, R.B.; Dweik, D.; Janka, Z.; Kozinszky, Z.; Keresztúri, A. Validation of the Edinburgh Postnatal Depression Scale as a screening tool for postpartum depression in a clinical sample in Hungary. *Midwifery* **2014**, *30*, 911–918. [CrossRef]
17. Gollan, J.K.; Wisniewski, S.R.; Luther, J.F.; Eng, H.F.; Dills, J.L.; Sit, D.; Ciolino, J.D.; Wisner, K.L. Generating an efficient version of the Edinburgh Postnatal Depression Scale in an urban obstetrical population. *J. Affect. Disord.* **2017**, *15*, 615–620. [CrossRef]
18. Odalovic, M.; Tadic, I.; Lakic, D.; Nordeng, H.; Lupattelli, A.; Tasic, L. Translation and factor analysis of structural models of Edinburgh Postnatal Depression Scale in Serbian pregnant and postpartum women—Web-based study. *Women Birth* **2016**, *28*, 31–35. [CrossRef]
19. Coates, R.; Ayers, S.; de Visser, R.O. Factor structure of the Edinburgh Postnatal Depression Scale in a population-based sample. *Psychol. Assess.* **2017**, *29*, 1016–1027. [CrossRef]
20. Kozinszky, Z.; Töreki, A.; Hompoth, E.A.; Dudas, R.; Németh, G. A more rational, theory-driven approach to analysing the factor structure of the Edinburgh Postnatal Depression Scale. *Psychiatry Res.* **2017**, *250*, 234–243. [CrossRef]
21. Vivilaki, V.G.; Dafermos, V.; Kogevinas, M.; Bitsios, P.; Lionis, C. The Edinburgh Postnatal Depression Scale: Translation and validation for a Greek sample. *BMC Public Health* **2009**, *9*, 329. [CrossRef]
22. Petrozzi, A.; Gagliardi, L. Anxious and depressive components of Edinburgh Postnatal Depression Scale in maternal postpartum psychological problems. *J. Perinat. Med.* **2013**, *41*, 343–348. [CrossRef]
23. Jardri, R.; Pelta, J.; Maron, M.; Thomas, P.; Delion, P.; Codaccioni, X.; Goudemand, M. Predictive validation study of the Edinburgh Postnatal Depression Scale in the first week after delivery and risk analysis for postnatal depression. *J. Affect. Disord.* **2006**, *93*, 169–176. [CrossRef]
24. Dennis, C.L.; Merry, L.; Stewart, D.; Gagnon, A.J. Prevalence, continuation, and identification of postpartum depressive symptomatology among refugee, asylum-seeking, non-refugee immigrant, and Canadian-born women: Results from a prospective cohort study. *Arch. Womens Ment. Health* **2016**, *19*, 959–967. [CrossRef]
25. Zanardo, V.; Volpe, F.; de Luca, F.; Giliberti, L.; Giustardi, A.; Parotto, M.; Straface, G.; Soldera, G. Maternity blues: A risk factor for anhedonia, anxiety, and depression components of Edinburgh Postnatal Depression Scale. *J. Matern.-Fetal Neonatal Med.* **2019**, *33*, 3962–3968. [CrossRef]
26. Cox, J.L.; Holden, J.M.; Sagovsky, R. Detection of postnatal depression. Development of the 10-item Edinburgh Postnatal Depression Scale. *Br. J. Psychiatry* **1987**, *150*, 782–786. [CrossRef]
27. Zung, W.; Durham, N.C. A Self-Rating Depression Scale. *Arch. Gen. Psychiatry* **1965**, *12*, 63–70.
28. Ruiz-Grosso, P.; de Mola, C.L.; Vega-Dienstmaier, J.M.; Arevalo, J.M.; Chavez, K.; Vilela, A.; Lazo, M.; Huapaya, J. Validation of the Spanish Center for Epidemiological StudiesDepression and Zung Self-Rating Depression Scales: A Comparative Validation Study. *PLoS ONE* **2012**, *7*, e45413.
29. Sedighi, S.; Najarzadegan, M.; Ghasemzadeh, H.; Khodabandeh, M.; Khazaei, M.; Mirzadeh, M.; Babakhanian, M.; Rokni, A.; Ghazanfarpour, M. Factor Structure and Psychometric Properties of Zung Self-Rating Depression Scale in Women with a Sick Child. *Int. J. Pediatrics* **2020**, *8*, 11581–11586.
30. R Core Team. *A Language and Environment for Statistical Computing*; R Foundation for Statistical Computing: Vienna, Austria, 2018; Available online: https://www.R-project.org/ (accessed on 18 October 2020).
31. Rosseel, Y. Lavaan: An R Package for Structural Equation Modeling. *J. Stat. Softw.* **2012**, *48*, 1–36. [CrossRef]
32. Epskamp, S.; Stuber, S. SemPlot: Path Diagrams and Visual Analysis of Various SEM Packages' Output. R Package Version 1.1. 2017. Available online: https://CRAN.R-project.org/package=semPlot (accessed on 25 October 2020).
33. Kline, R.B. *Principles and Practice of Structural Equation Modeling*, 3rd ed.; Guilford Press: London, UK, 2011.
34. Brown, T. *Confirmatory Factor Analysis for Applied Research*, 2nd ed.; Guilford Press: New York, NY, USA, 2015.
35. Matthey, S. Does an early postpartum Edinburgh Postnatal Depression Scale (EPDS) really detect the majority of women with elevated EPDS scores at 16-weeks postpartum? *Arch. Womens Ment. Health* **2017**, *20*, 811–812. [CrossRef]
36. Nagy, E.; Molnar, P.; Pal, A.; Orvos, H. Prevalence rates and socioeconomic characteristics of post-partum depression in Hungary. *Psychiatry Res.* **2011**, *185*, 113–120. [CrossRef] [PubMed]
37. Lyubenova, A.; Neupane, D.; Levis, B.; Wu, Y.; Sun, Y.; He, C.; Krishnan, A.; Bhandari, P.M.; Negeri, Z.; Imran, M.; et al. Depression prevalence based on the Edinburgh Postnatal Depression Scale compared to Structured Clinical Interview for DSM DIsorders classification: Systematic review and individual participant data meta-analysis. *Int. J. Methods Psychiatry Res.* **2020**, *30*, e1860. [CrossRef] [PubMed]
38. Cox, J. Thirty years with the Edinburgh Postnatal Depression Scale: Voices from the past and recommendations for the future. *Br. J. Psychiatry* **2019**, *214*, 127–129. [CrossRef] [PubMed]
39. NHIC-National Health Information Center. Starostlivosť o Rodičku a Novorodenca v Slovenskej Republike 2018 (Mother-Infant Healthcare in Slovak Republic 2018). Available online: http://www.nczisk.sk/Statisticke_vystupy/Tematicke_statisticke_vystupy/Gynekologia_Porodnictvo_Potraty/Porodnictvo/Pages/default.aspx (accessed on 10 November 2020).
40. Romera, I.; Delgado-Cohen, H.; Perez, T.; Caballero, L.; Gilaberte, I. Factor analysis of the Zung self-rating depression scale in a large sample of patients with major depressive disorder in primary care. *BMC Psychiatry* **2008**, *8*, 4. [CrossRef]

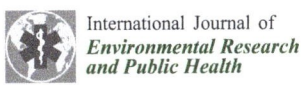

International Journal of
Environmental Research and Public Health

Article

Screening for Perinatal Anxiety Using the Childbirth Fear Questionnaire: A New Measure of Fear of Childbirth

Nichole Fairbrother [1,*], Fanie Collardeau [2], Arianne Albert [3] and Kathrin Stoll [1]

1 Department of Family Practice, Faculty of Medicine, University of British Columbia, Vancouver, BC V6T 1Z4, Canada; kathrin.stoll@ubc.ca
2 Department of Psychology, Faculty of Social Sciences, University of Victoria, Victoria, BC V8P 5C2, Canada; faniecol@uvic.ca
3 Women's Health Research Institute, Vancouver, BC V6H 2N9, Canada; arianne.albert@cw.bc.ca
* Correspondence: nicholef@uvic.ca

Abstract: Fear of childbirth affects as many as 20% of pregnant people, and has been associated with pregnancy termination, prolonged labour, increased risk of emergency and elective caesarean delivery, poor maternal mental health, and poor maternal-infant bonding. Currently available measures of fear of childbirth fail to fully capture pregnant people's childbirth-related fears. The purpose of this research was to develop a new measure of fear of childbirth (the Childbirth Fear Questionnaire; CFQ) that would address the limitations of existing measures. The CFQ's psychometric properties were evaluated through two studies. Participants for Study 1 were 643 pregnant people residing in Canada, the United States, and the United Kingdom, with a mean age of 29.0 (SD = 5.1) years, and 881 pregnant people residing in Canada, with a mean age of 32.9 (SD = 4.3) years for Study 2. In both studies, participants completed a set of questionnaires, including the CFQ, via an online survey. Exploratory factor analysis in Study 1 resulted in a 40-item, 9-factor scale, which was well supported in Study 2. Both studies provided evidence of high internal consistency and convergent and discriminant validity. Study 1 also provided evidence that the CFQ detects group differences between pregnant people across mode of delivery preference and parity. Study 2 added to findings from Study 1 by providing evidence for the dimensional structure of the construct of fear of childbirth, and measurement invariance across parity groups (i.e., the measurement model of the CFQ was generalizable across parity groups). Estimates of the psychometric properties of the CFQ across the two studies provided evidence that the CFQ is psychometrically sound, and currently the most comprehensive measure of fear of childbirth available. The CFQ covers a broad range of domains of fear of childbirth and can serve to identify specific fear domains to be targeted in treatment.

Keywords: childbirth; fear; assessment; birth; questionnaire development; caesarean; vaginal

1. Introduction

Worldwide, approximately 137 million births occur each year, with over 300,000 babies born in Canada alone [1]. Maternal mortality is lowest in high income countries [2]. Specifically, in 2017 the maternal mortality ratio (MMR: the number of maternal deaths per 100,000 live births, and a measure of the overall quality of maternal health and reproductive care) was 11 per 100,000 live births in high income countries [2]. The MMR is estimated at 10 for Canada and 19 for the United States [3]. In low-income countries, maternal mortality is higher, with 462 death per 100,000 live births [2]. Globally, from 2000 to 2017, the MMR dropped by 38% [2]. However, despite the relative safety of childbirth in developed nations, many pregnant people nevertheless experience high levels of fear of childbirth.

Pregnancy and childbirth are significant, emotionally powerful life events. For many childbearing people, pregnancy follows a complex emotional trajectory characterized by both positive and negative feelings in anticipation of their due date [4,5]. Mental health

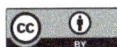

difficulties are common among perinatal people, with pre- and postnatal depression, and postpartum psychosis the most studied [6].

Until recently, perinatal anxiety had received limited attention [7]. We now know that the anxiety and their related disorder are the most common mental health conditions to affect pregnant and postpartum people [8]. Specifically, one in five pregnant and postpartum people suffer from one or more anxiety or anxiety-related disorders during the perinatal period [8]. This is much greater than the prevalence of depression affecting approximately six to twelve percent of perinatal people [9,10]. The anxiety disorders include all of the core anxiety conditions (generalized anxiety disorder, panic disorder, agoraphobia, social anxiety disorder and specific phobias) as well as obsessive-compulsive disorder and posttraumatic stress disorder. These latter conditions were, until recently also considered anxiety disorders, and many investigators continue to include them among the anxiety and anxiety-related disorders [11]. Among perinatal people, the content of one's anxiety often orients towards the health and wellbeing of the pregnancy and childbirth (for both the mother and the unborn child), and the health and wellbeing of one's new-born. For example, worries in generalized anxiety disorder may often involve these areas of concern, and perinatal obsessive-compulsive disorder is often characterized by unwanted, intrusive thoughts of infant-related harm [12–17]. A key domain of anxious concern among both nulliparous and multiparous pregnant people is childbirth. Childbirth related fears (e.g., fear of pain, medical interventions, potential harm to one's infant) are common and can be intense [18].

While positive feelings usually outweigh negative feelings, including worries about childbirth, for some, negative emotions, including fear related to giving birth, predominate (6). Despite the relative safety of childbirth in high income settings, pregnant people may experience fear about being unable to prepare for the unpredictable, the amount of pain they will experience during labour and birth, the possible medical procedures that may be required (e.g., caesarean), as well as concerns for the health and wellbeing of themselves and their new-born (4,6). In a recent, large-scale systematic review and meta-analyses the global pooled prevalence of FoB in pregnant women was estimated at 14% (95% CI 0.12–0.16) [19]. Twenty-nine primary studies conducted in middle- and high-income countries were included in this analysis. Significant between-study heterogeneity was reported, with prevalence estimates ranging from 3.7 to 43%, likely due to variability in methodological quality, measurement tools and cut-scores [19]. All but one [20] of the included studies employed self-report questionnaires as a measure of FoB. When measured using diagnostic interviews, clinically significant levels of fear of childbirth have been found to be much lower. To our knowledge, only three studies have taken this approach, reporting prevalence estimates of 2.4 [21], 4.5 [20], and 8.5% [22] for FoB. This is not surprising, as prevalence estimates are often higher when mental health difficulties are measured using self-report questionnaires, compared to when formal diagnostic criteria are employed [23–25]. Of note, studies employing diagnostic criteria to investigate FoB have only been carried out in high-income countries. Therefore, our knowledge of clinically significant levels of FoB in middle- or low-income countries remains limited.

With one exception [20], levels of fear of childbirth have typically been found to be higher among nulliparous people [19,21,26] compared with multiparous people. Fear of childbirth has also been associated with a range of negative outcomes including: avoidance of pregnancy, termination of pregnancy, higher levels of perceived pain during childbirth, increased length of labour, increased likelihood of emergency and elective caesarean birth, postnatal depression and posttraumatic stress disorder, increased parenting stress, and poor maternal-infant bonding [26–30]. There are, however, opportunities to mitigate these negative effects. Previous research has shown that psychotherapy and educational interventions, such as counselling delivered by maternity care providers or education on childbirth at the hospital, can reduce pregnant people's fears of childbirth [31]. Additionally, although medical indications for caesarean birth have been well-established, to our knowledge, there are few established psychosocial indications. Persistent, untreated fear of childbirth, which is clinically distressing or impairing, may justifiably be one such indication.

1.1. Measurements of Fear of Childbirth

Although numerous measures of childbirth fear have been reported in the literature ranging in length from a single item to 53 items, each of them either: (a) assesses only a subset of the content domains relevant to fear of childbirth [4,32–42]; (b) includes only one or two items for some of the domains assessed [4,43]; (c) includes non-fear-related items [4,32–35,41,44]; (d) are specific to a particular subpopulation (e.g., adolescents, those who have already given birth) [32,41]; or (e) are single or double item measures only [40,45]. See Table 1 for details.

Table 1. Measurements of fear of childbirth.

Name of Instrument	# of Items	Subscales Include at Least Three Items?	Complete Content Coverage	Excludes Non-Fear Content	For Use with Pregnant People?
Melender (2002)—unnamed [4]	53	NO	MED	NO	YES
Slade-Pais Expectations of Childbirth Scale (SPECS) [44]	50	YES	HIGH	NO	YES
Wijma Delivery Expectancy/Experience Questionnaire—Version A (W-DEQ-A) [33]	33	YES	LOW	NO	YES
Eriksson et al. (2005)—unnamed [34]	29	YES	LOW	NO	NO
Tokophobia Severity Scale (TSS) [46]	13	N/A	MED	NO	YES
Fear of Vaginal Delivery Scale [32]	10	N/A	MED	NO	NO
Birth Experiences Questionnaire (BEQ) [41]	10	N/A	LOW	NO	NO
Oxford Worries about Labour Scale (OWLS) [43]	9	Not all	HIGH	YES	YES
Birth Anticipation Scale (BAS) [36]	6	N/A	LOW	YES	YES
Prelog et al. (2019)—unnamed [42]	6	N/A	-	-	-
Fear of Birth Scale (FOBS) [45]	2	N/A	LOW	YES	YES
Visual Analogue Scale (VAS) [40]	1	N/A	LOW	YES	YES
Hildingsson et al. (2011)—unnamed [38]	1	N/A	LOW	YES	YES
Laursen et al. (2008)—unnamed [39]	1	N/A	LOW	YES	YES

In our opinion, one or two item measures are insufficient to produce a stable estimate of childbirth fear, nor can they encompass the possible range of concerns experienced by people who are pregnant, or may become pregnant (e.g., fear of harm, medical interventions, or pain). Further, evidence suggests that fear of childbirth is multidimensional [4,44,47]. Among the longer scales developed [4,33,36] each, either fails to assess key domains of childbirth fears (e.g., pain, harm to self or infant), includes non-fear relevant items, or under-samples content domains (i.e., have only one or two items for a particular content domain, whereas a minimum of three is needed to produce a stable measure).

By far the most commonly used measure of fear of childbirth is the Wijma Delivery Expectancy/Experience Questionnaire Version A (W-DEQ-A) [33]. The W-DEQ-A has been used in several countries [28,48–56]. The W-DEQ-A has been found to possess good psychometric properties [28,33,57]. Although psychometrically sound [28,33], the W-DEQ-A is not limited to an assessment of fear, but rather assesses a wide range of perceptions of labour and delivery (e.g., during labour and delivery, do you think you will feel: lonely; strong; confident; afraid; deserted; weak; safe; independent; desolate; tense; happy, etc.). In factor analytic studies of the W-DEQ-A, fear has been found to emerge as one of four, or one of six factors, strongly suggesting that the W-DEQ-A is not only a measure of fear [28,33]. Further, many aspects of fear of childbirth are not addressed in this measure (e.g., pain; perceptions of social embarrassment; pressure to receive/avoid pain medication; mother's safety; changes to the body and sexual function; fear of medical interventions). The W-DEQ-A may limit researchers' ability to assess whether specific aspects of fear of childbirth are predicated by different life experiences and/or result in differing outcomes. At the same time, the broad nature of W-DEQ-A items may still capture participants' experience of fear of childbirth albeit in a general way (i.e., still report fear, even if the exact content of their fear of childbirth would not be known).

Accurate measurement of fear of childbirth is important in correctly identifying those experiencing high levels of fear of childbirth, as well as identifying targets for treatment. At present, currently available measures of fear of childbirth do not fully meet this standard.

1.2. The Present Studies

We sought to develop a self-report measure of fear of childbirth that recognizes the complexity of childbirth fear and assesses fear of birth regardless of the planned or preferred mode of delivery. The purpose of this research was to evaluate the psychometric properties of a newly developed measure of FoB: Childbirth Fear Questionnaire (CFQ).

In Study 1, we sought to establish the factor structure of the CFQ (i.e., ascertain the appropriate number of factors and items per factor, and remove items that fail to load sufficiently on any factor). We also sought to conduct a preliminary evaluation of the resulting measure's reliability and construct validity. In view of these objectives, we conducted an exploratory factor analysis of the initial item pool and identified the items and subscales for Study 2. We also assessed the reliability, and convergent and discriminant validity of the measure. Specifically, we predicted that the CFQ would correlate more strongly with another measure of FoB (W-DEQ-A full scale and the W-DEQ-A fear scale) than with measures of blood and injury fears (the MQ) or depressed mood (the EPDS) [58]. To further assess the construct validity of the CFQ we also compared participants who reported a preference for a vaginal birth to those who reported a preference for a caesarean birth. We predicted that participants who reported a preference for a caesarean birth would also report higher levels of fear of pain from a vaginal birth, fear of harm to baby, fear of mum or baby dying, fear of insufficient pain medication, and fear of damage to one's body from a vaginal birth, but lower levels of fear of caesarean delivery and fear of medical interventions, compared with those who reported a preference for a vaginal birth.

In Study 2, we evaluated the replicability and generalizability of the factor structure of the CFQ and conducted further reliability, and convergent and discriminant validity evaluations. We tested the convergent/discriminant validity of the CFQ by comparing the relationship between the CFQ and the W-DEQ-A with the relationships between the CFQ and measures of depressed mood (the EPDS) and symptoms of posttraumatic stress disorder (the PDS-5). We predicted that the CFQ would correlate more strongly with both the W-DEQ-A full and fear scale [58] than with either the EPDS or the PDS-5.

2. Study 1

2.1. Materials and Methods

2.1.1. Participants

We recruited a convenience sample of English speaking, pregnant people who were over the age of 18 (mean = 29.0 years, SD = 5.1) and who were residing in Canada, the United Kingdom, or the United States to participate, via online forums frequented by pregnant people (e.g., pregnancy-related web sites and blogs). We planned for a sample size of approximately 500 individuals, following the recommendations of MacCallum et al. [59] for the sample size needs of an exploratory factor analysis (EFA). Our final sample consisted of 643 pregnant people.

2.1.2. Procedures

In order to complete the survey, participants were required to acknowledge that they had read the study cover sheet/consent form and agreed to participate. Consenting participants completed the online survey between 3 and 42 weeks' gestation. For each survey completed, $0.50 was donated to the Children's Health Foundation of Vancouver Island, British Columbia. The study was approved by the Behavioural Research Ethics Board of the University of British Columbia.

2.1.3. Measures

Background Questions. Participants completed a set of demographic questions (e.g., age, marital status, education, income, country of residence, and race and ethnicity), questions about the current pregnancy (e.g., method of conception, and number of foetuses), and previous pregnancies (if applicable) (e.g., the number of prior pregnancies, births, miscarriages, and vaginal and caesarean deliveries).

Birth Preferences. Using a 7-point Likert-type scale (ranging from a very strong preference for a vaginal birth to a very strong preference for a caesarean birth), participants were asked about mode of delivery preference (i.e., vaginal versus caesarean).

Childbirth Fear Questionnaire (CFQ)—Initial Item Pool. The initial pool of CFQ items and item domains were developed by a team of perinatal researchers from the fields of psychology, midwifery and nursing, and based on earlier work in this area, including our own [60]. Our group of investigators collaborated in reviewing the extant FoB measurement literature, generating items for inclusion in the CFQ, reviewing item wording, and ensuring that all domains of fear deemed relevant to childbirth had been included in the initial pool of items. In recognition of the likelihood that the CFQ would include both a total scale score and subscale scores, we developed multiple items for each fear domain (a minimum of three items per subscale are needed to ensure a reasonable degree of internal consistency reliability). To be able to reduce the overall number of items, and develop subscales with high internal consistency and reliability, each content domain initially included five or more items.

This process resulted in an initial pool of 49 items covering the following domains of childbirth-related fears: social embarrassment (e.g., fear of losing control), pain (i.e., fear of pain), pain medication (e.g., fear of not receiving the pain medication one is hoping for), mode of delivery (e.g., fear of a caesarean delivery), baby's and mother's physical safety (e.g., fear that one's infant may be harmed or die during labour/delivery), changes to one's body (e.g., scarring), sexual functioning (e.g., enjoying sexual activity less following delivery), and medical interventions (e.g., fear of having an episiotomy). The CFQ items are scored on a 0 (not at all) to 4 (extremely) point, Likert-type scale.

These initial fear domains represent content areas of fear and concerns commonly reported by pregnant people, such as fear of pain and fear that harm might come to the baby [47,61]. In earlier work [60], maternal complications, feelings of embarrassment, fear of medical interventions/surgery, scarring, sexual functioning, and body damage, were also identified as areas of childbirth related fear and concern, and were considered when developing the initial pool of items for the CFQ.

Wijma Delivery Expectancy Questionnaire (W-DEQ-A). The W-DEQ-A is a 33-item questionnaire, with items scored on a 0–5 Likert type scale, and a range of possible scores from 0 to 165. The psychometric properties of this assessment tool have been well established [28,33]. In the current sample, the internal consistency reliability for the W-DEQ-A was 0.92. In addition to the W-DEQ-A total score, there are also data to support the use of a 6-item fear scale [58].

In this study, in error, we administered the W-DEQ-A using a 0–4 Likert type scale (rather than the usual 0–5 scale). We then prorated the W-DEQ-A scores to the more standard 0–5 point scale as follows: original W-DEQ-A score was divided by four, then multiplied by 5. Our rescaled mean W-DEQ-A (M = 55.9) score was consistent with those found in the literature, which range from 52.9 to 68.3 [62]. Our mean scores for both nulliparous (60.7) and multiparous people (50.2) were consistent with those reported in the literature (i.e., 54.1 to 68.51 and 50.3 to 60.7, respectively), as was the percentage of participants scoring above 85 (i.e., 7.5% to 15.6% in the literature, and 9.8% in the current study) [62]. We are confident that our prorated W-DEQ-A scores are a valid estimate of correctly scaled W-DEQ-A items and were valid to use as the main measure of convergent validity.

Edinburgh Postnatal Depression Scale (EPDS). The EPDS is a 10-item self-report screening tool for pre and postnatal depression. The sensitivity and specificity of the EPDS are in acceptable ranges (65–100%, and 49–100%, respectively) [63]. The EPDS is the most widely used screening tool for perinatal depression [64]. It was included in this study as a measure of discriminant validity for the CFQ; childbirth fear should be no more than moderately correlated with depression. In the current sample, the internal consistency reliability of the EPDS was 0.88.

Mutilation Questionnaire (MQ). The MQ is a 30-item measure of blood and injury fears. Internal consistency for the MQ ranges from 0.75 to 0.86 [65]. In the current sample, the internal consistency reliability was 0.87. High MQ scores are associated with fainting at the sight of blood and injury [65,66]. The MQ was included as a second measure of discriminant validity for the CFQ; blood-injury fears should be no more than moderately correlated with fear of childbirth.

2.1.4. Data Analysis Strategy

Factor analyses were performed in R (v. 3.3.2) [67] using the psych() package (v. 1.6.9) [68] for fitting exploratory factor analysis models. Accompanying visualizations were created using the ggplot2() package (v. 2.2.1) [69]. Differences between correlations were tested using a test provided by Lee and Preacher [70], and standardized mean-difference effect sizes for t-tests (ds) were estimated using the calculator provided by Lakens [71]. All other analyses were carried out using IBM SPSS Statistics (v23) (IBM, Chicago, IL, USA).

Exploratory Factor Analysis. We followed the recommendations of Sakaluk and Short [72] and others (e.g., [73]) for conducting exploratory factor analysis on all CFQ items. Specifically, all solutions extracted common factors via maximum likelihood estimation, to facilitate the calculation of model fit indices. We determined the number of factors to retain through a combination of criteria, including: (1) parallel analysis [74]; (2) the minimum average partial (MAP) criterion [75]; (3) interpretations of absolute and relative indexes of model fit (the root mean square error of approximation [RMSEA], and Tucker-Lewis Index [TLI], respectively) [76]; (4) interpretations of the Bayesian Information Criterion (BIC); (5) nested model comparisons using likelihood-ratio tests between competing models; and (6) factor solution interpretability. All solutions were rotated to achieve simple structure and estimate factor correlations, using the oblique Oblimin method to allow for factor correlation.

We considered items that loaded onto a factor at ≥ 0.35 to be substantive indicators of the underlying latent construct. Items that did not load onto any factor beyond this threshold were determined to be poor indicators and were removed from the final version of the CFQ.

Convergent/Discriminant Validity. The convergent/discriminant validity of the CFQ was assessed via correlation analyses. We compared the correlations between the CFQ and the W-DEQ-A with the correlations between the CFQ and measures of depressed mood (the EPDS) and blood and injury fears (the MQ). We further conducted t-tests to compare mean subscale scores between participants with a strong desire for a vaginal birth to participants with a strong desire for a caesarean birth.

Reliability and Validity Analyses. The remaining analyses involved descriptive data (means, standard deviations, and percentages), Cronbach alpha reliability coefficients, correlations, and independent-samples t-tests. Differences between correlations were tested using a test of the difference between two dependent correlations with one variable in common [70].

Exploratory Analyses. We also conducted t-test analyses to compared CFQ subscale scores across parity and country (Canada and the United States) groups.

2.2. Results

2.2.1. Demographics

Participant demographic and reproductive information is presented in Table 2. Note that complications in the current pregnancy were reported by participants (22.9%), and ranged broadly in severity (e.g., early spotting, anaemia, pre-eclampsia). In this sample, 21.3% of participants scored a 12 or greater (common cut-score for depression) on the EPDS.

Table 2. Participant demographic and reproductive information. M, mean; SD, standard deviation.

Demographic Variables	Study 1 (n = 643)		Study 2 (n = 881)	
Age of Participants in Years	18–45 (M = 29.0, SD = 5.1)		19–49 (M = 32.9, SD = 4.3)	
	Percentage	n	Percentage	n
Married or cohabitating	93.0%	598	93.3%	819
Some postsecondary education	85.9%	520	96.8%	829
Country of residence				
Canada	63.6%	409	100%	881
United States	30.8%	198	N/A	N/A
United Kingdom	2.6%	17	N/A	N/A
European heritage	92.7%	596	72.5%	636
Asian heritage	4.0%	26	10.1%	89
English spoken at home	94.1%	605	94.3%	826
Current pregnancy				
Singleton pregnancy	97.4%	626	97.3%	854
Weeks pregnant: M (SD)	22.2 (10.4)	643	34.9 (2.5)	870
Pregnancy complications	22.9%	147	33.4%	293
Reproductive history				
Prior births	76.3%	n = 296	65.9%	n = 324
Vaginal	80.7%	239	81.8%	251
Caesarean	25.7%	76	31.0%	85
Prior pregnancy loss < 20 weeks	50.3%	195	39.2%	193
Prior pregnancy loss > 20 weeks	3.9%	15	1.6%	8
Questionnaire data	M	SD	M	SD
W-DEQ-A	55.9	23.5	58.2	23.0
EPDS	7.8	5.1	7.7	5.0
MQ	11.1	6.4	N/A	N/A
PDS-5	N/A	N/A	9.9	11.9

2.2.2. Exploratory Factor Analysis of the CFQ

Results of our parallel analysis (see Figure 1) suggested a maximum of 13 factors ought to be retained, whereas the MAP test suggested 9 factors was sufficient. We then proceeded to evaluate indexes of model fit, information criteria, and nested model comparisons for 1–13 factor solutions (see Table 3).

Each additionally extracted factor significantly improved the fit of our model. Adequate model fit based on the RMSEA was achieved from a 6-factor model onward, whereas adequate model fit based on the TLI was achieved near the 9- to 10-factor models. The BIC indicated that our models became unnecessarily complex after the 11-factor solution, and our 13-factor solution failed to converge. We therefore examined the pattern matrixes of loadings for the 9-, 10-, and 11-factor solutions.

The 9-factor solution was supported by the MAP test and had acceptable fit according to the RMSEA, and near-acceptable fit according to the TLI1; it was also the most conceptually interpretable of the three solutions we investigated in detail. The 10-factor solution, though acceptably fitting according to both the RMSEA and TLI, yielded a tenth factor that was not conceptually coherent. The 11-factor solution, finally, was also acceptably fitting, but the extracted eleventh factor had no substantially loading items. We therefore selected the 9-factor solution as the best fitting and conceptually interpretable model of the CFQ items.

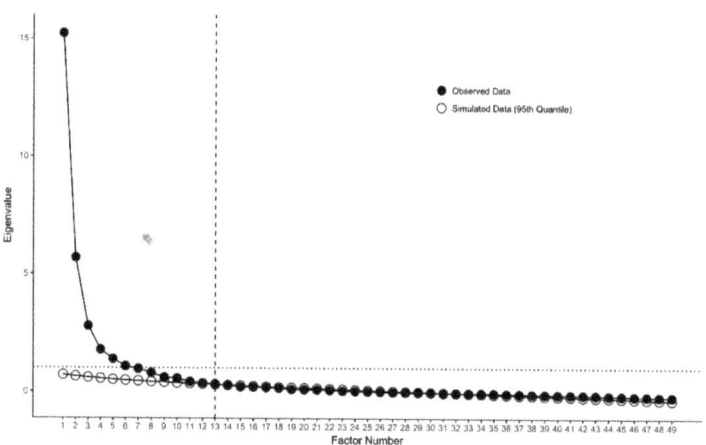

Figure 1. Parallel analysis of 49 CFQ items. Vertical dashed line indicates maximum recommended number of factors (last observed eigenvalue that is larger than 95th quantile of simulated eigenvalues). Horizontal dotted line indicates eigenvalue of 1.

Table 3. Study 1. Model fit indexes, information criteria, and model comparisons for 1–13 factor EFA solutions.

# of Factors	χ^2	df	RMSEA	TLI	BIC	$\Delta\chi^2$	Δdf
1	14,390.42 ***	1127	0.137	0.405	7103.07	—	—
2	10,789.4 ***	1079	0.116	0.544	3812.43	3601.02 ***	48
3	7965.64 ***	1032	0.104	0.659	1292.58	2823.76 ***	47
4	5796.91 ***	986	0.089	0.752	−578.71	2168.73 ***	46
5	4959.07 ***	941	0.083	0.783	−1125.57	837.84 ***	45
6	4332.69 ***	897	0.079	0.805	−1467.44	626.38 ***	44
7	3712.56 ***	854	0.074	0.830	−1809.53	620.13 ***	43
8	2923.31 ***	812	0.065	0.867	−2327.2	789.25 ***	42
9	**2448.91 *** **	**771**	**0.060**	**0.889**	**−2536.49**	**474.40 *** **	**41**
10	2092.93 ***	731	0.055	0.905	−2633.83	355.98 ***	40
11	1766.84 ***	692	0.051	0.921	−2707.73	326.09 ***	39
12	1549.77 ***	654	0.048	0.930	−2679.09	217.07 ***	38
13 [a]	1318.40 ***	617	0.044	0.942	−2671.21	231.37 ***	37

[a] Model did not converge. *** $p < 0.001$.

Factor loadings for the final nine factors are presented in Table 4, and represent: (1) Fear of loss of sexual pleasure/attractiveness (SEX), (2) Fear of pain from a vaginal birth (PAIN), (3) Fear of medical interventions (INT), (4) Fear of embarrassment (SHY), (5) Fear of harm to baby (HARM), (6) Fear of caesarean birth (CS), (7) Fear of mum or baby dying (DEATH), (8) Fear of insufficient pain medication (MEDS), and (9) Fear of body damage from a vaginal birth (DAMAGE). Correlations between the nine CFQ factors ranged from weak (r = −0.01) to strong (r = 0.84), with approximately one third equal to or greater than 0.50 (see Table 5 for details). Correlations at or above 0.50 were for: Fear of loss of sexual pleasure/attractiveness with Fear of pain from a vaginal birth, Fear of embarrassment, Fear of insufficient pain medication and Fear of body damage from a vaginal birth; Fear of pain from a vaginal birth with Fear of insufficient pain medication and Fear of body damage from a vaginal birth; Fear of medical interventions with Fear of caesarean birth; Fear of embarrassment with Fear of body damage from a vaginal birth, and Fear of harm to baby with Fear of mom or baby dying and Fear of body damage from a vaginal birth.

Table 4. Oblimin-rotated factor loadings from pattern matrix of 9-Factor CFQ solution.

Item Content	F1	F2	F3	F4	F5	F6	F7	F8	F9
Factor 1: Fear of Loss of Sexual Pleasure/Attractiveness (SEX)									
Vaginal stretching from vaginal birth	**0.659**	0.102	−0.020	0.027	0.055	−0.005	0.000	0.032	0.184
Body look less attractive following birth	**0.541**	0.099	−0.042	0.094	−0.004	0.089	−0.058	0.122	0.039
Vagina look less attractive following birth	**0.823**	0.037	−0.018	0.094	−0.048	0.038	−0.002	0.047	−0.003
Enjoying sex less b/c of stretching	**0.894**	−0.026	0.024	−0.032	0.002	−0.068	0.091	−0.055	−0.002
Partner enjoy sex less b/c of stretching	**0.902**	0.020	−0.030	0.065	0.017	0.049	−0.018	−0.009	−0.054
Enjoying sex less b/c of pain	**0.710**	−0.024	0.044	−0.058	0.129	−0.033	0.025	−0.013	0.062
Factor 2: Fear of Pain from a Vaginal Birth (PAIN)									
Experiencing pain during contractions	0.015	**0.957**	0.029	−0.002	0.020	0.010	0.007	0.012	−0.062
Experiencing pain during vaginal birth	0.019	**0.795**	−0.018	0.041	0.016	−0.033	0.020	0.020	0.110
Experiencing pain during labour	0.018	**0.974**	0.032	−0.022	0.021	0.002	−0.005	0.022	−0.030
Experiencing pain pushing baby out	0.002	**0.835**	−0.047	0.046	0.002	−0.003	0.032	0.016	0.085
Having a vaginal birth	−0.063	**0.359**	0.020	0.079	0.017	−0.196	0.041	0.138	0.277
Factor 3: Fear of Medical Interventions (INT)									
Experiencing pain during caesarean birth	−0.003	0.109	**0.580**	−0.049	−0.009	0.148	0.094	0.104	0.013
Harmed because of incompetent care	0.014	−0.116	**0.602**	0.087	0.166	0.048	0.085	−0.022	−0.031
Being left with scars from caesarean birth	0.201	−0.081	**0.451**	−0.105	−0.062	0.214	−0.062	0.163	0.064
Being administered injections	−0.055	0.051	**0.559**	0.146	0.001	0.039	−0.024	−0.169	0.038
Having catheter inserted	0.056	0.050	**0.504**	0.150	0.008	0.069	−0.013	−0.073	0.101
Having general anaesthetic	0.015	−0.004	**0.440**	0.020	0.060	0.187	−0.109	−0.092	0.134
Being administered epidural	−0.014	0.152	**0.446**	0.063	−0.011	0.126	−0.068	−0.319	0.099
Factor 4: Fear of Embarrassment (SHY)									
Being watched by strangers	−0.016	−0.089	0.351	**0.520**	−0.031	−0.015	0.029	0.006	0.034
Losing emotional control	0.167	0.101	0.016	**0.446**	0.071	−0.003	−0.140	0.036	0.066
Others seeing me urinate	0.049	-0.015	0.025	**0.766**	-0.008	−0.008	0.063	0.011	0.052
Others seeing me bowel	0.098	0.071	-0.103	**0.681**	0.066	0.049	0.007	0.085	0.002
Others seeing me naked	0.033	0.067	0.011	**0.755**	0.009	-0.079	0.038	0.045	-0.025
Factor 5: Fear of Harm to Baby (HARM)									
Baby being harmed during labour/birth	0.001	0.058	-0.039	0.013	**0.924**	−0.015	0.044	0.018	-0.001
Baby being damaged during labour/birth	0.058	0.041	−0.062	0.011	**0.886**	−0.002	0.046	0.010	−0.008
Baby being hurt by medical intervention	−0.014	−0.089	0.249	−0.011	**0.654**	0.095	0.108	0.012	0.055
Factor 6: Fear of Caesarean Birth (CS)									
Not being able to have birth I want	0.002	−0.052	−0.025	0.028	0.077	**0.792**	0.015	0.116	0.043
Not being able to have vaginal birth	0.004	−0.008	−0.038	−0.036	0.001	**0.932**	0.014	−0.034	−0.021
Having a caesarean birth	0.021	0.104	0.331	−0.046	−0.084	**0.581**	0.056	−0.034	0.000
Factor 7: Fear of Baby or Mum Dying (DEATH)									
Baby dying during labour/birth	0.000	0.030	0.000	0.006	0.071	0.025	**0.899**	−0.012	−0.013
Baby suffocating during labour/birth	0.013	0.001	−0.037	0.005	−0.001	0.006	**0.955**	0.015	0.041
Dying during labour/birth	0.129	0.007	0.277	0.072	0.089	−0.048	**0.377**	0.146	−0.135
Factor 8: Fear of Insufficient Pain Medication (MEDS)									
Not getting needed pain meds	0.016	0.097	0.044	0.078	0.048	0.033	0.033	**0.794**	0.002
Not having epidural during labour	0.000	0.059	−0.027	0.040	0.026	0.027	0.043	**0.790**	0.050
Not being able to have c-section	0.033	−0.093	0.030	0.083	0.068	−0.149	0.030	**0.297**	0.201
Factor 9: Fear of Body Damage (DAMAGE)									
Vaginal tearing during birth	0.107	0.135	−0.150	0.044	0.053	0.010	0.074	0.028	**0.685**
Rectal tearing during birth	0.061	0.025	0.011	0.140	0.151	0.005	0.112	0.065	**0.553**
Having an episiotomy	0.012	0.083	0.263	−0.002	−0.024	0.075	0.024	−0.012	**0.496**
Requiring vacuum or forceps	−0.008	−0.019	0.220	0.020	0.297	0.155	−0.045	0.035	**0.394**
Needing stitches	0.207	0.122	0.057	0.068	−0.078	0.037	0.130	0.028	**0.483**

Table 4. Cont.

Item Content	F1	F2	F3	F4	F5	F6	F7	F8	F9
			Discarded Items						
Not being strong	0.109	0.182	−0.112	0.340	0.129	0.241	−0.044	0.043	0.024
Receiving unwanted pain meds	−0.007	−0.115	0.322	0.164	0.121	0.294	0.024	−0.271	0.119
Feeling pressure to receive pain meds	−0.053	−0.008	0.217	0.159	−0.004	0.332	0.096	−0.314	0.106
Feeling pressure to have natural birth	0.005	0.149	−0.044	0.185	−0.043	0.033	0.121	0.289	−0.036
Baby contract illness during labour/birth	0.104	−0.065	0.088	−0.015	0.195	−0.055	0.338	0.118	0.039
Bleeding too much during labour/birth	0.156	0.066	0.258	0.105	0.155	−0.087	0.177	0.121	−0.047
Being left with scars from vaginal birth	0.323	0.047	0.192	−0.096	0.090	−0.124	−0.056	0.209	0.334
Having scars/wounds not healing	0.218	−0.029	0.238	0.104	0.116	0.060	0.049	0.168	0.153
Vomiting during labour/birth	0.050	0.139	−0.005	0.239	−0.012	−0.028	0.170	−0.022	0.184

Bold: the factor loadings of each item belonging to each subscale.

Table 5. Correlations among the CFQ subscales and total score for Study 1 (S1) and Study 2 (S2).

Fear of ...	SEX		PAIN		INT		SHY		HARM		CS		DEATH		MEDS		DAMAGE	
	S1	S2	S1	S2	S1	S2	S1	S2	S1	S2	S1	S2	S1	S2	S1	S2	S1	S2
1. SEX	–																	
2. PAIN	0.53 **	0.48 **	–															
3. INT	0.22 **	0.34 **	0.08	0.34 **	–													
4. SHY	0.59 **	0.51 **	0.49 **	0.50 **	0.34 **	0.40 **	–											
5. HARM	0.49 **	0.38 **	0.33 **	0.38 **	0.30 **	0.50 **	0.40 **	0.35 **	–									
6. CS	0.13 *	0.11 **	−0.01	0.11 *	0.60 **	0.59 **	0.16 **	0.18 **	0.27 **	0.31 **	–							
7. DEATH	0.45 **	0.38 **	0.35 **	0.38 **	0.23 **	0.45 **	0.42 **	0.36 **	0.78 **	0.79 **	0.20 **	0.22 **	–					
8. MEDS	0.50 **	0.37 **	0.59 **	0.62 **	−0.03	0.25 **	0.40 **	0.41 **	0.43 **	0.36 **	−0.04	−0.03	0.43 **	0.35 **	–			
9. DAMAGE	0.62 **	0.55 **	0.56 **	0.64 **	0.45 **	0.54 **	0.54 **	0.51 **	0.57 **	0.59 **	0.31 **	0.34 **	0.47 **	0.50 **	0.42 **	0.47 **	–	
Total	0.78 **	0.69 **	0.66 **	0.74 **	0.58 **	0.74 **	0.73 **	0.68 **	0.73 **	0.73 **	0.43 **	0.46 **	0.68 **	0.69 **	0.56 **	0.58 **	0.84 **	0.84 **

Note. ** = $p < 0.001$; * = $p < 0.01$.

2.2.3. Descriptive, Reliability, and Validity Analyses

Descriptive Analyses. Means and standard deviations for the 9 subscales, and the CFQ Total scale scores are presented in Table 6.

Table 6. CFQ total and subscale means (M) and standard deviations (SD).

Subscale	Study 1 (n = 643)	Study 2 (n = 874)
Fear of ...	M (SD)	M (SD)
loss of sexual pleasure/attractiveness (SEX)	1.20 (1.10)	0.82 (0.78)
pain from a vaginal birth (PAIN)	1.65 (1.10)	1.36 (1.02)
medical interventions (INT)	1.72 (.97)	1.05 (0.74)
embarrassment (SHY)	1.15 (0.95)	0.64 (0.66)
harm to baby (HARM)	2.25 (1.32)	1.57 (1.04)
caesarean birth (CS)	2.29 (1.23)	1.69 (1.09)
mum or baby dying (DEATH)	1.68 (1.30)	1.34 (1.14)
insufficient pain medication (MEDS)	0.80 (0.94)	0.60 (0.76)
body damage from a vaginal birth (DAMAGE)	1.89 (1.05)	1.52 (0.89)
CFQ Total Mean Scores	1.59 (0.73)	1.14 (0.61)

Note. All scores are mean item scores with a possible range of 0 (not at all) to 4 (extremely).

Reliability Analyses. The Cronbach alpha for the overall 40-item scale was 0.94. Cronbach alphas for the individual subscales ranged from 0.76 to 0.94. Specifically, Cronbach's alphas were 0.93 for Fear of loss of sexual pleasure/attractiveness, 0.94 for Fear or pain from a vaginal birth, 0.82 for Fear of medical interventions, 0.84 for Fear of embarrassment, 0.93 for Fear of harm to baby, 0.85 for CS, 0.86 for Fear of mum of baby dying, 0.76 for Fear of insufficient pain medication, and 0.85 for Fear of body damage from a vaginal birth.

Convergent/Discriminant Validity. The correlations between the CFQ and the W-DEQ-A (full and fear scales) were 0.41 ($p < 0.001$) and 0.57 ($p < 0.001$) respectively. The correlation between the CFQ and the EPDS was 0.35 ($p < 0.001$), and the correlation between the CFQ and the MQ was 0.28 ($p < 0.001$). The CFQ-W-DEQ-A (full scale) correlation was significantly greater than the CFQ-MQ correlation, $z = 2.73$, $p = 0.006$, but not the CFQ-EPDS correlation, $z = 1.60$, $p = 0.109$. The CFQ-W-DEQ-A (fear scale) correlation was significantly greater than both the CFQ-MQ correlation, $z = 7.17$, $p < 0.001$, and the CFQ-EPDS correlation, $z = 6.61$, $p < 0.001$.

Birth Preferences. Most people in our sample indicated a strong or a very strong preference for a vaginal childbirth (83.8%, $n = 539$), whereas only a small proportion indicated a strong or a very strong preference for a caesarean delivery (5.1%, $n = 33$). Consistent with the above hypotheses, compared with those who strongly preferred a vaginal birth, people who strongly preferred a caesarean delivery reported higher scores on the Fear of pain from a vaginal birth, $t (34.08) = -2.83$, $p = 0.008$, ds = 0.68, Fear of harm to baby, $t (570) = -2.84$, $p = 0.005$, ds = 0.51, Fear of mum or baby dying, $t (570) = -2.81$, $p = 0.005$, ds = 0.50, and Fear of insufficient pain medication, $t (33.50) = -5.54$, $p < 0.001$, ds = 1.53, subscales of the CFQ, but lower scores on the Fear of caesarean birth, $t (37.22) = 6.64$, $p < 0.001$, ds = -1.07, and the Fear of medical interventions, $t (570) = 2.15$, $p = 0.032$, ds = -0.39, subscales of the CFQ. However, our prediction that those who strongly preferred a caesarean birth would report higher scores on the Fear of damage to one's body from a vaginal birth was not supported, ds = 0.04. The means and standard deviations by mode of delivery preference are presented in Table 7.

Table 7. CFQ subscale means (M) and standard deviations (SD): by delivery preference and country.

Subscale	Birth Preferences		Parity		Nationality	
	Vaginal ($n = 539$)	Caesarean ($n = 33$)	Nulliparous ($n = 347$)	Multiparous ($n = 296$)	Canada ($n = 409$)	USA ($n = 198$)
Fear of …	M (SD)	M (SD)	M (SD)	M (SD)	M (SD)	M (SD)
loss of sexual pleasure/attractiveness (SEX)	1.1 (1.1)	1.4 (1.3)	1.4 (1.10)	0.9 (1.0) ***	1.2 (1.1)	1.2 (1.1)
pain from a vaginal birth (PAIN)	1.5 (1.0)	2.3 (1.4) **	2.0 (1.1)	1.3 (1.0) ***	1.6 (1.1)	1.7 (1.1)
medical interventions (INT)	1.8 (1.0)	1.4 (0.9) *	1.7 (0.9)	1.7 (1.0)	1.7 (1.0)	1.9 (1.0) *
embarrassment (SHY)	1.1 (0.9)	1.2 (1.1)	1.4 (1.0)	0.9 (0.9) ***	1.1 (0.9)	1.2 (.9)
harm to baby (HARM)	2.2 (1.3)	2.9 (1.5) **	2.4 (1.3)	2.1 (1.3) **	2.3 (1.3)	2.1 (1.3)
caesarean birth (CS)	2.5 (1.1)	1.3 (1.0) ***	2.2 (1.2)	2.4 (1.26)	2.2 (1.2)	2.5 (1.2) **
mum or baby dying (DEATH)	1.6 (1.3)	2.3 (1.2) **	1.7 (1.3)	1.7 (1.3)	1.6 (1.3)	1.8 (1.3)
insufficient pain medication (MEDS)	0.7 (0.8)	2.0 (1.4) ***	0.9 (1.0)	0.6 (0.9) ***	0.8 (0.9)	0.8 (1.0)
body damage from a vaginal birth (DAMAGE)	1.9 (1.0)	1.9 (1.5)	2.1 (1.0)	1.6 (1.0) ***	1.9 (1.1)	1.8 (1.0)
CFQ Total Mean Scores	1.6 (0.7)	1.8 (1.0)	1.7 (0.7)	1.4 (0.7) ***	1.6 (0.7)	1.6 (.7)

Note. All scores are mean item scores with a possible range of 0 (not at all) to 4 (extremely). * $p < 0.05$; ** $p < 0.01$; *** $p < 0.001$, based on t-tests for independent samples comparing women who: (a) prefer a vaginal birth to those who prefer a caesarean birth, (b) are nulliparous to women who are multiparous, and (c) are resident of Canada to those who are resident of the United States of America.

Parity. Nulliparous and multiparous participants differed significantly on six of the nine CFQ subscales, and the CFQ Total scales. In each case, nulliparous participants scored higher than multiparous participants. Specifically, nulliparous participants scored higher than multiparous participants on the following CFQ factors: Fear of loss of sexual pleasure/attractiveness, $t (639.43) = 6.34$, $p < 0.001$, ds = 0.50, Fear of pain from a vaginal birth, $t (641) = 8.70$, $p < 0.001$, ds = 0.69, Fear of embarrassment, $t (640.80) = 6.29$, $p < 0.001$, ds = 0.50, Fear of harm to baby $t (641) = 2.88$, $p = 0.004$, ds = 0.23, Fear of insufficient pain medication $t\,(639.22) = 3.98$, $p < 0.001$, $ds = 0.31$, and Fear of body damage from a vaginal birth $t\,(641) = 6.49$, $p < 0.001$, $ds = 0.51$, and CFQ Total scores $t\,(641) = 5.83$, $p < 0.001$, $ds = 0.45$. Nulliparous and multiparous participants did not differ significantly on the Fear of medical interventions, $ds = 0.01$, Fear of caesarean birth, $ds = 0.13$, or the Fear of mum or baby dying subscales, $ds = 0.03$. Means and standard deviations by parity, are presented in Table 7.

Country. Canadian and American participants differed on only two of nine CFQ subscales, Fear of medical interventions, $t\,(605) = -2.40$, $p = 0.017$, $ds = 0.21$, and Fear of caesarean birth, $t\,(605) = -3.00$, $p = 0.003$, $ds = 0.26$. In both instances, American participants reported higher levels of fear, though the magnitude of these nationality differences were generally smaller than those between birth preference and parity groups. Means and standard deviations by country for Canada and the US are presented in Table 7.

2.2.4. Summary

In our initial psychometric evaluation and development study of the initial 49 CFQ items, involving 643 pregnant people, exploratory factor analysis resulted in a 9-factor scale, supported by MAP test with acceptable fit based on RMSEA. The resulting 9 factors represent: (1) Fear of loss of sexual pleasure/attractiveness (SEX), (2) Fear of pain from a vaginal birth (PAIN), (3) Fear of medical interventions (INT), (4) Fear of embarrassment (SHY), (5) Fear of harm to baby (HARM), (6) Fear of caesarean birth (CS), (7) Fear of mum or baby dying (DEATH), (8) Fear of insufficient pain medication (MEDS), and (9) Fear of body damage from a vaginal birth (DAMAGE). Subscales were weakly to moderately correlated with a few strong correlations (Fear of loss of sexual pleasure/attractiveness with Fear of body damage from a vaginal birth, Fear of harm to baby with Fear of mom or baby dying, and Fear of caesarean birth with Fear of medical interventions). Cronbach alpha coefficients for the total scale and individual subscales were all above 0.76, providing evidence of high internal consistency reliability. Strong evidence of convergent/discriminant validity was found when comparing the 9-factor CFQ with another measure of fear of childbirth and measures of blood, injury injection fears and depressed mood. The CFQ subscale means were also compared across subgroups (e.g., preferred mode of delivery) with hypothesized differences supported by the data.

3. Study 2

3.1. Methods

3.1.1. Participants

We recruited a convenience sample of 881 English-speaking, pregnant people living in Canada, and over the age of 18 (mean = 32.9 yrs, SD = 4.3). Participants were located via Facebook and other online forums frequented by pregnant people (e.g., pregnancy-related web sites and blogs).

3.1.2. Procedures

Consenting participants completed an online survey between 11 and 46 weeks' gestation with an average of 35 weeks. Participants were eligible to win one of seven $150 prizes. The research was approved by the Behavioural Research Ethics Board of the University of British Columbia.

3.1.3. Measures

Participants completed an online survey. Similar to Study 1, the online survey included the same background and demographics questions, the 40 CFQ items retained from Study 1, the W-DEQ-A (without the scoring error described in Study 1), and the EPDS. We also administered a measure of PTSD (see below) [77]. The MQ was not administered to this sample.

Posttraumatic Diagnostic Scale for DSM-5 (PDS-5). The PDS-5 is a self-report tool used to assess post-traumatic stress disorder (PTSD) based on the DSM-5 diagnostic criteria. The

PDS-5, one of the most used self-report measures of PTSD, has been found to show good sensitivity and specificity, internal consistency and test-retest reliability, and convergent and discriminant validity [77,78]. A significantly elevated PDS-5 score (i.e., ≥28) yields a sensitivity of 79% and specificity of 78%, allowing for probable prediction of a PTSD diagnosis [77].

3.1.4. Data Analysis Strategy

Confirmatory Factor Analysis and Invariance Testing. We used confirmatory factor analysis (CFA) to test the replicability of our exploratory measurement model from Study 1; we also specified two additional methods factors that we anticipated shared variance on account of the repeated use of the terms "vaginal" (items 8, 19, 20, 31, 35, and 37) and "caesarean" (items 9, 21, and 34). Given the limited number of response options for the CFQ and that our indicators failed to meet assumptions of multivariate normality (Multivariate Skewness $p < 0.001$, Multivariate Kurtosis $p < 0.001$, univariate nonnormality for all indicators $p < 0.001$) for the default maximum-likelihood estimator, we opted instead to use a robust unweighted least squares estimator (ULSM). The model was identified, and the scale of latent variables was set, using a fixed-factor method, whereby latent variances were fixed to a value of 1 and all loadings were freely estimated. We evaluated models using conventional recommended cut offs for absolute and relative indexes of model fit [76,79], including the RMSEA and standardized root mean square residual (SRMR; both recommended to be <0.08), and the TLI and Comparative Fit Index (CFI; both recommended to be >0.90), being mindful of how model reliability can impact the appropriateness of these cut offs (see [80]). We conducted our CFA using the Lavaan() package (v. 0.5-23.1097) [81] for R [82].

Multi-Group Measurement Invariance Testing. We then tested the generalizability of our CFA model by examining measurement invariance across participants based on their experience of pregnancy as primiparous ($n = 208$) or multiparous ($n = 683$) mothers. Establishing measurement invariance is a necessary precursor to group comparisons of factor correlations or means, in order to rule out the possibility that differences from such comparisons simply reflect divergences in the way groups think about the constructs under consideration [79,83]. Specifically, groups must demonstrate the same number of factors and general pattern of loadings (i.e., configural invariance) and factor loadings of comparable magnitude (i.e., weak invariance) for group comparisons of correlations involving the factors to be valid. Moreover, groups must demonstrate configural and weak invariance, alongside intercepts of comparable magnitude (i.e., strong invariance) for group comparisons of factor means to be valid.

We began the process of testing measurement invariance by fitting and evaluating a configural invariance model. We then used a combination of nested model comparisons and examining the change in model fit indexes to determine whether the constraints imposed by the subsequent levels of invariance (i.e., weak and strong) were supported, e.g., (66); (67). We fitted and evaluated our invariance models using the semTools() package (v. 0.4-14) [84] for R [82], using the same scale-setting, and identification selections from our CFA analysis.

However, because of convergence issues with the USLM estimator for our invariance testing, we reverted to using a robust maximum-likelihood estimator for specifying invariance models. As a consequence, our invariance models appeared worse fitting than they would have been under the more appropriate USLM estimator (e.g., there was nearly a 0.10 CFI difference between base models depending on estimator selection). We think this compromise is acceptable, given that with these invariance tests we were primarily concerned with relative changes in model fit as we imposed more stringent invariance constraints.

Taxometric Analyses. Our final analysis regarding the measurement structure of the CFQ involved examining whether—as our factor analysis models presumed—the CFQ was best understood as reflecting some continuous dimension(s) or rather, some number of discrete categories, using taxometric analyses [85] (for reviews see [86,87]). In essence, taxometric analyses function by calculating indexes that ostensibly evidence continuity vs.

categorical-ness for a set of observed indicators (e.g., Mean Above Minus Below A Cut, MAMBAC), and then comparing the values of those indexes against those of the same indexes when coming from simulated populations in which a dimensional or categorical structure is specified. Specifically, a comparison curve fit index (CCFI) is computed as the ratio of the degree of misfit for the observed data to a dimensional population compared to a categorical population, with CCFI values less than 0.45 evidencing support for a dimensional model, values greater than 0.55 evidencing support for a categorical model, and values in between indicating an ambiguous outcome. Further, multiple taxometric indexes can be used to compute CCFIs in this fashion; in fact, it is recommended to do so as a form of consistency testing, in order to ensure interpretations are robust to the idiosyncrasies of each index [86]. We therefore evaluated CCFIs from three standardly reported taxometric indexes: MAMBAC, MAXEIG (maximum eigenvalue), and L-MODE (latent mode).

In order to conduct a taxometric analysis, we had to determine two additional analytic features: the indicators that we would include in the analysis, and the plausible size of a taxon (i.e., the first extracted category) underlying the CFQ, were a categorical solution to be supported [86]. Unlike other forms of latent variable modelling, taxometrics works best when using an efficient (i.e., limited, non-exhaustive) non-redundant (i.e., spanning the conceptual breadth of the construct) set of indicators from a larger measure; in particular Ruscio et al. [88] recommended somewhere between 3–5 indicators (as cited in [87]). As the CFQ contains many more items, we therefore conducted our taxometric analyses three times, using a different sampling of items across the subscales of the CFQ for each stance (Analysis 1: items 2, 8, 34, 39; Analysis 2: items 13, 21, 24, 26, and 40; and Analysis 3: items 3, 7, 9, and 37), which provided us another opportunity to evaluate the consistency of our analyses across different analytic specifications.

Next, taxometric model fitting requires the specification of a plausible taxon base rate (see [86]) in order to compute the desired CCFI values. As a recently developed alternative to subjectively determining this base rate (e.g., by consulting previous literature, guestimating, etc.) Ruscio et al. [88] developed a method of creating CCFI profiles, in which taxometric analyses were performed iteratively across a range of specified base-rates. The CCFI profile method, though computationally more intensive, is advantageous in that it provides a reliable means of determining whether the underlying measurement model is dimensional or categorical, and, when in fact categorical, CCFI profiles provide the most accurate estimate of the true underlying base rate. We therefore used the CCFI profile method, evaluating of CCFI values (and their average) across the broadest range of taxon base rates (2.5% to 97.5%).

We conducted all taxometric analyses using the RTaxometrics package [89] in R [82].

Descriptive, Reliability, and Validity Analyses. The remaining analyses involved descriptive data (means, standard deviations, and percentages), Cronbach alpha reliability coefficients, and correlations. Differences between correlations were tested using a test of the difference between two dependent correlations with one variable in common [70].

3.2. Results

3.2.1. Demographics

Participant demographic and reproductive information is presented in Table 2.

3.2.2. CFA and Invariance of the CFQ

Our CFA of the exploratory measurement model from Study 1 suggested that our model fit the data extremely well, (676) = 4300.63, $p < 0.001$, CFI = 0.977, TLI = 0.974, RMSEA = 0.064 (90% CI: 0.062, 0.066), SRMR = 0.055. Parameter estimates (see Table 8) suggest that our proposed model fit cut-offs were reasonable for detecting model misspecification, as most standardized factor loadings were near or greater than the population values specified in Hu and Bentler's simulation study [80].

Table 8. Model fit indexes for CFA model and invariance between nationality (Canada vs. USA) and parity (primiparous vs. multiparous) groups.

Model	χ^2	df	CFI	TLI	RMSEA 90% CI	SRMR	$\Delta\chi^2$	Δdf	ΔCFI
CFA	1981.26 ***	683	0.93	0.92	0.056, 0.062	0.05	–	–	–
Invariance (Nationality)									
Configural	2799.21 ***	1366	0.92	0.91	0.059, 0.065	0.06	–	–	–
Weak	2874.15 ***	1418	0.92	0.91	0.058, 0.065	0.06	76.69 *	52	0.001
Strong	2927.91 ***	1449	0.92	0.91	0.055, 0.061	0.06	52.65 **	31	0.001
Invariance (Parity)									
Configural	2790.74 ***	1366	0.91	0.90	0.059, 0.065	0.06	–	–	–
Weak	2864.79 ***	1418	0.91	0.90	0.058, 0.065	0.06	76.67 *	52	0.001
Strong	2943.60 ***	1449	0.91	0.90	0.058, 0.065	0.06	80.08 ***	31	0.003

Note. χ^2 is Yuan-Bentler corrected version, based on robust MLR estimation; $\Delta\chi^2$ is therefore computed using scaled Satorra-Bentler (2001) method. * $p < 0.05$; ** $p < 0.01$; *** $p < 0.001$

Our measurement invariance analyses, meanwhile, suggested that our measurement model was generalizable across parity status. Model fit was virtually unchanged moving from the non-grouped CFA model to the multi-group configural invariance model, and changes in model fit indexes between the configural invariance and loading invariant models (ΔFI = 0.000, ΔTLI = 0.004, ΔRMSEA = −0.001, ΔSRMR = −0.002, ΔBIC = −204.51) and loading invariant and intercept invariant models (ΔCFI = −0.002, ΔTLI = 0.001, ΔRMSEA = 0.000, ΔSRMR = 0.001, ΔBIC = −127.65) suggested that the added constraints on measurement parameters were reasonable.

Parity. Using structural equation modelling and comparing against the intercept-invariance model of the CFQ, we again found differences in CFQ scores based on parity, $\Delta 2 (9) = 60.73$, $p < 0.001$. As in Study 1, nulliparous participants scored higher than multiparous participants on seven of the nine CFQ factors, including the Fear of loss of sexual pleasure/attractiveness, $z = 4.78$, $p < 0.001$, ds = 0.52, Fear of pain from a vaginal birth, $z = 2.47$, $p = 0.01$, ds = 0.19, Fear of medical intervention, $z = 2.68$, $p = 0.007$, ds = 0.26, Fear of embarrassment, $z = 3.77$, $p < 0.001$, ds = 0.41, Fear of harm to baby $z = 3.67$, ds = 0.32, Fear of mom or baby dying, $z = 2.27$, $p = 0.02$, ds = 0.20, and Fear of body damage, $z = 4.50$, $p < 0.011$, ds = 0.37. Nulliparous and multiparous participants did not differ significantly on the Fear of caesarean birth, ds = 0.09, Fear of insufficient pain medication, d = 0.05.

In sum, our CFA-related analyses allow us to infer that the measurement model of the CFQ is both replicable, and generalizable across parity groups, indicating that it is appropriate for use within (and comparisons between) samples of participants who are expecting with different levels of pregnancy experience.

3.2.3. Taxometric Structure of the CFQ

Our three selected samplings of CFQ items generally exhibited excellent properties for candidate indicators in taxometric analyses, in terms of distributional characteristics, validity coefficients, and within-taxon and within-compliment correlations, see [86,87]. All three CCFI profiles (see Figure 2) strongly supported a dimensional structure for the CFQ and its subscales, as all individual CCFIs (with the exception of one CCFI from in one CCFI profile, MAXEIG in CCFI Profile 2) and their averages, across all three analyses, unambiguously supported dimensional structure (CCFIs < 0.45). We take the consistency of these effects as compelling evidence that the fear of childbirth is best understood as interrelated factors on which individuals differ in degree, not kind [85].

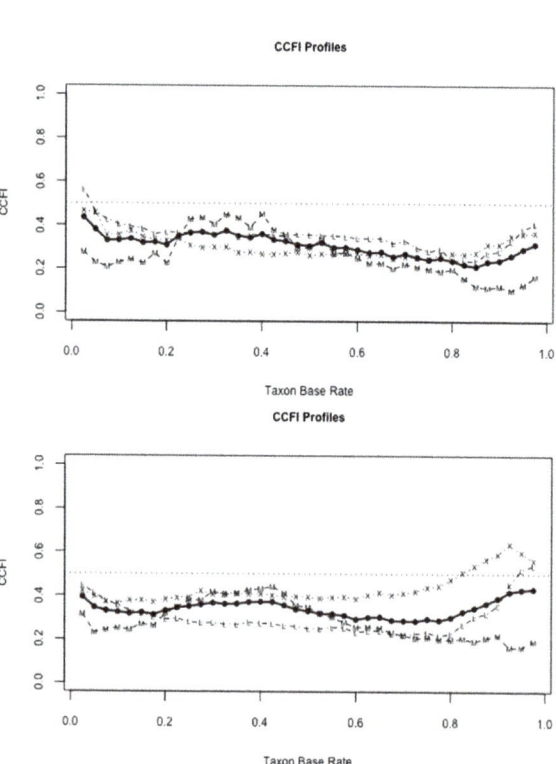

Figure 2. CCFI profiles from taxometric analyses of three unique sets of CFQ indicators. M = MAMBAC, X = MAXEIG, L = L-MODE, and solid dots = the average CCFI.

3.2.4. Descriptive, Reliability, and Validity Analyses

Descriptive Analyses. Means and standard deviations for each of the 9 subscales, and the CFQ Total scale scores are presented in Table 6.

Reliability Analyses. The Cronbach alpha for the overall 40-item scale was 0.94, and the Cronbach alphas for the individual subscales ranged from 0.71 to 0.94 (i.e., Fear of loss of sexual pleasure/attractiveness = 0.90; Fear of pain from a vaginal birth = 0.94; Fear of medical interventions = 0.78; Fear of embarrassment = 0.79; Fear of harm to baby = 0.84; Fear of caesarean birth = 0.87; Fear of mum or baby dying = 0.88; Fear or insufficient pain medication = 0.71; Fear of body damage from a vaginal birth = 0.85).

Convergent/Discriminant Validity. The correlations between the CFQ and the W-DEQ-A (full and fear scales) were 0.58 ($p < 0.001$) and 0.62 ($p < 0.001$) respectively. The correlation between the CFQ and the EPDS was 0.34 ($p < 0.001$), and the correlation between the CFQ and the PDS-5 was 0.24 ($p = 0.001$). The CFQ-W-DEQ-A (full scale) correlation was significantly greater than the CFQ-EPDS correlation, $z = 7.59$, $p < 0.001$, and the CFQ-PDS-5 correlation, $z = 6.97$, $p < 0.001$. The CFQ-W-DEQ-A (fear scale) correlation was significantly greater than both the CFQ-EPDS ($z = 9.00$, $p < 0.001$), and the CFQ-PDS-5 ($z = 7.97$, $p < 0.001$) correlations. See Table 5 for a full list of correlations.

3.3. Summary

Study 2 supported the 9-factor structure of the CFQ, and provided evidence of measurement invariance across parity groups. Specifically, those who had previously given birth understood and responded to CFQ items in the same way as participants who had not previously given birth. Additionally, further tests of the CFQ's latent structure strongly supported a dimensional structure. Thus, fear of childbirth is a construct on which individuals differ in degree rather than in kind (i.e., higher fear of childbirth is not qualitatively different from a lower fear of childbirth). As in Study 1, based on the results from Study 2, it can be inferred that the CFQ demonstrates high reliability, and convergent and discriminant validity. As was true in Study 1 also, overall, nulliparous participants scored higher on CFQ subscales compared to multiparous participants.

4. Discussion

The purpose of this research was to develop a new measure of fear of childbirth in pregnant people, that would encompass the breadth of such fears and overcome some of the limitations of commonly used methods to measure them. Exploratory factor analysis of the CFQ resulted in a 40-item, nine-factor questionnaire. Our nine-factor model was supported by a MAP test, exhibited reasonable model fit and good simple structure, and our factors were readily conceptually interpretable. The 9-factor structure of the CFQ was further supported in Study 2, in a larger sample of pregnant participants. Based on psychometric testing across the two studies, we can infer that the CFQ total scale and the nine subscales demonstrated good internal consistency, and convergent and discriminant validity across both studies.

The taxometric analyses strongly supported a dimensional structure. Thus, fear of childbirth is a construct on which individuals differ in degree rather than in kind (i.e., higher fear of childbirth is not qualitatively different from a lower fear of childbirth). It also suggests that multiple causal influences with small additive effects may best explain more intense fear of childbirth (i.e., rather than a larger single causal factor). While diagnostic categories are frequently used in psychology and might be helpful for clinicians and health authorities to prioritize individuals' access to treatment, diagnostic categories hypothesize a categorical latent structure. Given the dimensional latent structure of fear of childbirth, it will be important to bear in mind that any cut-off score will be arbitrary and result in a loss of information. It is thus better for future studies to keep the full continuum of scores and respect the dimensional latent structure of the data [90].

Second, our nine-factor model showed initial evidence of measurement invariance between parity groups. Thus, those who had previously given birth understood and responded to CFQ items in the same way as participants who had not previously given birth. Any variations in responses between those two groups will be due to real world differences, rather than to a misspecification of the measurement model for one or the other group. This is especially important, provided our finding that nulliparous participants scored higher than multiparous participants on several of the nine CFQ factors.

Data from both studies provide excellent support for the convergent and discriminant validity of the CFQ. As predicted, the CFQ correlated most strongly with another measure of fear of childbirth (W-DEQ-A), and less so with measures of depressed mood (EPDS), trauma symptoms (PDS-5) and blood, injury, injection fears (MQ). In addition, correlations with the CFQ were stronger for the W-DEQ-A (fear subscale) compared with the W-DEQ-A (full scale). This was expected and supports our contention that the W-DEQ-A is not strictly a measure of fear (i.e., includes multiple items more relevant to feelings of depressed mood and other positive and negative emotions). Although the W-DEQ-A fear subscale contains six items, only three truly reflect fear (i.e., afraid, tense and panic). The other three (hopelessness, pain and lose control of myself) are not specifically fear items. The weaker correlation between the CFQ and the W-DEQ-A (full scale) provides support for the CFQ as a novel measure of fear of childbirth, with an emphasis on fear, and distinct from the W-DEQ-A.

Furthermore, the nine factors of the CFQ have the potential to significantly add to our knowledge about fear of childbirth. For example, the nine subscales of the CFQ, identified through factor analysis, make it evident that pregnant people's concerns about childbirth encompass a broad range of potential fears, and that pregnant people who prefer a caesarean birth have different concerns than those who prefer a vaginal birth. Findings regarding the association of CFQ domains and mode of delivery preferences are consistent with our predictions that those who strongly prefer a caesarean birth are especially fearful of (a) the pain from a vaginal birth, and the possibility that they may not receive sufficient pain medication during labour/delivery, and (b) the possibility that something may go terribly wrong during labour/birth, and they or their infant may be harmed or die. Conversely, pregnant people who strongly prefer a vaginal birth are, as expected, more fearful of caesarean delivery and labour/birth related medical interventions in general. The same pattern of results can also be observed in the intercorrelations among the CFQ subscales. However, in contrast with our predictions, those who strongly prefer a caesarean birth did not report higher levels of fear of damage to one's body from a vaginal birth was not supported.

In both studies, the lowest CFQ-W-DEQ-A subscale correlation was for the Fear of caesarean birth subscale. The Fear of medical interventions subscale also correlated weakly with the W-DEQ-A in both studies, although less so in study two (i.e., r = 0.33 and 0.38 in study two, and r = 0.10 and 0.03 in study one). This weak relationship between the W-DEQ-A and these two CFQ subscales is likely a function of the fact that the CFQ is unique among measures of fear of childbirth in its assessment of fears related to operational (i.e., caesarean) delivery.

These finding highlight an interesting phenomenon, not easily assessed by previously available measures of fear of childbirth: that some pregnant people strongly prefer a caesarean birth and are predominantly fearful of the perceived pain and/or danger associated with vaginal delivery, whereas others strongly prefer a vaginal birth and are predominantly fearful of medical interventions in general, and caesarean birth in particular. The link between fear of labour pain and a preference for caesarean delivery is well-documented [60,91]. Very little is known about fears specific to those who prefer vaginal birth. In this regard, the CFQ fills an important gap in our knowledge of the childbirth fears most relevant to pregnant people who prefer a vaginal birth.

The only between-country (Canada and the United States) differences were for the Fear of medical interventions and the Fear of caesarean birth subscales. This is an expected finding as childbirth is a more medicalized experience in the United States in comparison with Canada [92]. Previous research has shown that those who experience pregnancy in a more medicalized birth culture report heightened fear of interventions and other fears that are specific to hospital settings [93]. Consequently, one would expect pregnant people's fears of medical experiences in childbirth to be heightened.

Another example, and a novel and important aspect of the CFQ, is the inclusion of subscales measuring (a) pregnant people's fears about negative, childbirth-related changes to their appearance and sexual functioning, including Fear of loss of sexual pleasure/attractiveness, and (b) Fear of embarrassment because of events occurring during labour/delivery (e.g., fear of urinating in front of others). It is well known that becoming a parent has a significant, and oftentimes negative, impact on one's romantic relationship, including one's sexual relationship [94,95]. That this is a concern for pregnant people appears well captured by the CFQ. That fears about a loss of sexual pleasure and attractiveness are associated with a fear of embarrassment during labour/delivery is not surprising in that both involve potential negative judgments by others, and potentially being seen in ways that are perceived as unattractive by typical standards. Our findings demonstrate that fears regarding embarrassment and sexual functioning/appearance are closely related to fears about childbirth pain and bodily damage in the context of a vaginal delivery, as well as harm or death to mum and baby during childbirth. It appears that pregnant people associate pain from a vaginal birth with vaginal damage, and correspondingly with negative changes to their sexual functioning and appearance, and embarrassing aspects of labour/delivery.

4.1. Clinical Implications

Current measures of fear of childbirth fail to assess the full spectrum of perinatal people's childbirth related fears. Given that fear of childbirth has been associated with several negative medical and social outcomes, an accurate assessment of these fears is important and has implications for pregnant individual's reproductive and mental health. The development of an effective self-report measure of fear of childbirth will facilitate: (a) the provision of appropriate treatment for those with these fears; (b) assessment of specific aspects of perinatal people's childbirth related fears; and (c) identification of fear of childbirth as a potential psychosocial indication for a caesarean delivery. The new CFQ will help to identify pregnant people's specific childbirth concerns, which may be amenable to education or a psychosocial intervention if more extreme.

4.2. Limitations

This study is limited by the fact that we collected data from two convenience samples of pregnant people. We did not collect prospective data, nor did we collect data from reproductive-aged people who were not pregnant. A further limitation is the fact that our sample was English-speaking only, highly educated, and predominantly married/common-law, and Caucasian. It is possible that responses to the CFQ may differ by culture, education, and marital status. Until psychometric evaluations of the CFQ have been undertaken in other cultural contexts, generalizability is, limited pregnant people similar to those in the two studies reported here. Finally, online survey administration prevents the calculation of response rates.

4.3. Future Directions

Future research would benefit from an evaluation of the CFQ among reproductive aged people who are not pregnant, but may one day become pregnant or give birth, those who are gender diverse, as well as reproductive-aged people who are biologically male. The attitudes of biologically male people towards birth and fears concerning childbirth have been shown to influence decision-making around mode of delivery [94]. Further, the validity of the measure should be assessed in other cultural contexts beyond predominantly Caucasian, English-speaking countries.

In our opinion, the most important next steps in the development of the CFQ are to: (a) evaluate the test-retest reliability and sensitivity to change of the CFQ, and (b) assess the CFQ as a screening tool for specific phobia of fear of childbirth (specific phobia is the diagnostic category which has been put forth as the most appropriate classification of fear of childbirth).

5. Conclusions

The Childbirth Fear Questionnaire (CFQ) is a promising new instrument for the multifactorial assessment of fear of childbirth. Evidence of its reliability and validity has been presented. We hope this new measure proves useful to identify pregnant people with elevated fear of childbirth, and for future research into the fear of childbirth.

Author Contributions: N.F. developed the manuscript concept and was responsible for the study design. N.F. and F.C. were responsible for study design, supervision of data collection, and interpretation of the data. A.A., K.S. in collaboration with N.F. and F.C., was responsible for data analyses. All authors were involved in manuscript drafting. All authors provided scientific input and edited and reviewed the manuscript content. All authors provided their final approval and agree to be accountable for all aspects of the work, ensuring integrity and accuracy. All authors have read and agreed to the published version of the manuscript.

Funding: This research was funded from the primary author's start-up funds via the Island Medical Program of the University of British Columbia.

Institutional Review Board Statement: This study was conducted in accordance with the Declaration of Helsinki. Ethical approval for this study was obtained from the Behavioural Ethics Board of the University of British Columbia (H15-03356). The University of British Columbia's Behavioural Research Ethics Board follows the Canadian Tri-Counsel Policy Statement (TCPS): Ethical Conduct for Research Involving Humans.

Informed Consent Statement: Informed consent was obtained from all subjects involved in the study.

Data Availability Statement: The datasets used and/or analysed during the current study are available from the corresponding author on reasonable request.

Acknowledgments: The authors would like to thank the study participants for their time and thoughtful engagement. We would especially like to Jessica Gaiptman and Stephanie Poje for their invaluable contribution to participant recruitment and data management.

Conflicts of Interest: The authors declare no conflict of interest.

References

1. Duffin, E. Number of Births in Canada 2021 | Statista n.d. Available online: https://www.statista.com/statistics/443051/number-of-births-in-canada/ (accessed on 3 January 2022).
2. World Health Organization. Maternal Mortality n.d. Available online: https://www.who.int/news-room/fact-sheets/detail/maternal-mortality (accessed on 3 January 2022).
3. The World Bank. Maternal Mortality Ratio (Modeled Estimate, per 100,000 Live Births) | Data n.d. Available online: https://data.worldbank.org/indicator/SH.STA.MMRT (accessed on 3 January 2022).
4. Melender, H.-L. Experiences of Fears Associated with Pregnancy and Childbirth: A Study of 329 Pregnant Women. *Birth* **2002**, *29*, 101–111. [CrossRef]
5. Larkin, P.; Begley, C.M.; Devane, D. Women's experiences of labour and birth: An evolutionary concept analysis. *Midwifery* **2009**, *25*, e49–e59. [CrossRef] [PubMed]
6. Howard, L.M. What does Excellence in Perinatal Mental Health Look Like? Meeting the NICE Guideline for Postnatal Mental Health. 2016. Available online: https://www.healthcareconferencesuk.co.uk/news/what-does-excellence-in-perinatal-mental-health-look-like-meeting-the-new-nice-guideline (accessed on 3 January 2022).
7. Matthey, S.; Barnett, B.; Howie, P.; Kavanagh, D. Diagnosing postpartum depression in mothers and fathers: Whatever happened to anxiety? *J. Affect. Disord.* **2003**, *74*, 139–147. [CrossRef]
8. Fawcett, E.J.; Fairbrother, N.; Cox, M.L.; White, I.; Fawcett, J.M. The Prevalence of Anxiety Disorders during Pregnancy and the Postpartum Period: A Multivariate Bayesian Meta-Analysis. *J. Clin. Psychiatry* **2019**, *80*, 1181. [CrossRef] [PubMed]
9. Reck, C.; Struben, K.; Backenstrass, M.; Stefenelli, U.; Reinig, K.; Fuchs, T.; Sohn, C.; Mundt, C. Prevalence, onset and comorbidity of postpartum anxiety and depressive disorders. *Acta Psychiatr. Scand.* **2008**, *118*, 459–468. [CrossRef]
10. Woody, C.A.; Ferrari, A.J.; Siskind, D.J.; Whiteford, H.A.; Harris, M.G. A systematic review and meta-regression of the prevalence and incidence of perinatal depression. *J. Affect. Disord.* **2017**, *219*, 86–92. [CrossRef]
11. American Psychiatric Association. *Diagnostic and Statistical Manual of Mental Disorders: DSM-5*, 5th ed.; American Psychiatric Publishing, Inc.: Arlington, VA, USA, 2013. [CrossRef]
12. Challacombe, F.L.; Bavetta, M.; DeGiorgio, S. Intrusive thoughts in perinatal obsessive-compulsive disorder. *BMJ* **2019**, *367*, l6574. [CrossRef]

13. Collardeau, F.; Corbyn, B.; Abramowitz, J.; Janssen, P.A.; Woody, S.; Fairbrother, N. Maternal unwanted and intrusive thoughts of infant-related harm, obsessive-compulsive disorder and depression in the perinatal period: Study protocol. *BMC Psychiatry* **2019**, *19*, 94. [CrossRef]
14. Sharma, V.; Mazmanian, D. Are we overlooking obsessive-compulsive disorder during and after pregnancy? Some arguments for a peripartum onset specifier. *Arch. Women's Ment. Health* **2020**, *24*, 165–168. [CrossRef]
15. Uguz, F.; Akman, C.; Kaya, N.; Çilli, A.S. Postpartum-onset obsessive-compulsive disorder: Incidence, clinical features, and related factors. *J. Clin. Psychiatry* **2007**, *68*, 14834. [CrossRef]
16. Goldfinger, C.; Green, S.M.; Furtado, M.; McCabe, R.E. Characterizing the nature of worry in a sample of perinatal women with generalized anxiety disorder. *Clin. Psychol. Psychother.* **2019**, *27*, 136–145. [CrossRef] [PubMed]
17. Buist, A.; Gotman, N.; Yonkers, K.A. Generalized anxiety disorder: Course and risk factors in pregnancy. *J. Affect. Disord.* **2011**, *131*, 277–283. [CrossRef] [PubMed]
18. O'Connell, M.A.; Leahy-Warren, P.; Khashan, A.S.; Kenny, L.C.; O'Neill, S.M. Worldwide prevalence of tocophobia in pregnant women: Systematic review and meta-analysis. *Acta Obstet. Gynecol. Scand.* **2017**, *96*, 907–920. [CrossRef] [PubMed]
19. Räisänen, S.; Lehto, S.M.; Nielsen, H.S.; Gissler, M.; Kramer, M.R.; Heinonen, S. Risk factors for and perinatal outcomes of major depression during pregnancy: A population-based analysis during 2002–2010 in Finland. *BMJ Open* **2014**, *4*, e004883. [CrossRef]
20. Zar, M.; Wijma, K.; Wijma, B. Relations between anxiety disorders and fear of childbirth during late pregnancy. *Clin. Psychol. Psychother.* **2002**, *9*, 122–130. [CrossRef]
21. Calderani, E.; Giardinelli, L.; Scannerini, S.; Arcabasso, S.; Compagno, E.; Petraglia, F.; Ricca, V. Tocophobia in the DSM-5 era: Outcomes of a new cut-off analysis of the Wijma delivery expectancy/experience questionnaire based on clinical presentation. *J. Psychosom. Res.* **2019**, *116*, 37–43. [CrossRef]
22. Clark, L.A.; Cuthbert, B.; Lewis-Fernández, R.; Narrow, W.E.; Reed, G.M. Three Approaches to Understanding and Classifying Mental Disorder: ICD-11, DSM-5, and the National Institute of Mental Health's Research Domain Criteria (RDoC). *Psychol. Sci. Public Interest* **2017**, *18*, 72–145. [CrossRef]
23. Eaton, W.W.; Neufeld, K.; Chen, L.-S.; Cai, G. A Comparison of Self-report and Clinical Diagnostic Interviews for Depression: Di-agnostic Interview Schedule and Schedules for Clinical Assessment in Neuropsychiatry in the Baltimore Epidemiologic Catchment Area Follow-Up. *Arch. Gen. Psychiatry* **2000**, *57*, 217–222. [CrossRef]
24. Thombs, B.D.; Kwakkenbos, L.; Levis, A.W.; Benedetti, A. Addressing overestimation of the prevalence of depression based on self-report screening questionnaires. *Can. Med. Assoc. J.* **2018**, *190*, E44–E49. [CrossRef]
25. Toohill, J.; Creedy, D.K.; Gamble, J.; Fenwick, J. A cross-sectional study to determine utility of childbirth fear screening in maternity practice–An Australian perspective. *Women Birth* **2015**, *28*, 310–316. [CrossRef]
26. Fisher, C.; Hauck, Y.; Fenwick, J. How social context impacts on women's fears of childbirth: A Western Australian example. *Soc. Sci. Med.* **2006**, *63*, 64–75. [CrossRef] [PubMed]
27. Johnson, R.; Slade, P. Does fear of childbirth during pregnancy predict emergency caesarean section? *BJOG Int. J. Obstet. Gynaecol.* **2002**, *109*, 1213–1221. [CrossRef] [PubMed]
28. Johnson, R.C.; Slade, P. Obstetric complications and anxiety during pregnancy: Is there a relationship? *J. Psychosom. Obstet. Gynecol.* **2003**, *24*, 1–14. [CrossRef]
29. Klusman, L.E. Reduction of pain in childbirth by the alleviation of anxiety during pregnancy. *J. Consult. Clin. Psychol.* **1975**, *43*, 162–165. [CrossRef] [PubMed]
30. Stoll, K.; Swift, E.M.; Fairbrother, N.; Nethery, E.; Janssen, P. A systematic review of nonpharmacological prenatal interventions for pregnancy-specific anxiety and fear of childbirth. *Birth* **2017**, *45*, 7–18. [CrossRef]
31. Areskog, B.; Kjessler, B.; Uddenberg, N. Identification of Women with Significant Fear of Childbirth during Late Pregnancy. *Gynecol. Obstet. Investig.* **1982**, *13*, 98–107. [CrossRef]
32. Wijma, K.; Wijma, B.; Zar, M. Psychometric aspects of the W-DEQ; a new questionnaire for the measurement of fear of childbirth. *J. Psychosom. Obstet. Gynecol.* **1998**, *19*, 84–97. [CrossRef]
33. Eriksson, C.; Westman, G.; Hamberg, K. Experiential factors associated with childbirth-related fear in Swedish women and men: A population based study. *J. Psychosom. Obstet. Gynecol.* **2005**, *26*, 63–72. [CrossRef]
34. Wootton, B.M.; Diefenbach, G.J.; Bragdon, L.B.; Steketee, G.; Frost, R.O.; Tolin, D.F. A contemporary psychometric evaluation of the Obsessive Compulsive Inventory—Revised (OCI-R). *Psychol. Assess.* **2015**, *27*, 874–882. [CrossRef]
35. Cnm, C.E.; Cnattingius, S.; Kjerulff, K.H. Birth Experience in Women with Low, Intermediate or High Levels of Fear: Findings from the First Baby Study. *Birth* **2013**, *40*, 289–296. [CrossRef]
36. Haines, H.M.; Rubertsson, C.; Pallant, J.F.; Hildingsson, I. The influence of women's fear, attitudes and beliefs of childbirth on mode and experience of birth. *BMC Pregnancy Childbirth* **2012**, *12*, 55. [CrossRef] [PubMed]
37. Hildingsson, I.; Nilsson, C.; Karlström, A.; Lundgren, I. A Longitudinal Survey of Childbirth-Related Fear and Associated Factors. *J. Obstet. Gynecol. Neonatal Nurs.* **2011**, *40*, 532–543. [CrossRef]
38. Laursen, M.; Hedegaard, M.; Johansen, C.H. Fear of childbirth: Predictors and temporal changes among nulliparous women in the Danish National Birth Cohort. *BJOG Int. J. Obstet. Gynaecol.* **2008**, *115*, 354–360. [CrossRef] [PubMed]
39. Rouhe, H.; Salmela-Aro, K.; Halmesmäki, E.; Saisto, T. Fear of childbirth according to parity, gestational age, and obstetric history. *BJOG Int. J. Obstet. Gynaecol.* **2008**, *116*, 67–73. [CrossRef] [PubMed]

40. Saxbe, D.; Horton, K.T.; Tsai, A.B. The Birth Experiences Questionnaire: A brief measure assessing psychosocial dimensions of childbirth. *J. Fam. Psychol.* **2018**, *32*, 262–268. [CrossRef] [PubMed]
41. Prelog, P.R.; Makovec, M.R.; Šimic, M.V.; Premru-Srsen, T.; Perat, M. Individual and contextual factors of nulliparas' levels of depression, anxiety and fear of childbirth in the last trimester of pregnancy: Intimate partner attachment a key factor? *Slov. J. Public Health* **2019**, *58*, 112–119. [CrossRef] [PubMed]
42. Redshaw, M.; Martin, C.; Rowe, R.; Hockley, C. The Oxford Worries about Labour Scale: Women's experience and measurement characteristics of a measure of maternal concern about labour and birth. *Psychol. Health Med.* **2009**, *14*, 354–366. [CrossRef]
43. Slade, P.; Pais, T.; Fairlie, F.; Simpson, A.; Sheen, K. The development of the Slade–Pais Expectations of Childbirth Scale (SPECS). *J. Reprod. Infant Psychol.* **2016**, *34*, 495–510. [CrossRef]
44. Haines, H.; Pallant, J.F.; Karlström, A.; Hildingsson, I. Cross-cultural comparison of levels of childbirth-related fear in an Australian and Swedish sample. *Midwifery* **2011**, *27*, 560–567. [CrossRef]
45. Geissbuehler, V.; Eberhard, J. Fear of childbirth during pregnancy: A study of more than 8000 pregnant women. *J. Psychosom. Obstet. Gynecol.* **2002**, *23*, 229–235. [CrossRef]
46. Bergström, M.; Rudman, A.; Waldenström, U.; Kieler, H. Fear of childbirth in expectant fathers, subsequent childbirth experience and impact of antenatal education: Subanalysis of results from a randomized controlled trial. *Acta Obstet. Gynecol. Scand.* **2013**, *92*, 967–973. [CrossRef] [PubMed]
47. Fairbrother, N.; Woody, S.R. Fear of childbirth and obstetrical events as predictors of postnatal symptoms of depression and post-traumatic stress disorder. *J. Psychosom. Obstet. Gynecol.* **2007**, *28*, 239–242. [CrossRef] [PubMed]
48. Fenwick, J.; Gamble, J.; Creedy, D.K.; Buist, A.; Turkstra, E.; Sneddon, A.; A Scuffham, P.; Ryding, E.L.; Jarrett, V.; Toohill, J. Study protocol for reducing childbirth fear: A midwife-led psycho-education intervention. *BMC Pregnancy Childbirth* **2013**, *13*, 190. [CrossRef]
49. A Hall, W.; Stoll, K.; Hutton, E.K.; Brown, H. A prospective study of effects of psychological factors and sleep on obstetric interventions, mode of birth, and neonatal outcomes among low-risk British Columbian women. *BMC Pregnancy Childbirth* **2012**, *12*, 78. [CrossRef] [PubMed]
50. Jespersen, C.; Hegaard, H.K.; Schroll, A.-M.; Rosthøj, S.; Kjærgaard, H. Fear of childbirth and emergency caesarean section in low-risk nulliparous women: A prospective cohort study. *J. Psychosom. Obstet. Gynecol.* **2014**, *35*, 109–115. [CrossRef]
51. Ryding, E.; Wijma, B.; Wijma, K.; Rydhström, H. Fear of childbirth during pregnancy may increase the risk of emergency cesarean section. *Acta Obstet. Gynecol. Scand.* **1998**, *77*, 542–547. [CrossRef] [PubMed]
52. Salomonsson, B.; Gullberg, M.T.; Alehagen, S.; Wijma, K. Self-efficacy beliefs and fear of childbirth in nulliparous women. *J. Psychosom. Obstet. Gynecol.* **2013**, *34*, 116–121. [CrossRef]
53. Storksen, H.T.; Eberhard-Gran, M.; Garthus-Niegel, S.; Eskild, A. Fear of childbirth; the relation to anxiety and depression. *Acta Obstet. Gynecol. Scand.* **2011**, *91*, 237–242. [CrossRef]
54. Wiklund, I.; Edman, G.; Ryding, E.-L.; Andolf, E. Expectation and experiences of childbirth in primiparae with caesarean section. *BJOG: Int. J. Obstet. Gynaecol.* **2008**, *115*, 324–331. [CrossRef]
55. Spielberger, C.D. State-Trait Anxiety Inventory. In *The Corsini Encyclopedia of Psychology*; John Wiley & Sons, Ltd.: Hoboken, NJ, USA, 2010. [CrossRef]
56. Garthus-Niegel, S.; Størksen, H.T.; Torgersen, L.; Von Soest, T.; Eberhard-Gran, M. The Wijma Delivery Expectancy/Experience Questionnaire—A factor analytic study. *J. Psychosom. Obstet. Gynecol.* **2011**, *32*, 160–163. [CrossRef]
57. MacCallum, R.C.; Widaman, K.F.; Zhang, S.; Hong, S. Sample size in factor analysis. *Psychol. Methods* **1999**, *4*, 84–99. [CrossRef]
58. Stoll, K.; Fairbrother, N.; Carty, E.; Jordan, N.; Miceli, C.; Vostrcil, Y.; Willihnganz, L. "It's All the Rage These Days": University Students' Attitudes Toward Vaginal and Cesarean Birth. *Birth* **2009**, *36*, 133–140. [CrossRef] [PubMed]
59. Maier, B. Women's worries about childbirth: Making safe choices. *Br. J. Midwifery* **2010**, *18*, 293–299. [CrossRef]
60. Toohill, J.; Fenwick, J.; Gamble, J.; Creedy, D.K. Prevalence of childbirth fear in an Australian sample of pregnant women. *BMC Pregnancy Childbirth* **2014**, *14*, 1–10. [CrossRef] [PubMed]
61. Eberhard-Gran, M.; Eskild, A.; Tambs, K.; Opjordsmoen, S.; Samuelsen, S.O. Review of validation studies of the Edinburgh Postnatal Depression Scale. *Acta Psychiatr. Scand.* **2001**, *104*, 243–249. [CrossRef]
62. Jomeen, J.; Martin, C.R. Confirmation of an occluded anxiety component within the Edinburgh Postnatal Depression Scale (EPDS) during early pregnancy. *J. Reprod. Infant Psychol.* **2005**, *23*, 143–154. [CrossRef]
63. Kleinknecht, R.A.; Thorndike, R.M. The Mutilation Questionnaire as a predictor of blood/injury fear and fainting. *Behav. Res. Ther.* **1990**, *28*, 429–437. [CrossRef]
64. Kleinknecht, R.A.; Morgan, M.P. Treatment of posttraumatic stress disorder with eye movement desensitization. *J. Behav. Ther. Exp. Psychiatry* **1992**, *23*, 43–49. [CrossRef]
65. R Core Team. R: A Language and Environment for Statistical Computing. 2017. Available online: https://www.R-project.org/ (accessed on 3 January 2022).
66. Revelle, W. Psych: Procedures for Personality and Psychological Research. 2016. Available online: https://CRAN.R-project.org/package=psych (accessed on 3 January 2022).
67. Wickham, H. *ggplot2: Elegant Graphics for Data Analysis*; Springer: New York, NY, USA, 2019.
68. Lee, I.A.; Preacher, K.J. Calculation for the Test of the Difference between Two Dependent Correlations with One Variable in Common. 2013. Available online: http://quantpsy.org (accessed on 3 January 2022).

69. Lakens, D. Calculating and reporting effect sizes to facilitate cumulative science: A practical primer for *t*-tests and ANOVAs. *Front. Psychol.* **2013**, *4*, 863. [CrossRef]
70. Sakaluk, J.K.; Short, S.D. A Methodological Review of Exploratory Factor Analysis in Sexuality Research: Used Practices, Best Practices, and Data Analysis Resources. *J. Sex Res.* **2017**, *54*, 398–408. [CrossRef]
71. Fabrigar, L.R.; Wegener, D.T. *Exploratory Factor Analysis*; Oxford University Press: Oxford, UK, 2011.
72. Horn, J.L. A rationale and test for the number of factors in factor analysis. *Psychometrika* **1965**, *30*, 179–185. [CrossRef] [PubMed]
73. Velicer, W.F. Determining the number of components from the matrix of partial correlations. *Psychometrika* **1976**, *41*, 321–327. [CrossRef]
74. Hu, L.-T.; Bentler, P.M. Cutoff criteria for fit indexes in covariance structure analysis: Conventional criteria versus new alternatives. *Struct. Equ. Model. Multidiscip. J.* **1999**, *6*, 1–55. [CrossRef]
75. Foa, E.B.; McLean, C.P.; Zang, Y.; Zhong, J.; Powers, M.B.; Kauffman, B.Y.; Rauch, S.; Porter, K.; Knowles, K. Psychometric properties of the Posttraumatic Diagnostic Scale for DSM–5 (PDS–5). *Psychol. Assess.* **2016**, *28*, 1166–1171. [CrossRef]
76. Mughal, A.Y.; Devadas, J.; Ardman, E.; Levis, B.; Go, V.F.; Gaynes, B.N. A systematic review of validated screening tools for anxiety disorders and PTSD in low to middle income countries. *BMC Psychiatry* **2020**, *20*, 211. [CrossRef] [PubMed]
77. Little, T.D. *Longitudinal Structural Equation Modeling*; Guilford Press: New York, NY, USA, 2013.
78. McNeish, D.; An, J.; Hancock, G.R. The Thorny Relation between Measurement Quality and Fit Index Cutoffs in Latent Variable Models. *J. Pers. Assess.* **2017**, *100*, 43–52. [CrossRef] [PubMed]
79. Rosseel, Y. lavaan: AnRPackage for Structural Equation Modeling. *J. Stat. Softw.* **2012**, *48*, 1–36. [CrossRef]
80. R Core Team. R: A Language and Environment for Statistical Computing 2020. Available online: http://www.r-project.org/index.html (accessed on 3 January 2022).
81. Vandenberg, R.J.; Lance, C.E. A Review and Synthesis of the Measurement Invariance Literature: Suggestions, Practices, and Recommendations for Organizational Research. *Organ. Res. Methods* **2000**, *3*, 4–70. [CrossRef]
82. semTools Contributors. semTools: Useful Tools for Structural Equation Modeling. 2016. Available online: https://rdrr.io/cran/semTools/ (accessed on 3 January 2022).
83. Meehl, P.E. Factors and Taxa, Traits and Types, Differences of Degree and Differences in Kind. *J. Pers.* **1992**, *60*, 117–174. [CrossRef]
84. Ruscio, J.; Haslam, N.; Ruscio, A.M. *Introduction to the Taxometric Method: A Practical Guide*; Routledge: New York, NY, USA, 2013. [CrossRef]
85. Sakaluk, J.K. Expanding Statistical Frontiers in Sexual Science: Taxometric, Invariance, and Equivalence Testing. *J. Sex Res.* **2018**, *56*, 475–510. [CrossRef]
86. Ruscio, J.; Carney, L.M.; Dever, L.; Pliskin, M.; Wang, S.B. Using the comparison curve fix index (CCFI) in taxometric analyses: Averaging curves, standard errors, and CCFI profiles. *Psychol. Assess.* **2018**, *30*, 744–754. [CrossRef] [PubMed]
87. Ruscio, J.; Wang, S. RTaxometrics: Taxometric Analysis. 2017. Available online: https://cran.r-project.org/web/packages/RTaxometrics/index.html (accessed on 3 January 2022).
88. A Structure-Based Approach to Psychological Assessment: Matching Measurement Models to Latent Structure—John Ruscio, Ayelet Meron Ruscio, 2002 n.d. Available online: https://journals.sagepub.com/doi/abs/10.1177/1073191102091002?casa_token=mbRPkjvqoM4AAAAA:T5-lV8oAODSQgqIzZ4KR82T7DHagC6d1RdUXNHt1sSCck7ilcDoUQbXIkHYWK98mYy_GZD51xdLB (accessed on 31 January 2022).
89. Stoll, K.; Hall, W. Attitudes and Preferences of Young Women with Low and High Fear of Childbirth. *Qual. Health Res.* **2013**, *23*, 1495–1505. [CrossRef]
90. Stoll, K.H.; Downe, S.; Edmonds, J.; Gross, M.M.; Malott, A.; Pm, J.M.; Sadler, M.; Thomson, G. The ICAPP Study Team A Survey of University Students' Preferences for Midwifery Care and Community Birth Options in 8 High-Income Countries. *J. Midwifery Women's Health* **2020**, *65*, 131–141. [CrossRef]
91. Christiaens, W.; Van De Velde, S.; Bracke, P. Pregnant Women's Fear of Childbirth in Midwife- and Obstetrician-Led Care in Belgium and the Netherlands: Test of the Medicalization Hypothesis. *Women Health* **2011**, *51*, 220–239. [CrossRef] [PubMed]
92. Gottman, J.M.; Notarius, C.I. Marital Research in the 20th Century and a Research Agenda for the 21st Century. *Fam. Process* **2002**, *41*, 159–197. [CrossRef] [PubMed]
93. Pacey, S. Couples and the first baby: Responding to new parents' sexual and relationship problems. *Sex. Relatsh. Ther.* **2004**, *19*, 223–246. [CrossRef]
94. Hildingsson, I. Swedish couples' attitudes towards birth, childbirth fear and birth preferences and relation to mode of birth—A longitudinal cohort study. *Sex. Reprod. Health* **2014**, *5*, 75–80. [CrossRef]
95. Wootton, B.M.; Davis, E.; Moses, K.; Moody, A.; Maguire, P. The development and initial validation of the Tokophobia Severity Scale. *Clin. Psychol.* **2020**, *24*, 267–275. [CrossRef]

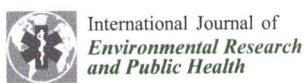

Article

The Childbirth Fear Questionnaire and the Wijma Delivery Expectancy Questionnaire as Screening Tools for Specific Phobia, Fear of Childbirth

Nichole Fairbrother [1,*], Arianne Albert [2], Fanie Collardeau [3] and Cora Keeney [1]

1. Department of Family Practice, University of British Columbia, Vancouver, BC V6T 1Z4, Canada; cora.keeney@ubc.ca
2. Women's Health Research Institute, Vancouver, BC V6H 2N9, Canada; arianne.albert@cw.bc.ca
3. Department of Psychology, University of Victoria, Victoria, BC V8P 5C2, Canada; faniecol@uvic.ca
* Correspondence: nicholef@uvic.ca; Tel.: +1-250-0519-5390 (ext. 36439)

Abstract: Background: Perinatal anxiety and related disorders are common (20%), distressing and impairing. Fear of childbirth (FoB) is a common type of perinatal anxiety associated with negative mental health, obstetrical, childbirth and child outcomes. Screening can facilitate treatment access for those most in need. Objectives: The purpose of this research was to evaluate the accuracy of the Childbirth Fear Questionnaire (CFQ) and the Wijma Delivery Expectations Questionnaire (W-DEQ) of FoB as screening tools for a specific phobia, FoB. Methods: A total of 659 English-speaking pregnant women living in Canada and over the age of 18 were recruited for the study. Participants completed an online survey of demographic, current pregnancy and reproductive history information, as well as the CFQ and the W-DEQ, and a telephone interview to assess specific phobia FoB. Results: Symptoms meeting full and subclinical diagnostic criteria for a specific phobia, FoB, were reported by 3.3% and 7.1% of participants, respectively. The W-DEQ met or exceeded the criteria for a "good enough" screening tool across several analyses, whereas the CFQ only met these criteria in one analysis and came close in three others. Conclusions: The W-DEQ demonstrated high performance as a screening tool for a specific phobia, FoB, with accuracy superior to that of the CFQ. Additional research to ensure the stability of these findings is needed.

Keywords: perinatal mental health; anxiety disorders; perinatal anxiety; fear of childbirth; screening

1. Introduction

Anxiety and anxiety-related conditions are the most prevalent of all psychiatric disorders [1,2]. A third of the adult population will suffer from one or more anxiety or anxiety-related disorder at some time in their life [1]. This is significantly greater than the prevalence of mood disorders (i.e., depressive and bipolar disorders) at 21.4% [1]. Women are also 1.5 times as likely as men to suffer from anxiety or anxiety-related condition [1,2]. A recent meta-analysis indicates that one in five pregnant and postpartum people suffer from one or more anxiety or anxiety-related disorder during pregnancy or postpartum [3]. This is significantly more than perinatal depression, where six to twelve percent of pregnant and postpartum people suffer from an episode of major depression during the perinatal period [4,5].

Anxiety and anxiety-related disorders are associated with substantial indirect costs related to functional impairment (e.g., diminished work capacity, unemployment) [4]. People with these conditions are significantly more impaired with respect to social, emotional and physical functioning compared with non-anxious individuals [6]. Anxiety and its related disorders are associated with high levels of health care service utilization [7–11].

Some level of maternal prenatal anxiety (i.e., dimensional anxiety not necessarily associated with a diagnosis) is a normal aspect of pregnancy for many, if not most, pregnant people and unlikely to negatively impact fetal or obstetric outcomes [12]. Maternal prenatal anxiety has, despite various methodological challenges and limitations [12–15], been associated with a number of adverse pregnancy outcomes such as preterm delivery, miscarriage, preeclampsia and low birth weight [12,16–19], as well as some negative effects on the developing infant, including small differences in brain development and attention, and small effects on infant temperament and emotion-regulation [12–15,20–22]. Prenatal maternal anxiety is also a strong risk factor for postpartum depression, even after controlling for prenatal depression [23–26]. Anxiety and their related disorders, specifically, were also found to be associated with deleterious fetal, infant and maternal outcomes, including pregnancy complications and preterm birth, spontaneous abortions, neonatal morbidity and lower birth weight [27–31]. For example, mothers with postpartum obsessive-compulsive disorder were found to be less confident and sensitive in mother-infant interactions than mothers without obsessive-compulsive disorder [32]. Additionally, maternal postpartum social anxiety disorder was associated with reduced cognitive and language abilities in offspring [33]. Overall, maternal anxiety disorders are predictive of anxiety disorders in offspring [34].

There are a number of domains of anxiety (i.e., content areas) that are a particular focus among perinatal people. These include obsessive compulsive disorder (OCD), in which the focus of the obsessions (a core feature of OCD) is on harm coming to one's infant [35], post-traumatic stress disorder (PTSD) subsequent to traumatic childbirth [36], a fear of needles or other medical procedures (e.g., instrumental or surgical birth) [37], pregnancy-specific anxiety (i.e., high anxiety related to the wellbeing of one's pregnancy [38]) and fear of childbirth (FoB) [39]. FoB is the focus of the current study.

FoB is common among people with childbearing potential (i.e., people who are pregnant, may become pregnant or who have already given birth). In the most comprehensive systematic review and meta-analyses of FoB in pregnant women conducted to date, the worldwide pooled prevalence of FoB was estimated at 14% (95% CI 0.12–0.16) [40]. The study was based on data from 29 primary studies and included a total of 853,988 pregnant women. Prevalence estimates from individual studies varied significantly from 3.7 to 43%. Of concern is that there was a high level of between-study heterogeneity, not explained via sensitivity and subgroup analyses. Unexplained variability in prevalence estimates may be a result of the significant methodological variability across studies (e.g., variability in cut-scores and measurement tools). Historically, FoB was not conceptualized as a diagnosable mental health condition but rather a form of dimensional psychological distress characterized by fear and anxiety and assessed via a self-report inventory [40]. When mental health difficulties are assessed using self-report questionnaires, prevalence estimates tend to be much higher than when formal diagnostic criteria are employed [41–43]. For example, all of the studies included in this meta-analysis of prevalence employed self-report questionnaires and not diagnostic interviews. The one study in which diagnostic criteria were clearly employed also, as expected, reported a much lower prevalence of FoB (3.7%) compared with the meta-analysis as a whole [39].

FoB can be highly distressing and associated with various psychosocial, mental health, obstetrical, childbirth and child-related outcomes [44–47]. For some, FoB is so intense as to lead to delaying or avoiding pregnancy and pregnancy termination, even among those who wish to bear children [48–50]. Obstetrical and birth complications include increased requests for epidural anesthesia during labor [49,50], longer labors [51–53] and a higher likelihood of emergency and planned cesarean section (CS) [52,54–59]. For example, fear of vaginal birth is consistently associated with a preference for cesarean birth, and severe fear of vaginal birth has been associated with a greater likelihood of a cesarean birth without medical indications [52,60–62].

There is also a higher likelihood of negative birth experiences among women with a fear of childbirth [63,64], especially if the woman delivers by emergency CS or instrumental vaginal delivery [51,65]. There is also an association between FoB and mental health difficulties, including postnatal depression, specific phobia and PTSD [66–69]. In particular, there is a strong association between previous negative birth experiences and/or traumatic births and FoB [69]. History of prior operative or instrumental delivery was also associated with higher levels of FoB [57,58,70], with the odds of FoB increasing with the number of obstetric complications experienced during a previous pregnancy [65]. Women with a previous negative birth experience are five times more likely to experience FoB in a subsequent pregnancy [65]. Although most studies have found a positive relationship between parity and FoB, with higher levels of childbirth fear reported by nulliparous compared with multiparous women [45,47,50,58,70–73], there is some evidence that the most severe levels of FoB are experienced by multiparous women [39]. A range of socio-demographic variables are associated with higher levels of childbirth fear including lower educational attainment, younger age [74,75], low social support [61,76], dissatisfaction with partner or support received from partner [60,74], mental health variables such as higher anxiety and stress [54,57,60,72,74,76], history of depression and depression during pregnancy [61,74,77,78], low confidence in one's ability to cope with labour and birth [61,74,77,78] and history of abuse [45,76,79]. Higher levels of fatigue during pregnancy [80] and lower self-rated health [81] were also associated with higher levels of FoB.

The lack of a clear diagnostic classification for FoB is problematic because, in the absence of diagnostic criteria, it may be difficult to determine which questionnaire-based cut-scores may best represent clinically meaningful fear meriting treatment. Specifically, to merit the diagnosis of an anxiety disorder, symptoms must be clinically distressing or functionally impairing [82]. Although not yet fully established, a specific phobia may be the most appropriate diagnostic category for FoB, in particular for nulliparous people [54,83–85]. A specific phobia is a fear and avoidance of circumscribed objects and situations (e.g., insects, animals, heights, blood, injections). Given that FoB is a circumscribed fear with symptoms and features closely resembling those of other specific phobias, it was proposed as perhaps the most appropriate diagnostic classification for FoB [54,83–85]. Further, tokophobia (severe FoB) is classified in the *International Classification of Diseases-11* as a phobic anxiety disorder [86]. Although other candidate disorders include PTSD (among multiparous people), health anxiety disorder, social anxiety disorder and generalized anxiety disorder, at present, the extant evidence suggests that specific phobia is a very reasonable place to start. In the only study to evaluate this systematically (N = 106), 8.5% of study participants (a general sample of nulliparous pregnant women in Sweden) were found to meet the Diagnostic and Statistical Manual of Mental Disorders, fifth edition (DSM-5) diagnostic criteria for specific phobia FoB [83]. Although small (N = 106), this is also the only study published to date to assess any self-report measure of FoB as a potential screening tool for diagnosable FoB [83]. In this study, a Wijma Delivery Expectancy Questionnaire (W-DEQ) score of ≥ 85 was found to be the optimal cut-off score for identifying FoB, with excellent sensitivity (100%), specificity (93.8%) and agreement between the W-DEQ A and the SCID-5 (specific phobia; Cohen's Kappa coefficient, $\kappa = 0.720$). Determining appropriate cut-scores for self-report measures of FoB can be aided via studies in which diagnostic interviews for a specific phobia, FoB, were also employed, and screening metrics evaluated. In the absence of this, it is difficult to determine if cut-scores based on other approaches (e.g., the top 25% of scores) actually represent clinically meaningful distress and/or impairment in functioning. Given the above, we opted, in this study, to focus our attention on FoB diagnosable as a form of specific phobia.

Our study team recently developed a new measure of FoB: The Childbirth Fear Questionnaire (CFQ) [87]. The CFQ was designed to overcome the limitations of existing measures and as a screening tool for FoB. Existing measure frequently omit important domains of FoB [56,70,75,88–95], include non-fear related items [88,90,92,94–97], are too brief to encompass the full FoB experience (e.g., 1–2 items only) [56,70,75,91], or include too few items per subscale to achieve stability [92,98]. We developed the CFQ to cover the full range of domains of FoB with a view to enabling the identification of specific fear domains to be targeted in treatment. We also sought to develop a measure that would function well as a screening tool for diagnosable FoB. Screening represents a critical step in the pathway to treatment [99]. Although diagnostic assessments by trained professionals are the gold standard for providing mental health diagnoses, they are both expensive and time-consuming. Consequently, more rapid and cost-effective screening is essential for identifying those suffering from clinically meaningful FoB. Without screening, those suffering may fail to be identified and, as a result, fail to receive evidence-based care [100]. The CFQ was evaluated in two separate samples, with both an exploratory and a confirmatory factor analysis. The psychometric properties of the CFQ are strong, and two manuscripts pertaining to this measure were published, with a third currently under review [71,87,101].

The primary objective of this research was to evaluate the screening accuracy of the CFQ for subclinical and full criteria specific phobia, FoB. A secondary objective was to compare the screening accuracy of the CFQ to the screening accuracy of the W-DEQ. Given known differences in FoB between nulliparous and multiparous people [39,71,72], we also elected to report the screening accuracy of the CFQ and the W-DEQ separately for nulliparous and multiparous participants. As a further distinction, we also reported the accuracy of the CFQ and the W-DEQ separately for those primarily fearful of vaginal birth and those primarily fearful of cesarean birth. We hypothesized measures of FoB might perform differently for people whose primary fears relate to vaginal delivery compared to those whose primary fears relate to medical and surgical interventions (i.e., cesarean birth) [101]. We chose the W-DEQ as the comparator measure because: (a) the W-DEQ is the most commonly used measure to assess FoB and has broad international acceptance [46]; (b) the W-DEQ is the only measure of FoB to be evaluated as a screening tool for a specific phobia, FoB [46]; and (c) the CFQ was developed with a view of overcoming some of the limitations of the W-DEQ (i.e., the inclusion of non-fear-related items, and a failure to assess all of the relevant FoB content domains) [87]. In contrast with the W-DEQ, the CFQ assesses a broader range of FoB content areas, includes only fear-related items, and includes a measure of interference, making it more similar to a diagnostic measure (i.e., mental health diagnoses require either distress or interference in order for a diagnosis to be given).

2. Materials and Methods

This paper reports on a secondary analysis of a larger dataset, for which detailed methods were published [87].

2.1. Ethics

This research received ethical approval from the Behavioral Research Ethics Board of the University of British Columbia. All participants provided informed, written consent prior to participation.

2.2. Participants

All English-speaking, pregnant individuals over the age of 18 and residing in Canada were eligible to take part in this study. In total, 881 participants took part in the online questionnaire between 11- and 46-weeks' gestation (an average of 35 weeks). Primary data collection took place between August 2016 and November 2019.

2.3. Procedures

Perinatal people were directed to the online survey via the study advertisement posted on online forums and social media pages frequented by pregnant women (e.g., pregnancy-related Facebook groups and websites). Participants who completed the survey were entered into a draw with the chance to win one of seven CAD 150 prizes.

2.4. Measures

Demographic (e.g., age, education, marital status, income, race/ethnicity and country of residence), pregnancy (e.g., number of fetuses and method of conception) and reproductive history (e.g., the number of prior pregnancies, births, miscarriages and vaginal and cesarian deliveries) was collected via self-report. Participants were also asked about their delivery preferences using a single question. Scoring for this item was based on a 7-point Likert-type scale ranging from "I have a very strong desire for a vaginal birth" (0) to "I have a very strong desire for a cesarian birth" (6). The center of the scale (3) was "I have no preference either way".

The Childbirth Fear Questionnaire (CFQ) [87] is a recently developed, 40-item, self-report measure used to assess fear of childbirth. The 40 items are scored on a Likert-type scale ranging from 0 (no fear) to 4 (extreme fear), and measuring nine, frequently reported dimensions of FoB. The 40-item CFQ fear dimensions include (1) fear of loss of sexual pleasure or attractiveness (SEX), (2) fear of pain from a vaginal birth (PAIN), (3) fear of medical intervention (INT), (4) fear of embarrassment (SHY), (5) fear of harm to the baby (HARM), (6) fear of cesarean birth (CS), (7) fear of mom or baby dying (DEATH), (8) fear of insufficient pain medication (MEDS), (9) fear of body damage from a vaginal birth (DAMAGE). The dimensions are scored by taking the average of the item scores within that dimension (range = 0–4). The CFQ also includes an additional 8-item Interference scale with items covering multiple life domains. For the Interference scale, participants are asked to rate, from 0 (no interference) to 4 (extreme interference), how much their FoB interfered with various aspects of their life. Each of the eight items asked about interference with a different life domain (i.e., interference with one's relationships with one's partner/spouse, family members, prenatal caregivers and others, as well as interference with one's work life, leisure activities and preparation for the new baby). The CFQ total score includes only the 40 fear items and is scored as the mean of the subscale scores (range = 0–4). The Interference scale is scored separately. Consequently, the CFQ produces a fear score and an interference score. Initial validation of the CFQ produced a Cronbach's alpha reliability coefficient of 0.94 for the overall scale and a range between 0.76 and 0.94 for the individual subscales [71]. The CFQ demonstrated good convergent and discriminant validity when comparing the associations between the CFQ with other measures of FoB. Evidence suggests that the CFQ is accurate in detecting group differences between pregnant people in relation to delivery mode preference and parity.

The Wijma Delivery Expectancy Questionnaire (W-DEQ-A) [90]. The W-DEQ-A is a 33-item questionnaire. Items are scored on a 0–5 Likert type scale ranging from 0 (extremely) to 5 (not at all). The minimum and maximum scores of the questionnaires are 0 and 165, with higher scores reflecting higher levels of fear. The psychometric properties of the W-DEQ-A are well established [94,102]. The internal consistency reliability in the present sample was 0.92. In addition to the W-DEQ-A total score, there are data to support the administration of a 6-item fear scale, which were found to be highly correlated with the full scale and several other important outcomes [103].

The Diagnostic Assessment Research Tool (DART v1.03.16) [104]. The DART (v1.03.16) is a modular, semi-structured interview designed for the assessment of DSM-5 diagnoses. Although the DART remains early in its development, psychometric evidence to date strongly supports the interrater reliability and construct (convergent and discriminant) validity of the measure as a diagnostic interview for DSM-5 disorders [105]. We used the specific phobia section of the DART to assess specific phobia, fear of childbirth, in this study. Minor wording modifications were made to orient the interview exclusively to fear of childbirth. Interviewers were research assistants, graduate students in clinical psychology and the principal investigator, and were trained and supervised by the principal investigator. Participants' responses were classified as indicating full criteria diagnosis, a subclinical diagnosis, or no diagnosis of specific phobia, FoB. Subclinical diagnoses are those in which all disorder criteria are endorsed other than the distress/impairment criteria (i.e., the symptoms do not cause clinically significant distress or life impairment). In the context of specific phobia, FoB, this implies that those who reported symptoms meeting the criteria for a subclinical specific phobia reported high levels of consistent and persistent fear of childbirth, but these symptoms failed to cause clinically significant distress or impairment in functioning. Because FoB appears to exist on a continuum from mild (i.e., most pregnant people experience some, at least low levels, of FoB) to severe (for some, it may be debilitating), it may be important to identify and offer services to pregnant people with subclinical levels of specific phobia, FoB, as well as those who report symptoms meeting full diagnostic criteria.

2.5. Data Analysis Strategy

All analyses were carried out in R v.4.1.1 [106] and SPSS v.24 [107].

The precision of estimates of a diagnostic accuracy study depends on the prevalence of the condition in the sample [108]. The lower the prevalence, the larger the number of participants with cases needed to precisely estimate metrics such as sensitivity and specificity, as lower prevalence results in estimated metrics that can be unreliable and imprecise [109]. For these reasons, we conducted an assessment of screening accuracy for both subclinical and full criteria diagnoses of specific phobia, FoB. Specifically, we began by comparing cases with a diagnosis meeting the full criteria for a specific phobia, FoB, to the remainder of the sample. However, due to small numbers of cases meeting full criteria, we also compared cases of full and subclinical criteria to the remainder of the sample.

Given the data indicating that childbirth fears may differ among nulliparous and multiparous people [72], we felt it was important to provide information about screening accuracy for each group separately. We have also provided screening accuracy data for the CFQ (total scores) with and without the Interference subscale included. We sought to investigate whether the interference subscale would improve screening accuracy. Screening accuracy was determined by using cutpoints of the scales to identify participants likely to have a specific phobia, FoB, compared to the results of the Diagnostic Assessment Research Tool for each participant.

To determine optimal cutpoints, we used the "cutpointr" [110] package in R. Cutpoints were estimated by maximizing the Youden's J index using 1000 bootstrap replicates. The returned optimal cutpoint and its associated area under the curve (AUC), sensitivity, specificity, Youden's J index, negative predictive value (NPV) and positive likelihood ratio (LR+) were the means of these metrics across all 1000 replicates. This whole process was bootstrapped 100 times to validate the out-of-sample performance. These "out of bag" or oob estimates are reported in the Results. To evaluate if specific combinations of items might be better predictors, we also used logistic regressions of each outcome (subclinical and full criteria diagnoses of specific phobia, FoB, and for those primarily fearful of vaginal birth and those primarily fearful of a cesarean birth) against all of the CFQ subscales. Non-significant subscales ($p < 0.1$) were removed from the models, and model predictions in the form of probabilities between 0 and 1 were calculated for each participant. These predicted probabilities were then subjected to the same cutpoint analysis as the subscales described above. Predicted probabilities of FoB can be calculated from the estimated log-odds (β) using the formula below.

$$P(\text{FoB}) = \frac{1}{1 + e^{-(\beta_0 + \beta_1 x_1 + \ldots)}}$$

For all assessments of screening accuracy, we also sought to evaluate the screening accuracy of the CFQ and the W-DEQ against the criteria for a "good enough" screening tool proposed by Fairbrother and colleagues [111]. They propose that, in order for a screening tool to be deemed sufficiently accurate for use in clinical settings, it should meet certain minimum standards of accuracy, including an AUC of 0.8 or greater, a Youden's J index of 0.5 or more (J = 0.05 when sensitivity and specificity both equal 0.75), a NPV of 0.8 or greater, and a LR+ of 4.0 or more. An LR+ of 4.0 means that with a positive test result, one is 25% more likely to have the condition in question compared with the baseline probability of having the condition [112]. Any recommendations regarding the accuracy and clinical utility of the CFQ and the W-DEQ is based on how well they perform in relation to these criteria.

3. Results

3.1. Participants

A total of 659 pregnant people participated in Subclinical and full criteria diagnoses of specific phobia in this study. Participants ranged in age from 21 to 49 (M = 32.9, SD = 4.10). Of these, 270 (48%) were nulliparous at the time of participation, and 296 (52%) were multiparous. Information pertaining to participant demographics, current pregnancy and reproductive history is provided in Table 1. Means and standard deviations for the CFQ and the W-DEQ are reported in Table 2.

Table 1. Participant demographic information and reproductive information (N = 659).

Demographic Variables	Percentage	n
Married or cohabitating	93.3%	613
Cis-gender female	99.1%	652
Some postsecondary education	94.4%	623
European heritage	76.3%	502
English spoken at home	95.4%	629
Current Pregnancy		
Singleton pregnancy	97.7%	642
Weeks pregnant: M (SD)	34.6 (2.1)	497
Pregnancy complications	30.8%	202
Reproductive History		
Prior births	52.3%	296
Prior vaginal birth	51.2%	198
Prior cesarean birth	17.7%	66
Prior pregnancy loss < 20 weeks	40.6%	157
Prior pregnancy loss > 20 weeks	1.3%	5

Table 2. Means (M) and standard deviations (SD) for the Childrbith Fear Questionnaire (CFQ; total and subscales) and the Wijma Delivery Expectations Questionnaire (W-DEQ).

	Full Sample M (SD)	Nullips Only M (SD)	Multips Only M (SD)
CFQ Total	1.11 (0.59)	1.23 (0.61)	1.02 (0.56)
CFQ Interference	0.42 (0.47)	0.44 (0.47)	0.39 (0.45)
W-DEQ	55.44 (23.76)	59.07 (22.77)	52.8 (24.09)

Note: CFQ Total and CFQ Interference scores are mean items scores (i.e., out of a possible 0–4). W-DEQ scores are for the total out of 33 items.

3.2. Prevalence of Specific Phobia, Fear of Childbirth

Twenty-two (3.3%) participants reported symptoms meeting full diagnostic criteria for a specific phobia, fear of childbirth, and 47 (7.1%) reported symptoms meeting subclinical criteria for a specific phobia, fear of childbirth. When segregated by parity, fewer (1.9%) nulliparous participants met the full criteria for specific phobia compared with multiparous participants (5.1%). However, similar proportions of nulliparous and multiparous participants met subclinical criteria for a specific phobia, fear of childbirth (6.3 and 6.8%, respectively).

3.3. ROC Curves and Diagnostic Accuracy

We present the initial screening metrics for the CFQ and the W-DEQ in Tables 3–5, with corresponding ROC curves presented in Figures 1–3 in the manuscript with supplementary ROC curves presented in the Supplementary Material in Figures S1–S9 (see Supplementary Material).

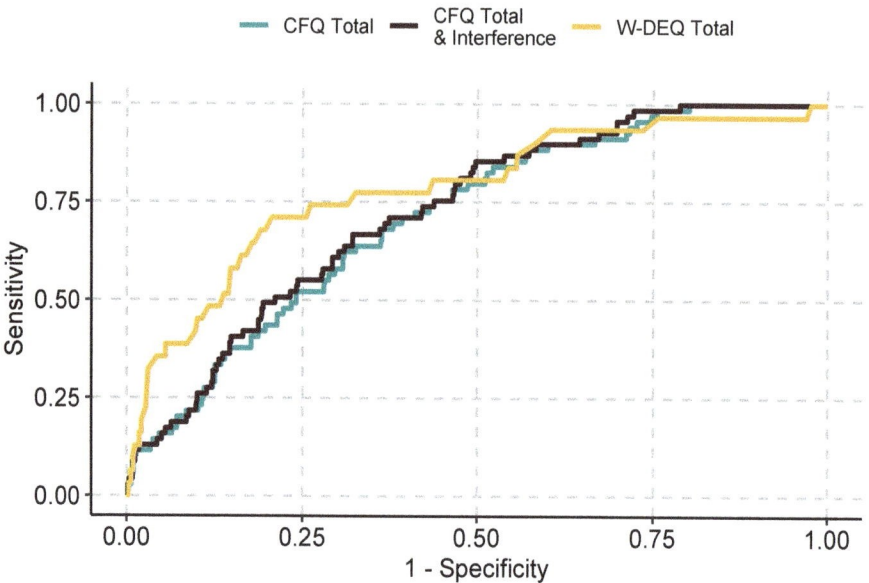

Figure 1. Receiver operating characteristic (ROC) curves for the Childbirth Fear Questionnaire (CFQ) and the Wijma Delivery Expectations Questionnaire (W-DEQ) for the full sample (full diagnostic criteria ONLY).

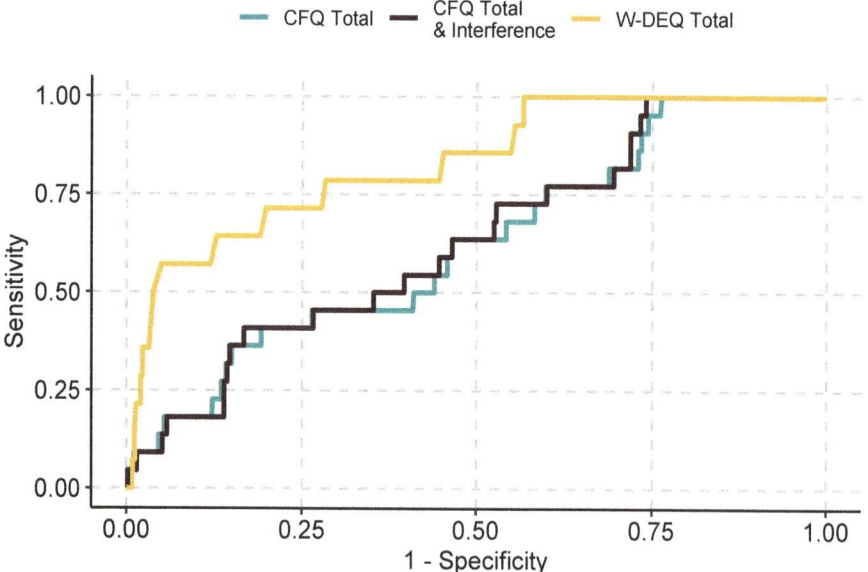

Figure 2. ROC curves for the CFQ and the W-DEQ for the full sample (subclinical and full diagnostic criteria combined).

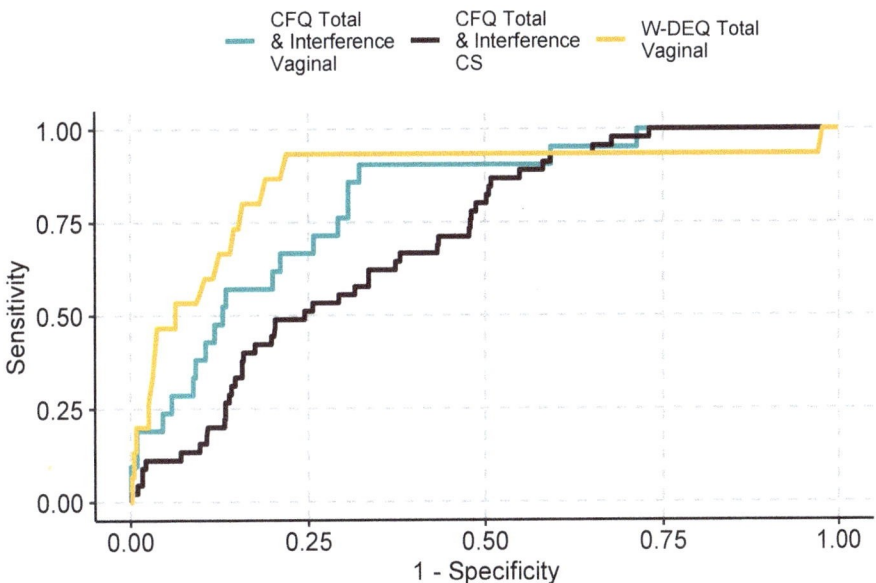

Figure 3. ROC curves for the CFQ (Total and Interference subscale scores) and the W-DEQ (subclinical and full diagnostic criteria combined).

In Table 3, screening metrics are provided for the CFQ (both with and without the Interference Subscale) and the W-DEQ for a specific phobia, FoB, full criteria across parity groups. In Table 4, we present the same findings, but for a specific phobia, FoB, full criteria and subclinical were combined. In Table 5, we present the screening metrics for the CFQ (including the Interference Subscale) and the W-DEQ across parity groups, separately for those primarily fearful of vaginal birth and those primarily fearful of cesarean birth. For this table, there were not enough cases to present the screening accuracy of the W-DEQ for fear of cesarean birth. Consequently, only the W-DEQ screening accuracy for fear of vaginal birth was provided. Given the smaller samples available for this final analysis, screening metrics are provided for subclinical and full diagnostic criteria cases combined.

Table 3. Receiver operating characteristic (ROC) results for the Childbirth Fear Questionnaire (CFQ) and the Wijma Delivery Expectations Questionnaire (W-DEQ) across parity (full diagnostic criteria ONLY).

		Prevalence	AUC	J	Cutpoint	Sensitivity	Specificity	NPV	LR+
CFQ Total Scores	Full sample	3.3%	0.63	0.11	1.17	0.56	0.55	0.97	1.24
	Nulliparous only	1.9%	0.45	0.45	1.34	0.60	0.45	0.98	1.09
	Multiparous only	5.0%	0.67	0.17	1.05	0.60	0.57	0.96	1.40
CFQ Total & Interference Subscale Scores	Full sample	3.3%	0.62	0.10	1.13	0.53	0.57	0.97	1.23
	Nulliparous only	1.9%	0.56	0.23	0.69	1.00	0.23	1.0	1.30
	Multiparous only	5.0%	0.69	0.35	1.63	0.47	0.89	0.97	4.27
W-DEQ	Full sample	3.9%	0.82	0.43	78.87	0.62	0.81	0.98	3.26
	Nulliparous only	*2.5%*	*0.88*	*0.69*	*95.37*	*0.75*	*0.94*	*0.99*	*12.50*
	Multiparous only	*5.9%*	*0.83*	*0.53*	*76.56*	*0.70*	*0.83*	*0.98*	*4.12*

Note: Cut scores for the CFQ are mean items scores (i.e., out of a possible 0–4). W-DEQ cut scores are for the total out of 33 items; AUC = Area under the curve; J = Youden's J Index; NPV = Negative predictive value; LR+ = Positive likelihood ratio.

Table 4. ROC Results for the Childbrith Fear Questionnaire (CFQ) and the Wijma Delivery Expectations Questionnaire (W-DEQ) across parity (subclinical and full diagnostic criteria combined).

		Prevalence	AUC	J	Cutpoint	Sensitivity	Specificity	NPV	LR+
CFQ Total Scores	Full sample	10.0%	0.72	0.29	1.18	0.29	0.69	0.90	0.94
	Nulliparous only	8.0%	0.75	0.30	1.46	0.66	0.64	0.96	1.83
	Multiparous only	12.0%	0.71	0.26	1.13	0.63	0.63	0.93	1.70
CFQ Total & Interference Subscale Scores	Full sample	10.0%	0.73	0.30	1.13	0.69	0.61	0.95	1.77
	Nulliparous only	8.0%	0.77	0.37	1.38	0.71	0.66	0.96	2.09
	Multiparous only	12.0%	0.73	0.30	1.05	0.67	0.63	0.93	1.81
W-DEQ Total Scores	Full sample	9.0%	0.79	0.47	73.59	0.68	0.79	0.96	3.24
	Nulliparous only	7.0%	0.68	0.26	81.51	0.44	0.82	0.95	2.44
	Multiparous only	*11.0%*	*0.88*	*0.53*	*70.62*	*0.74*	*0.79*	*0.96*	*3.52*

Note: Cut scores for the CFQ are mean items scores (i.e., out of a possible 0–4). W-DEQ cut scores are for the total out of 33 items; AUC = Area under the curve; J = Youden's J Index; NPV = Negative predictive value; LR+ = Positive likelihood ratio.

Table 5. ROC Results for the Childbrith Fear Questionnaire (CFQ; Total and Interference subscale scores) and the Wijma Delivery Expectations Questionnaire (W-DEQ), separately for fear of vaginal and fear of cesarean birth (subclinical and full diagnostic criteria combined).

CFQ Total & Interference Subscale Scores									
		Prevalence	AUC	J	Cutpoint	Sensitivity	Specificity	NPV	LR+
Fear of Vaginal Birth	Full sample	3.2%	0.81	0.43	1.38	0.71	0.72	0.99	2.54
	Nulliparous only	*1.5%*	*0.88*	*0.67*	*1.42*	*1.00*	*0.67*	*1.00*	*3.03*
	Multiparous only	4.1%	0.80	0.44	1.38	0.67	0.77	0.98	2.91
Fear of cesarean birth	Full sample	6.9%	0.71	0.27	1.04	0.73	0.54	0.96	1.59
	Nulliparous only	4.9%	0.78	0.49	1.51	0.77	0.72	0.98	2.75
	Multiparous only	8.6%	0.73	0.39	0.94	0.84	0.55	0.97	1.87
W-DEQ									
		Prevalence	AUC	J	Cutpoint	Sensitivity	Specificity	NPV	LR+
Fear of Vaginal Birth	Full sample	4.2%	0.86	0.56	78.87	0.74	0.83	0.99	4.35
	Nulliparous only	2.5%	0.73	0.70	96.36	0.75	0.95	0.99	15.0
	Multiparous only	*5.3%*	*0.92*	*0.70*	*75.24*	*0.89*	*0.81*	*0.99*	*4.68*

AUC = Area under the curve; J = Youden's J Index; NPV = Negative predictive value; LR+ = Positive likelihood ratio.

In these preliminary ROC analyses, the W-DEQ evidenced the highest level of screening accuracy, meeting or exceeding the criteria for a "good enough" screening tool across several analyses. Specifically, when comparing those reporting symptoms meeting full diagnostic criteria for a specific phobia, FoB compared to the remainder of the sample, the W-DEQ met or exceeded the "good enough" criteria for both nulliparous and multiparous participants and came close to meeting these criteria for the full sample. When comparing those who reported symptoms meeting full or subclinical diagnoses with the remainder of the sample, the W-DEQ exceeded the criteria for a "good enough" screening tool for multiparous participants (in general and among those primarily fearful of a vaginal birth), as well as for all participants primarily fearful for a vaginal birth.

The CFQ only met or exceeded the criteria for a "good enough" screening tool for nulliparous participants primarily fearful of vaginal birth. When comparing those reporting symptoms meeting full or subclinical diagnoses with the remainder of the sample, the CFQ came close to meeting the criteria for a "good enough" screening tool for nulliparous participants in general, for nulliparous participants primarily fearful of cesarean birth, and for those primarily fearful of a vaginal birth (full sample).

However, cutpoints from the predicted probabilities of the logistic regressions performed much better for the sample as a whole and across nulliparous and multiparous participants separately. Specifically, among nulliparous participants, the INT, CS and Interference subscale emerged as significant predictors, resulting in screening metrics that exceeded the criteria for a "good enough screening tool". The logistic regression predicting fear of vaginal birth (nulliparous participants only) included too few positive cases (n = 4) to accurately estimate logistic regression parameters. Fear of cesarean birth was predicted by the INT and CS subscales, with screening metrics again exceeding those required for a "good enough" measure. Among multiparous participants, diagnostic status was predicted by the CFQ SEX, PAIN and the Interference subscales. In this analysis, findings fell very slightly below those of a "good enough" measure (i.e., AUC = 0.84; Youden's J Index = 0.42). Among multiparous participants with predominantly a fear of vaginal birth, SEX, PAIN, HARM, CS, DEATH and the Interference scale significantly predicted diagnostic status. In this case, the screening metrics exceeded the requirements of a "good enough" screening tool. In the case of participants primarily fearful of cesarean birth, only SEX and the Interference subscale significantly predicted diagnostic status. Screening metrics fell slightly below that required for a "good enough" screening tool (i.e., AUC = 0.79; Youden's index = 0.41). Findings from these analyses are presented in Tables 6 and 7 and Figure 3.

Table 6. Results of logistic regressions on Chidbirth Fear Questionnaire (CFQ) subscales for nulliparous participants.

Predictors	SP Diagnostic Status Dichotomized (FULL&SUB versus NOT)–Reduced Model			Fear of CS Birth Dichotomized (FULL&SUB versus NOT)–Reduced Model		
	Log-Odds	CI	p	Log-Odds	CI	p
(Intercept)	−6.23	−8.18−−4.69	<0.001	−8.96	−13.09−−6.18	<0.001
INT	1.31	0.48–2.22	0.003	1.31	0.32–2.43	0.01
CS	0.62	0.09–1.19	0.03	1.57	0.68–2.71	0.002
INTERFERENCE	1.01	0.08–1.97	0.03			
Observations	267			267		
R^2 Tjur	0.25			0.27		
AUC	0.87			0.94		
Optimal cutpoint	0.10	Cases correctly classified:		0.12	Cases correctly classified:	
Youden's index	0.51	• 16/22 positive cases		0.65	• 11/13 positive cases	
Sensitivity	0.69	• 206/245 negative cases		0.80	• 214/254 negative cases	
Specificity	0.82			0.85		

Note: Formulas for predicted probability for individual (i): $P(FoB_i) = \frac{1}{1+e^{-i}}$, $P(FoCB_i) = \frac{1}{1+e^{-i}}$; Full = Full clinical diagnostic criteria; SUB = Subclinical diagnostic criteria; SP = Specific phobia; CI = Confidence interval; AUC = Area under the curve; FoB = Fear of childbrith; FoCB = Fear of cesarean birth; INT = Fear of medical intervention; CS = Fear of ceserean section.

Table 7. Results of logistic regressions on CFQ subscales for multiparous participants.

Predictors	SP Diagnostic Status Dichotomized (FULL&SUB versus NOT)–Reduced Model			Fear of Vaginal Birth Dichotomized (FULL&SUB versus NOT)–Reduced Model			Fear of Cesarean Birth Dichotomized (FULL&SUB versus NOT)–Reduced Model		
	Log-Odds	CI	p	Log-Odds	CI	p	Log-Odds	CI	p
(Intercept)	−3.83	−4.86−−2.96	<0.001	−5.89	−8.38−−4.02	<0.001	−3.25	−4.07−−2.54	<0.001
SEX	−1.1	−1.96−−0.36	0.007				−0.72	−1.59−0.01	0.074
PAIN	0.76	0.33–1.21	0.001	1.03	0.39–1.75	0.003			
HARM				1.29	0.08–2.61	0.044			
CS				−0.79	−1.65−−0.05	0.049			
DEATH				−1.02	−2.18−−0.01	0.063			
INTERFERENCE	2.48	1.66–3.39	<0.001	2.43	1.09–4.00	0.001	2.31	1.48–3.21	<0.001
Observations	291			291			291		
R^2 Tjur	0.24			0.239			0.16		

Table 7. Cont.

Predictors	SP Diagnostic Status Dichotomized (FULL&SUB versus NOT)–Reduced Model			Fear of Vaginal Birth Dichotomized (FULL&SUB versus NOT)–Reduced Model			Fear of Cesarean Birth Dichotomized (FULL&SUB versus NOT)–Reduced Model		
	Log-Odds	CI	p	Log-Odds	CI	p	Log-Odds	CI	p
AUC	0.84	Cases correctly classified: • 21/34 positive cases • 215/257 negative cases		0.92	Cases correctly classified: • 9/12 positive cases • 249/279 negative cases		0.79	Cases correctly classified: • 17/25 positive cases • 214/266 negative cases	
Optimal cutpoint	0.15			0.07			0.10		
Youden's index	0.42			0.67			0.41		
Sensitivity	0.62			0.77			0.61		
Specificity	0.82			0.90			0.80		

Formula for predicted probability for individual (i): $P(FoB_i) = \frac{1}{1+e^{-(-3.83-1.1 \cdot SEX_i + 0.76 \cdot PAIN_i + 2.48 \cdot Interference_i)}}$, $P(FoVB_i) = \frac{1}{1+e^{-(-5.89+1.03 \cdot PAIN_i + 1.29 \cdot HARM_i - 0.79 \cdot CS_i - 1.02 \cdot DEATH_i + 2.43 \cdot Interference_i)}}$, $P(FoCB_i) = \frac{1}{1+e^{-(-3.25-0.72 \cdot SEX_i + 2.31 \cdot Interference_i)}}$; Full = Full clinical diagnostic criteria; SUB = Subclinical diagnostic criteria; SP = Specific phobia; CI = Confidence interval; AUC = Area under the curve; FoB = Fear of childbirth; FoVB = Fear of vaginal birth; FoCB = Fear of ceserean birth; INT = Fear of medical intervention; SEX = fear of loss of sexual pleasure or attractiveness; PAIN = fear of pain from a vaginal birth; HARM = fear of harm to the baby; CS = Fear of cesarean section; DEATH = fear of mom or baby dying.

4. Discussion

4.1. FoB: General Comments

The current study contributes to our general understanding of FoB. First, while similar proportions of nulliparous and multiparous participants met subclinical criteria for a specific phobia, a higher proportion of multiparous participants (5.1%) met full criteria for specific phobia compared to nulliparous participants (1.9%). Thus, a greater proportion of multiparous birthing people reported more distress and impairment related to their FoB symptoms than nulliparous birthing people. Previous research suggests that, overall, nulliparous women may experience higher levels of FoB than multiparous women but that the most severe levels of FoB are experienced by multiparous women [39,47,50,71,72,113]. Furthermore, a history of prior birth experiences, and specifically negative birth experiences, may increase the likelihood of women experiencing more severe FoB in a subsequent pregnancy [39,57,69,70].

Additionally, our study points to important differences between the fear domains most relevant to multiparous and nulliparous birthing individuals. Specifically, for nulliparous participants, fear of cesarean birth and other medical interventions predominated. For multiparous participants, however, a fear of harm to one infant and fear of pain during a vaginal birth emerged. It is likely that the specific fears experienced by multiparous birthing people stem from their previous childbirth experiences. Thus, psychoeducation and interventions given to birthing people suffering from distressing and/or impairing levels of FoB need to take parity into account. Additional research is necessary to further understand how multiparous birthing people's FoB may be based on realistic fears and experiences (e.g., a knowledge that they are more sensitive to pain or traumatic vaginal birth experiences).

4.2. Screening for FoB

In the current study, strong support was found for both the CFQ and the W-DEQ as screening tools for a specific phobia, FoB. Specifically, the CFQ (once specific subscales were identified via logistic regression) and the W-DEQ either met or exceeded the criteria for a "good enough" screening tool across multiple comparisons. These findings provide encouraging support for the CFQ and the W-DEQ as screening tools for diagnosable FoB.

In the first set of analyses of the full measure, the CFQ performed less well than the W-DEQ. However, once the CFQ subscales were selected, using logistic regression, findings strongly supported the use of the CFQ as a screening tool to identify birthing people with subclinical and clinical levels of FoB. Specifically, the findings from individual logistic regression analyses showed the CFQ to perform very well as a screening tool for a specific phobia, FoB. The findings from ROC analyses based on logistic regression showed that the CFQ either fell only slightly short or met or exceeded the criteria for a "good enough" screening tool in all cases. The one exception was for nulliparous participants who were predominantly fearful of vaginal birth. In this case, there were too few positive cases ($n = 4$) for the regression to produce meaningful findings. The full CFQ also met the criteria for a "good enough" screening tool (excluding the positive likelihood ratio) for nulliparous participants primarily fearful of vaginal birth. The CFQ came close to meeting these criteria in three other comparisons: for nulliparous participants in general, for those primarily fearful of cesarean birth, and for those primarily fearful of a vaginal birth (nulliparas and multiparas together).

A number of interesting findings emerged from the logistic regressions of CFQ subscales. Specifically, the CFQ Interference subscale was found to be a robust predictor of specific phobia, FoB across all analyses other than for nulliparous participants primarily fearful of cesarean birth. The CFQ Interference subscale is not part of the Full CFQ, as it specifically assesses impairment and does not measure the intensity of a specific fear domain. It nevertheless appears to be a crucial addition to the measure, allowing for a more sensitive assessment of impairment. The Interference subscale of the CFQ improved the measure's screening accuracy. This pattern was consistent across evaluations of the CFQ when comparing participants who reported symptoms meeting full diagnostic criteria against all other participants, as well as when comparisons were made with participants reporting symptoms meeting full or subclinical diagnostic criteria against all other participants. This trend remained the case also for analyses examining the full CFQ as well as those employing a subset of the CFQ subscale scores. For any clinical applications of the CFQ as a screening tool for a specific phobia, FoB should include this component of the measure.

Further, the fears of nulliparous participants appear to differ from those of multiparous participants. Specifically, for nulliparous participants, fear of cesarean birth and other medical interventions predominated. For multiparous participants, however, a fear of harm to one infant and fear of pain during a vaginal birth emerged. Among multiparous participants, fear of changes to one's appearance and sexual functioning, fear of cesarean birth and fear of mom or baby dying were all inversely related to reporting symptoms meeting the criteria for a specific phobia, FoB. Given the multifactorial nature of the CFQ, it appears that specific CFQ subscales or content areas are more relevant to some subgroups of pregnant people based on parity and whether one is more fearful of a vaginal or cesarean birth.

The full CFQ measure performed best when comparing both subclinical and full criteria diagnoses to participants without a diagnosis. The performance of the full CFQ when comparing those who reported symptoms meeting full diagnostic criteria for a specific phobia, FoB, to those who did not report symptoms meeting these criteria was mediocre and felt well below the criteria for a "good enough" screening tool. The screening accuracy of the CFQ was dramatically improved following the use of logistic regression to select a specific CFQ subscale for each subgroup (e.g., nulliparous and multiparous participants). Using specific CFQ subscales to predict diagnostic status resulted in screening metrics that would generally be considered good to excellent. Again, additional research is needed to improve subscales selection for birthing people ONLY meeting full criteria for FoB (as opposed to birthing people experiencing subclinical and clinical symptoms).

Study findings are also consistent with, and build upon, findings from the only other study of the W-DEQ as a screening tool for a specific phobia, FoB [83]. In that previous small (N = 106) study of the screening accuracy of the W-DEQ for a specific phobia, FoB, among nulliparous pregnant people, the W-DEQ evidenced an AUC of 0.96 and a Youden's index of 0.93. The optimal cut score was determined to be 85. The authors compared participants reporting symptoms meeting full criteria for a specific phobia, FoB, to those who did not. In the present study, the same analysis (i.e., full diagnostic criteria for nulliparous participants only) produced an AUC of 0.88, a Youden's J index of 0.69, and an optimal cut score of 95.4.

Together, these two studies support the screening accuracy of the W-DEQ for a specific phobia, FoB (full criteria). A note of caution regarding these findings is merited given the small numbers of positive cases in both studies, in particular the smaller study by Calderani and colleagues [83].

Our findings suggest that the W-DEQ performs best when comparing pregnant people who have reported symptoms meeting full diagnostic criteria for FoB to those who did not report symptoms meeting these criteria. A note of caution here is also merited due to the fact that the number of participants meeting the full criteria was small, rendering estimates of performance unstable. Additional research involving larger samples is needed to fully clarify the merits and disadvantages of screening for a specific phobia, FoB full criteria versus full or subclinical, and to ensure the stability and replicability of estimates of performance, especially for comparisons of specific phobia, FoB full diagnostic criteria to all other participants.

Interestingly, when we compared participants who reported symptoms meeting full or subclinical diagnostic criteria for a specific phobia, FoB, to the remainder of the sample, the W-DEQ performed best when limiting these analyses to participants who were primarily fearful of vaginal birth. It may be that the W-DEQ performs best for people who are most fearful of vaginal birth, but additional research will be needed to clarify this. Of note, when limiting the analysis to those primarily fearful of vaginal birth, the W-DEQ performed best for multiparous participants. This is counter-intuitive in that one might expect the fears of multiparous people to more closely resemble symptoms of post-traumatic stress disorder and not specific phobia [49,67].

4.3. Limitations and Future Directions

Although this study was adequately powered (N = 659), subsamples of participants reporting symptoms meeting full diagnostic criteria for a specific phobia, FoB, were much smaller. Consequently, we were unable to conduct all ROC analyses comparing participants whose symptoms met the full criteria for a specific phobia, FoB, against the remaining participants. For some ROC analyses, we compared those who reported symptoms meeting full or subclinical criteria against the remaining participants. This improved power but may not fully generalize to pregnant people with symptoms meeting full criteria for specific phobia FoB. Future research with larger samples will be able to refine some of the findings from the present research.

Given that specific phobia may not be the only diagnostic category most relevant for FoB, it would be extremely helpful to evaluate the ability of the CFQ and the W-DEQ to screen for any mental health diagnosis under which a particular person's FoB may fall. For example, for some people, FoB may be best characterized as a post-traumatic stress disorder, whereas for others, it may be best understood as a specific phobia or health anxiety. It would be helpful to know if the majority of people whose FoB is severe enough to merit a mental health diagnosis can be captured by the CFQ or the W-DEQ. Studies in which the screening ability of these two measures are assessed against a broader range of anxiety-related conditions will be able to answer this question.

Future research may benefit from efforts to replicate the regression analyses and resulting ROC findings of the CFQ subscales to ensure the stability of these findings. Future research will also be needed to ascertain the utility of the CFQ and W-DEQ in diverse cultural groups, social contexts (e.g., lower socio-economic status) and countries.

5. Conclusions

The W-DEQ performs well as a screening tool for a specific phobia, FoB, for pregnant people overall and across various subgroups (e.g., nulliparous and multiparous pregnant people). The CFQ performs less well as a screening tool for a specific phobia, FoB, but nevertheless holds promise. Additional research is needed to ensure replicability of findings and to further evaluate the potential of the CFQ to accurately screen for diagnosable FoB.

Supplementary Materials: The following supporting information can be downloaded at: https://www.mdpi.com/article/10.3390/ijerph19084647/s1, Figure S1: Receiver operating characteristic (ROC) curves for the Childbrith Fear Questionnaire (CFQ) across parity (full diagnostic criteria ONLY). Figure S2: ROC curves for the CFQ (Total and Interference Subscale scores) across parity (full diagnostic criteria ONLY). Figure S3: ROC curves for the Wijma Delivery Expectations Questionnaire (W-DEQ) across parity (full diagnostic criteria ONLY). Figure S4: ROC curves for the CFQ across parity (subclinical and full diagnostic criteria combined). Figure S5: ROC curves for the CFQ (Total and Interference Subscale scores) across parity (subclinical and full diagnostic criteria combined). Figure S6: ROC curves for the W-DEQ across parity (subclinical and full diagnostic criteria combined). Figure S7: ROC curves for the CFQ across parity, separately for fear of vaginal birth (subclinical and full diagnostic criteria combined). Figure S8: ROC curves for the CFQ across parity (Total and Interference Subscale scores), separately for fear of cesarean birth (CS; subclinical and full diagnostic criteria combined). Figure S9: ROC curves for the W-DEQ across parity, separately for fear of vaginal birth (subclinical and full diagnostic criteria combined).

Author Contributions: N.F. developed the manuscript concept and was responsible for the study design. N.F. and F.C. were responsible for the supervision of data collection and interpretation of the data. A.A., in collaboration with N.F. and F.C., was responsible for data analyses. All authors were involved in manuscript drafting. N.F., A.A., F.C. and C.K. were involved in manuscript drafting. N.F., A.A., F.C. and C.K. provided scientific input and edited and reviewed the manuscript content. N.F., A.A., F.C. and C.K. provided their final approval and agreed to be accountable for all aspects of the work, ensuring integrity and accuracy. All authors have read and agreed to the published version of the manuscript.

Funding: This research was funded from the primary author's start-up funds via the Island Medical Program of the University of British Columbia.

Institutional Review Board Statement: This study was conducted in accordance with the Declaration of Helsinki. Ethical approval for this study was obtained from the Behavioural Ethics Board of the University of British Columbia (H15-03356) and written informed consent was obtained from all participants. The University of British Columbia's Behavioural Research Ethics Board follows the Canadian Tri-Counsel Policy Statement (TCPS): Ethical Conduct for Research Involving Humans.

Informed Consent Statement: Informed consent was obtained from all subjects involved in the study.

Data Availability Statement: The datasets used and/or analyzed during the current study are available from the corresponding author on reasonable request.

Acknowledgments: The authors would like to thank the study participants for the generous gift of their time and thoughtful engagement. We would like to thank Jessica Gaiptman, Stephanie Poje, Rebecca Ferguson, Emily Friedrich, and Jennifer Suen for their invaluable contribution to participant recruitment and project management. We would also like to thank Rebecca Ferguson, Anika Brown, Sarah Ollerhead and Danielle Marwick for their contribution to participant interviewing.

Conflicts of Interest: The authors declare no conflict of interest.

References

1. Kessler, R.C.; Berglund, P.; Demler, O.; Jin, R.; Merikangas, K.R.; Walters, E.E. Lifetime Prevalence and Age-of-Onset Distributions of DSM-IV Disorders in the National Comorbidity Survey Replication. *Arch. Gen. Psychiatry* **2005**, *62*, 593–602. [CrossRef] [PubMed]
2. Kessler, R.C.; Petukhova, M.; Sampson, N.A.; Zaslavsky, A.M.; Wittchen, H.-U. Twelve-month and lifetime prevalence and lifetime morbid risk of anxiety and mood disorders in the United States. *Int. J. Methods Psychiatr. Res.* **2012**, *21*, 169–184. [CrossRef] [PubMed]
3. Fawcett, E.J.; Fairbrother, N.; Cox, M.L.; White, I.; Fawcett, J.M. The Prevalence of Anxiety Disorders during Pregnancy and the Postpartum Period: A Multivariate Bayesian Meta-Analysis. *J. Clin. Psychiatry* **2019**, *80*, 1181. [CrossRef] [PubMed]
4. Reck, C.; Struben, K.; Backenstrass, M.; Stefenelli, U.; Reinig, K.; Fuchs, T.; Sohn, C.; Mundt, C. Prevalence, onset and comorbidity of postpartum anxiety and depressive disorders. *Acta Psychiatr. Scand.* **2008**, *118*, 459–468. [CrossRef] [PubMed]
5. Woody, C.A.; Ferrari, A.J.; Siskind, D.J.; Whiteford, H.A.; Harris, M.G. A systematic review and meta-regression of the prevalence and incidence of perinatal depression. *J. Affect. Disord.* **2017**, *219*, 86–92. [CrossRef]
6. Fifer, S.K.; Mathias, S.D.; Patrick, D.L.; Mazonson, P.D.; Lubeck, D.P.; Buesching, D.P. Untreated Anxiety among Adult Primary Care Patients in a Health Maintenance Organization. *Arch. Gen. Psychiatry* **1994**, *51*, 740–750. [CrossRef]

7. Demers, M. Frequent users of ambulatory health care in Quebec: The case of doctor-shoppers. *Can. Med. Assoc. J.* **1995**, *153*, 37–42.
8. Fournier, L.; Lesage, A.D.; Toupin, J.; Cyr, M. Telephone Surveys as an Alternative for Estimating Prevalence of Mental Disorders and Service Utilization: A Montreal Catchment Area Study. *Can. J. Psychiatry* **1997**, *42*, 737–743. [CrossRef]
9. Horenstein, A.; Heimberg, R.G. Anxiety disorders and healthcare utilization: A systematic review. *Clin. Psychol. Rev.* **2020**, *81*, 101894. [CrossRef]
10. McCusker, J.; Boulenger, J.-P.; Boyer, R.; Bellavance, F.; Miller, J.-M. Use of health services for anxiety disorders: A multisite study in Quebec. *Can. J. Psychiatry* **1997**, *42*, 730–736. [CrossRef]
11. Ohayon, M.M.; Shapiro, C.M.; Kennedy, S. Differentiating DSM-IV Anxiety and Depressive Disorders in the General Population: Comorbidity and Treatment Consequences. *Can. J. Psychiatry* **2000**, *45*, 166–172. [CrossRef] [PubMed]
12. Matthey, S. Anxiety and Stress During Pregnancy and the Postpartum Period. In *The Oxford Handbook of Perinatal Psychology*; Oxford University Press: Oxford, UK, 2016. [CrossRef]
13. Korja, R.; Nolvi, S.; Grant, K.A.; McMahon, C. The Relations Between Maternal Prenatal Anxiety or Stress and Child's Early Negative Reactivity or Self-Regulation: A Systematic Review. *Child Psychiatry Hum. Dev.* **2017**, *48*, 851–869. [CrossRef] [PubMed]
14. Erickson, N.; Gartstein, M.; Dotson, J.A.W. Review of Prenatal Maternal Mental Health and the Development of Infant Temperament. *J. Obstet. Gynecol. Neonatal Nurs.* **2017**, *46*, 588–600. [CrossRef]
15. Rees, S.; Channon, S.; Waters, C.S. The impact of maternal prenatal and postnatal anxiety on children's emotional problems: A systematic review. *Eur. Child Adolesc. Psychiatry* **2019**, *28*, 257–280. [CrossRef] [PubMed]
16. Ding, X.-X.; Wu, Y.-L.; Xu, S.-J.; Zhu, R.-P.; Jia, X.-M.; Zhang, S.-F.; Huang, K.; Zhu, P.; Hao, J.-H.; Tao, F.-B. Maternal anxiety during pregnancy and adverse birth outcomes: A systematic review and meta-analysis of prospective cohort studies. *J. Affect. Disord.* **2014**, *159*, 103–110. [CrossRef]
17. Mulder, E.J.H.; de Medina, P.G.R.; Huizink, A.C.; Bergh, B.R.H.V.D.; Buitelaar, J.K.; Visser, G.H.A. Prenatal maternal stress: Effects on pregnancy and the (unborn) child. *Early Hum. Dev.* **2002**, *70*, 3–14. [CrossRef]
18. Schneider, M.L.; Moore, C.F.; Kraemer, G.W.; Roberts, A.D.; DeJesus, O.T. The impact of prenatal stress, fetal alcohol exposure, or both on development: Perspectives from a primate model. *Psychoneuroendocrinology* **2002**, *27*, 285–298. [CrossRef]
19. Wadhwa, P.D.; Glynn, L.; Hobel, C.J.; Garite, T.J.; Porto, M.; Chicz-DeMet, A.; Wiglesworth, A.K.; Sandman, C.A. Behavioral perinatology: Biobehavioral processes in human fetal development. *Regul. Pept.* **2002**, *108*, 149–157. [CrossRef]
20. Adamson, B.; Letourneau, N.; Lebel, C. Prenatal maternal anxiety and children's brain structure and function: A systematic review of neuroimaging studies. *J. Affect. Disord.* **2018**, *241*, 117–126. [CrossRef]
21. O'Connor, T.G.; Heron, J.; Golding, J.; Glover, V.; the ALSPAC Study Team. Maternal antenatal anxiety and behavioural/emotional problems in children: A test of a programming hypothesis. *J. Child Psychol. Psychiatry* **2003**, *44*, 1025–1036. [CrossRef]
22. O'Connor, T.G.; Heron, J.; Glover, V. Antenatal Anxiety Predicts Child Behavioral/Emotional Problems Independently of Postnatal Depression. *J. Am. Acad. Child Adolesc. Psychiatry* **2002**, *41*, 1470–1477. [CrossRef] [PubMed]
23. Grigoriadis, S.; Graves, L.; Peer, M.; Mamisashvili, L.; Tomlinson, G.; Vigod, S.N.; Dennis, C.-L.; Steiner, M.; Brown, C.; Cheung, A.; et al. A systematic review and meta-analysis of the effects of antenatal anxiety on postpartum outcomes. *Arch. Women's Ment. Health* **2019**, *22*, 543–556. [CrossRef] [PubMed]
24. Matthey, S.; Barnett, B.; Howie, P.; Kavanagh, D. Diagnosing postpartum depression in mothers and fathers: Whatever happened to anxiety? *J. Affect. Disord.* **2003**, *74*, 139–147. [CrossRef]
25. Robertson, E.; Grace, S.; Wallington, T.; Stewart, D.E. Antenatal risk factors for postpartum depression: A synthesis of recent literature. *Gen. Hosp. Psychiatry* **2004**, *26*, 289–295. [CrossRef]
26. Sutter-Dallay, A.; Giaconne-Marcesche, V.; Glatigny-Dallay, E.; Verdoux, H. Women with anxiety disorders during pregnancy are at increased risk of intense postnatal depressive symptoms: A prospective survey of the MATQUID cohort. *Eur. Psychiatry* **2004**, *19*, 459–463. [CrossRef]
27. Bánhidy, F.; Ács, N.; Puhó, E.; Czeizel, A.E. Association between maternal panic disorders and pregnancy complications and delivery outcomes. *Eur. J. Obstet. Gynecol. Reprod. Biol.* **2006**, *124*, 47–52. [CrossRef]
28. Chen, Y.-H.; Lin, H.-C.; Lee, H.-C. Pregnancy outcomes among women with panic disorder—Do panic attacks during pregnancy matter? *J. Affect. Disord.* **2010**, *120*, 258–262. [CrossRef]
29. Lilliecreutz, C.; Josefsson, A. Prevalence of blood and injection phobia among pregnant women. *Acta Obstet. Gynecol. Scand.* **2008**, *87*, 1276–1279. [CrossRef]
30. Seng, J.; Oakley, D.J.; Sampselle, C.M.; Killion, C.; Graham-Bermann, S.; Liberzon, I. Posttraumatic stress disorder and pregnancy complications. *Obstet. Gynecol.* **2001**, *97*, 17–22. [CrossRef]
31. Yonkers, K.A.; Blackwell, K.A.; Glover, J.; Forray, A. Antidepressant Use in Pregnant and Postpartum Women. *Annu. Rev. Clin. Psychol.* **2014**, *10*, 369–392. [CrossRef]
32. Challacombe, F.L.; Salkovskis, P.M.; Woolgar, M.; Wilkinson, E.L.; Read, J.; Acheson, R. Parenting and mother-infant interactions in the context of maternal postpartum obsessive-compulsive disorder: Effects of obsessional symptoms and mood. *Infant Behav. Dev.* **2016**, *44*, 11–20. [CrossRef] [PubMed]
33. Castelli, R.D.; de Ávila Quevedo, L.; da Cunha Coelho, F.M.; Lopez, M.A.; da Silva, R.A.; Böhm, D.M.; Souza, L.D.D.M.; de Matos, M.B.; Pinheiro, K.A.T.; Pinheiro, R.T. Cognitive and language performance in children is associated with maternal social anxiety disorder: A study of young mothers in southern Brazil. *Early Hum. Dev.* **2015**, *91*, 707–711. [CrossRef] [PubMed]

34. Martini, J.; Knappe, S.; Beesdo-Baum, K.; Lieb, R.; Wittchen, H.-U. Anxiety disorders before birth and self-perceived distress during pregnancy: Associations with maternal depression and obstetric, neonatal and early childhood outcomes. *Early Hum. Dev.* **2010**, *86*, 305–310. [CrossRef]
35. Fairbrother, N.; Collardeau, F.; Albert, A.; Challacombe, F.L.; Thordarson, D.S.; Woody, S.; Janssen, P.A. High prevalence and incidence of OCD among women across pregnancy and postpartum. *J. Clin. Psychiatry* **2021**, *82*, 30368. [CrossRef] [PubMed]
36. Nieminen, K.; Berg, I.; Frankenstein, K.; Viita, L.; Larsson, K.; Persson, U.; Spånberger, L.; Wretman, A.; Silfvernagel, K.; Andersson, G.; et al. Internet-provided cognitive behaviour therapy of posttraumatic stress symptoms following childbirth—A randomized controlled trial. *Cogn. Behav. Ther.* **2016**, *45*, 287–306. [CrossRef]
37. Searing, K.; Baukus, M.; Stark, M.A.; Morin, K.H.; Rudell, B. Needle Phobia during Pregnancy. *J. Obstet. Gynecol. Neonatal Nurs.* **2006**, *35*, 592–598. [CrossRef]
38. Arch, J.J. Pregnancy-specific anxiety: Which women are highest and what are the alcohol-related risks? *Compr. Psychiatry* **2013**, *54*, 217–228. [CrossRef]
39. Räisänen, S.; Lehto, S.; Nielsen, H.; Gissler, M.; Kramer, M.; Heinonen, S.; Lehto, S. Fear of childbirth in nulliparous and multiparous women: A population-based analysis of all singleton births in Finland in 1997–2010. *BJOG Int. J. Obstet. Gynaecol.* **2014**, *121*, 965–970. [CrossRef]
40. O'Connell, M.A.; Leahy-Warren, P.; Khashan, A.S.; Kenny, L.C.; O'Neill, S.M. Worldwide prevalence of tocophobia in pregnant women: Systematic review and meta-analysis. *Acta Obstet. Gynecol. Scand.* **2017**, *96*, 907–920. [CrossRef]
41. Clark, L.A.; Cuthbert, B.; Lewis-Fernández, R.; Narrow, W.E.; Reed, G.M. Three Approaches to Understanding and Classifying Mental Disorder: ICD-11, DSM-5, and the National Institute of Mental Health's Research Domain Criteria (RDoC). *Psychol. Sci. Public Interes.* **2017**, *18*, 72–145. [CrossRef]
42. Eaton, W.W.; Neufeld, K.; Chen, L.-S.; Cai, G. A Comparison of Self-report and Clinical Diagnostic Interviews for Depression: Diagnostic Interview Schedule and Schedules for Clinical Assessment in Neuropsychiatry in the Baltimore Epidemiologic Catchment Area Follow-Up. *Arch. Gen. Psychiatry* **2000**, *57*, 217–222. [CrossRef] [PubMed]
43. Thombs, B.D.; Kwakkenbos, L.; Levis, A.W.; Benedetti, A. Addressing overestimation of the prevalence of depression based on self-report screening questionnaires. *Can. Med. Assoc. J.* **2018**, *190*, E44–E49. [CrossRef] [PubMed]
44. Challacombe, F.L.; Nath, S.; Trevillion, K.; Pawlby, S.; Howard, L.M. Fear of childbirth during pregnancy: Associations with observed mother-infant interactions and perceived bonding. *Arch. Women's Ment. Health* **2020**, *24*, 483–492. [CrossRef] [PubMed]
45. Lukasse, M.; Schei, B.; Ryding, E.L. Prevalence and associated factors of fear of childbirth in six European countries. *Sex. Reprod. Health* **2014**, *5*, 99–106. [CrossRef]
46. Nilsson, C.; Hessman, E.; Sjöblom, H.; Dencker, A.; Jangsten, E.; Mollberg, M.; Patel, H.; Sparud-Lundin, C.; Wigert, H.; Begley, C. Definitions, measurements and prevalence of fear of childbirth: A systematic review. *BMC Pregnancy Childbirth* **2018**, *18*, 28. [CrossRef]
47. O'Connell, M.A.; Leahy-Warren, P.; Kenny, L.C.; O'Neill, S.M.; Khashan, A.S. The prevalence and risk factors of fear of childbirth among pregnant women: A cross-sectional study in Ireland. *Acta Obstet. Gynecol. Scand.* **2019**, *98*, 1014–1023. [CrossRef]
48. Möller, L.; Josefsson, A.; Lilliecreutz, C.; Gunnervik, C.; Bladh, M.; Sydsjö, G. Reproduction, fear of childbirth and obstetric outcomes in women treated for fear of childbirth in their first pregnancy: A historical cohort. *Acta Obstet. Gynecol. Scand.* **2019**, *98*, 374–381. [CrossRef]
49. Hofberg, K.; Ward, M.R. Fear of pregnancy and childbirth. *Postgrad. Med. J.* **2003**, *79*, 505–510. [CrossRef]
50. Zar, M.; Wijma, K.; Wijma, B. Pre- and Postpartum Fear of Childbirth in Nulliparous and Parous Women. *Scand. J. Behav. Ther.* **2001**, *30*, 75–84. [CrossRef]
51. Adams, S.; Eberhard-Gran, M.; Eskild, A. Fear of childbirth and duration of labour: A study of 2206 women with intended vaginal delivery. *BJOG Int. J. Obstet. Gynaecol.* **2012**, *119*, 1238–1246. [CrossRef]
52. Ryding, E.L.; Lukasse, M.; Van Parys, A.-S.; Wangel, A.-M.; Karro, H.; Kristjansdottir, H.; Schroll, A.-M.; Schei, B.; the Bidens Group. Fear of Childbirth and Risk of Cesarean Delivery: A Cohort Study in Six European Countries. *Birth* **2015**, *42*, 48–55. [CrossRef]
53. Takegata, M.; Haruna, M.; Matsuzaki, M.; Shiraishi, M.; Okano, T.; Severinsson, E. Does Antenatal Fear of Childbirth Predict Postnatal Fear of Childbirth? A Study of Japanese Women. *Open J. Nurs.* **2015**, *05*, 144–152. [CrossRef]
54. Sydsjö, G.; Bladh, M.; Lilliecreutz, C.; Persson, A.-M.; Vyöni, H.; Josefsson, A. Obstetric outcomes for nulliparous women who received routine individualized treatment for severe fear of childbirth—A retrospective case control study. *BMC Pregnancy Childbirth* **2014**, *14*, 126. [CrossRef] [PubMed]
55. Fuglenes, D.; Aas, E.; Botten, G.; Øian, P.; Kristiansen, I.S. Why do some pregnant women prefer cesarean? The influence of parity, delivery experiences, and fear. *Am. J. Obstet. Gynecol.* **2011**, *205*, 45.e1–45.e9. [CrossRef] [PubMed]
56. Haines, H.M.; Rubertsson, C.; Pallant, J.F.; Hildingsson, I. The influence of women's fear, attitudes and beliefs of childbirth on mode and experience of birth. *BMC Pregnancy Childbirth* **2012**, *12*, 55. [CrossRef] [PubMed]
57. Handelzalts, J.E.; Fisher, S.; Lurie, S.; Shalev, A.; Golan, A.; Sadan, O. Personality, fear of childbirth and cesarean delivery on demand. *Acta Obstet. Gynecol. Scand.* **2011**, *91*, 16–21. [CrossRef]
58. Nieminen, K.; Stephansson, O.; Ryding, E.L. Women's fear of childbirth and preference for cesarean section—A cross-sectional study at various stages of pregnancy in Sweden. *Acta Obstet. Gynecol. Scand.* **2009**, *88*, 807–813. [CrossRef] [PubMed]

59. Wiklund, I.; Edman, G.; Andolf, E. Cesarean section on maternal request: Reasons for the request, self-estimated health, expectations, experience of birth and signs of depression among first-time mothers. *Acta Obstet. Gynecol. Scand.* **2007**, *86*, 451–456. [CrossRef]
60. Saisto, T.; Salmela-Aro, K.; Nurmi, J.-E.; Halmesmäki, E. Psychosocial characteristics of women and their partners fearing vaginal childbirth. *Br. J. Obstet. Gynaecol.* **2001**, *108*, 492–498. [CrossRef]
61. Salomonsson, B.; Gullberg, M.T.; Alehagen, S.; Wijma, K. Self-efficacy beliefs and fear of childbirth in nulliparous women. *J. Psychosom. Obstet. Gynecol.* **2013**, *34*, 116–121. [CrossRef]
62. Stoll, K.; Hauck, Y.; Downe, S.; Edmonds, J.; Gross, M.M.; Malott, A.; McNiven, P.; Swift, E.; Thomson, G.; Hall, W. Cross-cultural development and psychometric evaluation of a measure to assess fear of childbirth prior to pregnancy. *Sex. Reprod. Health* **2016**, *8*, 49–54. [CrossRef]
63. Otley, H. Fear of childbirth: Understanding the causes, impact and treatment. *Br. J. Midwifery* **2011**, *19*, 215–220. [CrossRef]
64. Waldenström, U.; Hildingsson, I.; Ryding, E.L. Antenatal fear of childbirth and its association with subsequent caesarean section and experience of childbirth. *BJOG Int. J. Obstet. Gynaecol.* **2006**, *113*, 638–646. [CrossRef]
65. Størksen, H.T.; Garthus-Niegel, S.; Vangen, S.; Eberhard-Gran, M. The impact of previous birth experiences on maternal fear of childbirth. *Acta Obstet. Gynecol. Scand.* **2012**, *92*, 318–324. [CrossRef]
66. Alipour, Z.; Lamyian, M.; Hajizadeh, E. Anxiety and fear of childbirth as predictors of postnatal depression in nulliparous women. *Women Birth* **2012**, *25*, e37–e43. [CrossRef]
67. Ayers, S. Fear of childbirth, postnatal post-traumatic stress disorder and midwifery care. *Midwifery* **2014**, *30*, 145–148. [CrossRef]
68. Nath, S.; Busuulwa, P.; Ryan, E.G.; Challacombe, F.L.; Howard, L.M. The characteristics and prevalence of phobias in pregnancy. *Midwifery* **2020**, *82*, 102590. [CrossRef]
69. Storksen, H.T.; Eberhard-Gran, M.; Garthus-Niegel, S.; Eskild, A. Fear of childbirth; the relation to anxiety and depression. *Acta Obstet. Gynecol. Scand.* **2012**, *91*, 237–242. [CrossRef]
70. Rouhe, H.; Salmela-Aro, K.; Halmesmäki, E.; Saisto, T. Fear of childbirth according to parity, gestational age, and obstetric history. *BJOG Int. J. Obstet. Gynaecol.* **2008**, *116*, 67–73. [CrossRef]
71. Fairbrother, N.; Thordarson, D.S.; Stoll, K. Fine tuning fear of childbirth: The relationship between Childbirth Fear Questionnaire subscales and demographic and reproductive variables. *J. Reprod. Infant Psychol.* **2018**, *36*, 15–29. [CrossRef]
72. Jokić-Begić, N.; Žigić, L.; Radoš, S.N. Anxiety and anxiety sensitivity as predictors of fear of childbirth: Different patterns for nulliparous and parous women. *J. Psychosom. Obstet. Gynecol.* **2014**, *35*, 22–28. [CrossRef]
73. Poikkeus, P.; Saisto, T.; Unkila-Kallio, L.; Punamaki, R.L.; Repokari, L.; Vilska, S.; Tiitinen, A.; Tulppala, M. Fear of Childbirth and Pregnancy-Related Anxiety in Women Conceiving with Assisted Reproduction. *Obstet. Gynecol.* **2006**, *108*, 70–76. [CrossRef]
74. Gao, L.-L.; Liu, X.J.; Fu, B.L.; Xie, W. Predictors of childbirth fear among pregnant Chinese women: A cross-sectional questionnaire survey. *Midwifery* **2015**, *31*, 865–870. [CrossRef]
75. Laursen, M.; Hedegaard, M.; Johansen, C.H. Fear of childbirth: Predictors and temporal changes among nulliparous women in the Danish National Birth Cohort. *BJOG Int. J. Obstet. Gynaecol.* **2008**, *115*, 354–360. [CrossRef]
76. Nerum, H.; Halvorsen, L.; Straume, B.; Sørlie, T.; Øian, P. Different labour outcomes in primiparous women that have been subjected to childhood sexual abuse or rape in adulthood: A case-control study in a clinical cohort. *BJOG Int. J. Obstet. Gynaecol.* **2013**, *120*, 487–495. [CrossRef]
77. Gourounti, K.; Kouklaki, E.; Lykeridou, K. Validation of the Childbirth Attitudes Questionnaire in Greek and psychosocial characteristics of pregnant women with fear of childbirth. *Women Birth* **2015**, *28*, e44–e51. [CrossRef]
78. Lowe, N.K. Self-efficacy for labor and childbirth fears in nulliparous pregnant women. *J. Psychosom. Obstet. Gynecol.* **2000**, *21*, 219–224. [CrossRef]
79. Heimstad, R.; Dahloe, R.; Laache, I.; Skogvoll, E.; Schei, B. Fear of childbirth and history of abuse: Implications for pregnancy and delivery. *Acta Obstet. Gynecol. Scand.* **2006**, *85*, 435–440. [CrossRef]
80. Hall, W.A.; Hauck, Y.L.; Carty, E.M.; Hutton, E.K.; Fenwick, J.; Stoll, K. Childbirth Fear, Anxiety, Fatigue, and Sleep Deprivation in Pregnant Women. *J. Obstet. Gynecol. Neonatal Nurs.* **2009**, *38*, 567–576. [CrossRef]
81. Qiu, L.; Sun, N.; Shi, X.; Zhao, Y.; Feng, L.; Gong, Y.; Yin, X. Fear of childbirth in nulliparous women: A cross-sectional multicentre study in China. *Women Birth* **2020**, *33*, e136–e141. [CrossRef]
82. American Psychiatric Association. *Diagnostic and Statistical Manual of Mental Disorders: DSM-5*, 5th ed.; American Psychiatric Publishing, Inc.: Arlington, VA, USA, 2013. [CrossRef]
83. Calderani, E.; Giardinelli, L.; Scannerini, S.; Arcabasso, S.; Compagno, E.; Petraglia, F.; Ricca, V. Tocophobia in the DSM-5 era: Outcomes of a new cut-off analysis of the Wijma delivery expectancy/experience questionnaire based on clinical presentation. *J. Psychosom. Res.* **2019**, *116*, 37–43. [CrossRef]
84. Hofberg, K.; Brockington, I.F. Tokophobia: An unreasoning dread of childbirth: A series of 26 cases. *Br. J. Psychiatry* **2000**, *176*, 83–85. [CrossRef] [PubMed]
85. Zar, M.; Wijma, K.; Wijma, B. Relations between anxiety disorders and fear of childbirth during late pregnancy. *Clin. Psychol. Psychother.* **2002**, *9*, 122–130. [CrossRef]
86. World Health Organization. ICD-11. ICD-11 Classif Ment Behav Disord Clin Descr Diagn Guidel 2019. Available online: https://icd.who.int/en (accessed on 13 March 2022).

87. Fairbrother, N.; Collardeau, F.; Albert, A.; Thordarson, D.S.; Stoll, K. Screening for Perinatal Anxiety Using the Childbirth Fear Questionnaire: A New Measure of Fear of Childbirth. *Int. J. Environ. Res. Public Health* **2022**, *19*, 2223. [CrossRef] [PubMed]
88. Areskog, B.; Kjessler, B.; Uddenberg, N. Identification of Women with Significant Fear of Childbirth during Late Pregnancy. *Gynecol. Obstet. Investig.* **1982**, *13*, 98–107. [CrossRef]
89. Elvander, C.; Cnattingius, S.; Kjerulff, K.H. Birth Experience in Women with Low, Intermediate or High Levels of Fear: Findings from the First Baby Study. *Birth* **2013**, *40*, 289–296. [CrossRef] [PubMed]
90. Eriksson, C.; Westman, G.; Hamberg, K. Experiential factors associated with childbirth-related fear in Swedish women and men: A population based study. *J. Psychosom. Obstet. Gynecol.* **2005**, *26*, 63–72. [CrossRef]
91. Hildingsson, I.; Nilsson, C.; Karlström, A.; Lundgren, I. A Longitudinal Survey of Childbirth-Related Fear and Associated Factors. *J. Obstet. Gynecol. Neonatal Nurs.* **2011**, *40*, 532–543. [CrossRef]
92. Melender, H.-L. Experiences of Fears Associated with Pregnancy and Childbirth: A Study of 329 Pregnant Women. *Birth* **2002**, *29*, 101–111. [CrossRef]
93. Prelog, P.R.; Makovec, M.R.; Šimic, M.V.; Premru-Srsen, T.; Perat, M. Individual and contextual factors of nulliparas' levels of depression, anxiety and fear of childbirth in the last trimester of pregnancy: Intimate partner attachment a key factor? *Slov. J. Public Health* **2019**, *58*, 112–119. [CrossRef]
94. Wijma, K.; Wijma, B.; Zar, M. Psychometric aspects of the W-DEQ; a new questionnaire for the measurement of fear of childbirth. *J. Psychosom. Obstet. Gynecol.* **1998**, *19*, 84–97. [CrossRef] [PubMed]
95. Wootton, B.M.; Davis, E.; Moses, K.; Moody, A.; Maguire, P. The development and initial validation of the Tokophobia Severity Scale. *Clin. Psychol.* **2020**, *24*, 267–275. [CrossRef]
96. Saxbe, D.; Horton, K.T.; Tsai, A.B. The Birth Experiences Questionnaire: A brief measure assessing psychosocial dimensions of childbirth. *J. Fam. Psychol.* **2018**, *32*, 262–268. [CrossRef] [PubMed]
97. Slade, P.; Pais, T.; Fairlie, F.; Simpson, A.; Sheen, K. The development of the Slade-Pais Expectations of Childbirth Scale (SPECS)*. *J. Reprod. Infant Psychol.* **2016**, *34*, 495–510. [CrossRef]
98. Redshaw, M.; Martin, C.; Rowe, R.; Hockley, C. The Oxford Worries about Labour Scale: Women's experience and measurement characteristics of a measure of maternal concern about labour and birth. *Psychol. Health Med.* **2009**, *14*, 354–366. [CrossRef]
99. Austin, M.P.; Highet, N.; *Expert Working Group. Mental Health Care in the Perinatal Period: Australian Clinical Practice Guideline 2017*; Centre of Perinatal Excellence: Melbourne, Australia, 2017.
100. Hart, K.; Flynn, H.A. Screening, Assessment, and Diagnosis of Mood and Anxiety Disorders During Pregnancy and the Postpartum Period. In *The Oxford Handbook of Perinatal Psychology*; Oxford University Press: New York, NY, USA, 2016; pp. 319–340. [CrossRef]
101. Stoll, K.; Fairbrother, N.; Thordarson, D.S. Childbirth Fear: Relation to Birth and Care Provider Preferences. *J. Midwifery Women's Health* **2018**, *63*, 58–67. [CrossRef]
102. Johnson, R.; Slade, P. Does fear of childbirth during pregnancy predict emergency caesarean section? *BJOG Int. J. Obstet. Gynaecol.* **2002**, *109*, 1213–1221. [CrossRef]
103. Garthus-Niegel, S.; Størksen, H.T.; Torgersen, L.; Von Soest, T.; Eberhard-Gran, M. The Wijma Delivery Expectancy/Experience Questionnaire—A factor analytic study. *J. Psychosom. Obstet. Gynecol.* **2011**, *32*, 160–163. [CrossRef]
104. McCabe, R.E.; Milosevic, I.; Rowa, K.; Shnaider, P.; Pawluk, E.J.; Antony, M.M. Diagnostic Assessment Research Tool (DART) 2017. Available online: https://healthsci.mcmaster.ca/docs/librariesprovider122/pdf/dart-instructions-current.pdf?sfvrsn=b95b406e_2 (accessed on 13 March 2022).
105. Schneider, L.H.; Pawluk, E.J.; Milosevic, I.; Shnaider, P.; Rowa, K.; Antony, M.M.; Musielak, N.; McCabe, R.E. The Diagnostic Assessment Research Tool in action: A preliminary evaluation of a semistructured diagnostic interview for DSM-5 disorders. *Psychol. Assess.* **2022**, *34*, 21–29. [CrossRef]
106. R Core Team. *R: A Language and Environment for Statistical Computing*; Foundation for Statistical Computing: Vienna, Austria, 2021.
107. IBM Corp. *IBM SPSS Statistics for Windows*; Version 24.0; IBM Corp: Armonk, NY, USA, 2016.
108. Bujang, M.A.; Adnan, T.H. Requirements for Minimum Sample Size for Sensitivity and Specificity Analysis. *J. Clin. Diagn. Res.* **2016**, *10*, YE01–YE06. [CrossRef]
109. Holtman, G.A.; Berger, M.Y.; Burger, H.; Deeks, J.; Donner-Banzhoff, N.; Fanshawe, T.R.; Koshiaris, C.; Leeflang, M.M.; Oke, J.L.; Perera, R.; et al. Development of practical recommendations for diagnostic accuracy studies in low-prevalence situations. *J. Clin. Epidemiol.* **2019**, *114*, 38–48. [CrossRef] [PubMed]
110. Thiele, C. Cutpointr: Determine and Evaluate Optimal cutpoints in Binary Classification Tasks. R Package Version 1.0.32 2020:158. Available online: https://cran.r-project.org/web/packages/cutpointr/cutpointr.pdf (accessed on 13 March 2022).
111. Fairbrother, N.; Corbyn, B.; Thordarson, D.S.; Ma, A.; Surm, D. Screening for perinatal anxiety disorders: Room to grow. *J. Affect. Disord.* **2019**, *250*, 363–370. [CrossRef] [PubMed]
112. Sackett, D.L.; Rosenberg, W.; Gray, J.A.M.; Haynes, R.B.; Richardson, W.S. Evidence based medicine: What it is and what it isn't. *BMJ* **1996**, *312*, 71–72. [CrossRef] [PubMed]
113. Räisänen, S.; Lehto, S.M.; Nielsen, H.S.; Gissler, M.; Kramer, M.R.; Heinonen, S. Risk factors for and perinatal outcomes of major depression during pregnancy: A population-based analysis during 2002–2010 in Finland. *BMJ Open* **2014**, *4*, e004883. [CrossRef] [PubMed]

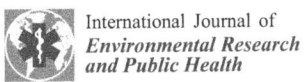

Article

The Relevance of Insomnia in the Diagnosis of Perinatal Depression: Validation of the Italian Version of the Insomnia Symptom Questionnaire

Lavinia De Chiara [1], Cristina Mazza [2], Eleonora Ricci [2], Alexia Emilia Koukopoulos [3], Georgios D. Kotzalidis [1], Marco Bonito [4], Tommaso Callovini [5], Paolo Roma [6,*] and Gloria Angeletti [1]

[1] Department of Neurosciences, Mental Health, Sensory Functions (NESMOS), Sant'Andrea University Hospital, Faculty of Medicine and Psychology, Sapienza University of Rome, Via Grottarossa 1035-1039, 00189 Rome, Italy; lavinia.dechiara@uniroma1.it (L.D.C.); giorgio.kotzalidis@uniroma1.it (G.D.K.); gloria.angeletti@uniroma1.it (G.A.)

[2] Department of Neuroscience, Imaging and Clinical Sciences, G. d'Annunzio University of Chieti-Pescara, Via dei Vestini 31, 66100 Chieti, Italy; cristina.mazza@unich.it (C.M.); eleonora.ricci@unich.it (E.R.)

[3] Department of Neuroscience/Mental Health, UOC Psichiatria, Psicofarmacologia Clinica, Azienda Ospedaliera Universitaria Policlinico Umberto I, Viale Regina Elena, 328, 00161 Rome, Italy; alexia.koukopoulos@uniroma1.it

[4] Dipartimento Materno Infantile, San Pietro Fatebenefratelli Hospital, Via Cassia, 600, 00189 Rome, Italy; bonitomarco@libero.it

[5] Department of Medicine and Surgery, University of Milano Bicocca, Via Cadore 48, 20900 Monza, Italy; t.callovini@campus.unimib.it

[6] Department of Human Neurosciences, Sapienza University of Rome, Viale Regina Elena 334, 00161 Rome, Italy

* Correspondence: paolo.roma@uniroma1.it

Abstract: Background. Sleep disorders are common in perinatal women and may underlie or trigger anxiety and depression. We aimed to translate and validate and evaluate the psychometric properties of the Italian version of the Insomnia Symptom Questionnaire (ISQ), in a sample of women during late pregnancy and 6-months postpartum according to the DSM-5 criteria. Methods. The ISQ was administered to 292 women prenatally along with other measures of sleep quality, depression, and anxiety, to examine its construct and convergent validity. Women were readministered the ISQ six months postdelivery to assess test–retest reliability. Women were divided into DSM-5 No-Insomnia (N = 253) and Insomnia (N = 39) groups. Results. The insomnia group had received more psychopharmacotherapy, had more psychiatric family history, increased rates of medically assisted reproduction, of past perinatal psychiatric disorders, and scored higher on almost all TEMPS-A dimensions, on the EPDS, HCL-32, PSQI, and on ISQ prenatally and postnatally. ISQ scores correlated with all scales, indicating adequate convergent and discriminant validity; furthermore, it showed antenatal–postnatal test–retest reliability, 97.5% diagnostic accuracy, 79.5% sensitivity, 94.9% specificity, 70.5% positive predictive power, and 92.8% negative predictive power. Conclusions. The ISQ is useful, valid, and reliable for assessing perinatal insomnia in Italian women. The Italian version showed equivalent properties to the original version.

Keywords: Insomnia Symptom Questionnaire; sleep disorders; perinatal period; internal consistency; convergent validity

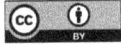

1. Introduction

The DSM-5 [1] defined insomnia as dissatisfaction with sleep quantity or quality, associated with one or more of the following symptoms: difficulty initiating sleep, difficulty maintaining sleep, frequent awakenings, or problems returning to sleep after awakenings. Sleep difficulties occur despite adequate opportunity for sleep, at least 3 nights per week, for at least 3 months. The sleep disturbance causes clinically significant distress or impairment in social, occupational, educational, academic, behavioral, or other important areas of functioning. In contrast to the DSM-IV-TR [2], the DSM-5 makes no distinction between primary and comorbid insomnia, and dissatisfaction with sleep quantity or quality were included as prerequisites for diagnosing insomnia. When assessing sleep quality, the accuracy of the definition of sleep quality itself is a fundamental issue. The International Classification of Sleep Disorders-Third Edition (ICSD-3) criteria [3] are consistent with the DSM-5. The updated version of the DSM does not conflict with the former version for what concerns symptom identification and assigning the diagnosis.

Sleep disturbances are highly prevalent during pregnancy [4,5]. Their trajectories may affect pregnancy and birth outcomes [6,7]. A recent meta-analysis indicated that 45.7% of expectant mothers experienced poor sleep quality [8], and another meta-analysis focusing on insomnia, reported a general mean of 38.2% which peaked during the last trimester [9]. Women experience dramatic physical changes during the perinatal period; while many adapt well to being pregnant, some become severely distressed [10–12]. Physical discomfort during pregnancy may involve possible chronic sleep disruption and fragmentation [13]. Sleep deprivation may predict mental disorders [14]. Therefore, it appears that anxiety, depression, and sleep disorders are related bidirectionally, independently of which one is the initial trigger [15].

Insomnia during pregnancy is a risk factor for postpartum depressive symptoms [16–19]. Conversely, mothers with depression have a higher risk of developing sleep disturbance [20,21]. Perinatal depression, defined as a major depressive episode during pregnancy or within the first year postpartum, is the most common complication of childbirth and a major public health problem affecting all members of the family while too often escaping detection and treatment.

Recent studies highlight the critical role of screening, early diagnosis, and suitable insomnia treatment during pregnancy in reducing depressive symptoms [22]. The association between poor sleep and perinatal psychiatric disorders has important clinical implications [23]; pregnant women who suffer from poor sleep quality can be identified easily by midwives or obstetricians during routine prenatal checkups, thus potentiating mood disorder prevention [24]. Given women's reluctance to take psychotropic medications during pregnancy [25], sleep protection as nonpharmacological means to prevent and reduce postpartum mental illness has been advocated [26].

There are currently several self-reported questionnaires available for assessing sleep quality and insomnia in the general population. The Pittsburgh Sleep Quality Index (PSQI) [27,28] and the Insomnia Severity Index (ISI) [29,30] are the most widely used tools in Italy. Few tools are available in Italian to assess the prevalence of insomnia during the perinatal period. The Insomnia Symptom Questionnaire (ISQ) [31] is a 13-item self-report instrument designed to identify insomnia and validated to recognize insomnia in pregnant women [20]. ISQ questions are based on DSM-IV-TR criteria for primary insomnia. The questionnaire is a short and cost-effective tool that can be quickly employed in large observational studies or in clinical practice.

During pregnancy, sleep quality assessment should be advised to guide possible preventative and therapeutic interventions [23]. The aim of the present study was to translate and validate the ISQ and evaluate the psychometric properties of its Italian version in a sample of women during late pregnancy and 6 months postpartum according to the DSM-5 criteria.

2. Materials and Methods

2.1. Research Setting

The study was developed in the context of a collaborative screening effort between the Gynaecology and Obstetrics unit of San Pietro Fatebenefratelli Hospital of Rome, Italy, and the Center for Prevention and Treatment of Women's Mental Health Problems, Psychiatry Unit, Sapienza University, Faculty of Medicine and Psychology, Sant'Andrea Hospital, Rome, Italy.

2.2. Participants

We recruited 304 women at the Gynaecology and Obstetrics unit of San Pietro Fatebenefratelli Hospital in Rome, a large maternity unit, between July and December 2018 during their routine third-trimester screening. The women included in the study were screened once during their third trimester of pregnancy (T0) and again six months postpartum (T1). We recruited 39 women with DSM-5 insomnia. Exclusion criteria were age less than 18 years old, failure to provide free informed consent, and incomplete comprehension of the Italian language that prevented participants from completing the questionnaires. Participants with an incomplete ISQ were also excluded from the final analysis ($N = 12$). Antenatal participants who had consented to be contacted in the postnatal period were called by two trained psychologists of our Centre for Prevention and Treatment of Women's Mental Health, 6 months following the birth of their baby, and invited to complete the questionnaires again through an online system (Google Form).

The final study sample comprised 292 women, aged 19–46 years (mean = 33.26, SD = 5.04); 95% of participants ($N = 278$) were in a stable relationship, most of them held a university degree ($N = 158$, 54.1%) and were employed ($N = 230$, 78.8%), 160 participants (54.8%) reported changes in sleep hours. The sample was split into Insomnia ($N = 39$) and a No-Insomnia samples ($N = 253$) according to whether they met or not DSM-5 criteria for insomnia. Descriptive statistics of the two subsamples are presented in Results and Table 1.

Table 1. Descriptive statistics of No-Insomnia and Insomnia samples.

	No-Insomnia Sample N (%)	Insomnia Sample N (%)		df	p
Continuous Variables			F		
Age					
M(SD)	33.13 (5.11)	34.10 (4.60)	1.254	1/289	0.264
Min-Max	19–46	22–42			
BMI Early Pregnancy					
M(SD)	22.59 (3.81)	22.92 (3.02)	0.197	1/245	0.658
Min-Max	15.63–42.52	17.44–28.98			
TEMPS-A Depressive					
M(SD)	5.49 (2.38)	8.70 (4.06)	**41.855**	1/248	**<0.001**
TEMPS-A Cyclothymic					
M(SD)	3.07 (2.94)	5.64 (3.66)	**20.226**	1/248	**<0.001**
TEMPS-A Hyperthymic					
M(SD)	10.73 (3.76)	9.73 (4.80)	1.889	1/245	0.171
TEMPS-A Irritable					
M(SD)	1.88 (2.21)	4.15 (3.29)	**26.140**	1/242	**<0.001**
TEMPS-A Anxious					
M(SD)	5.01 (4.04)	10.27 (5.35)	**43.933**	1/242	**<0.001**
EPDS					
M(SD)	5.26 (3.77)	10.46 (2.61)	**52.439**	1/289	**<0.001**
SAS					
M(SD)	33.51 (6.52)	39.94 (5.69)	**31.315**	1/271	**<0.001**
HCL-32					
M(SD)	11.68 (6.56)	15.43 (6.58)	**8.674**	1/254	**0.004**
PSQI Global Score					
M(SD)	5.75 (3.02)	12.29 (2.89)	**144.850**	1/276	**<0.001**
Categorical Variables			Chi-squared test		
Level of Education			0.691	2	0.708
Middle school	14 (5.6)	1 (2.6)			
High school	101 (40.1)	17 (43.6)			
University/Postgraduate	137 (54.4)	21 (53.8)			
N/A	1	-			

Table 1. Cont.

	No-Insomnia Sample N (%)	Insomnia Sample N (%)		df	p
Occupation			1.512	1	0.219
Unemployed	55 (21.8)	5 (13.2)			
Employed	197 (78.2)	33 (86.8)			
N/A	1	1			
Partner			0.474	1	0.491
No	3 (1.2)	0 (0)			
Yes	240 (98.8)	38 (100)			
N/A	10	1			
BMI cutoff			2.533	3	0.469
Underweight	20 (9.1)	2 (7.4)			
Normal weight	152 (69.1)	17 (63.0)			
Overweight	41 (18.6)	8 (29.6)			
Obese	7 (3.2)	0 (0)			
N/A	33	12			
BMI—Range Weight Gain			0.389	2	0.823
Under range	91 (44.0)	9 (39.1)			
Normal	81 (39.1)	9 (39.1)			
Above range	35 (16.9)	5 (21.7)			
N/A	46	16			
Medical Conditions			0.020	1	0.888
No	192 (75.9)	30 (76.9)			
Yes	61 (24.1)	9 (23.1)			
Psychiatric History			3.068	1	0.080
No	205 (81.3)	27 (69.2)			
Yes	47 (18.7)	12 (30.8)			
N/A	1	-			
Previous Psychopharmacological Therapy			16.772	1	<0.001
No	238 (94.1)	29 (74.4)			
Yes	15 (5.9)	10 (25.6)			
Current Psychopharmacological Therapy			0.058	1	0.810
No	248 (98.0)	38 (97.4)			
Yes	5 (2.0)	1 (2.6)			
Psychiatric Family History			10.287	1	0.001
No	192 (75.9)	20 (51.3)			
Yes	61 (24.1)	19 (48.7)			
Menstrual Cycle Regularity			0.446	1	0.504
No	49 (19.6)	9 (24.3)			
Yes	201 (80.4)	28 (75.7)			
N/A	4	2			
Premenstrual Syndrome			3.199	1	0.074
No	137 (55.0)	15 (39.5)			
Yes	112 (45.0)	23 (60.5)			
N/A	4	1			
Others Completed Pregnancies			0.118	1	0.731
No	156 (62.4)	22 (59.5)			
Yes	94 (37.6)	15 (40.5)			
N/A	3	2			
Abortions			1.746	1	0.186
No	181 (72.7)	23 (62.2)			
Yes	68 (27.3)	14 (37.8)			
N/A	4	2			

Table 1. Cont.

	No-Insomnia Sample N (%)	Insomnia Sample N (%)		df	p
Caffeine			1.576	1	0.209
No	126 (50.4)	15 (39.5)			
Yes	124 (49.6)	23 (60.5)			
N/A	3	1			
Tobacco			0.053	1	0.818
No	221 (90.2)	32 (91.4)			
Yes	24 (8.6)	3 (8.6)			
N/A	8	4			
Alcohol			0.202	1	0.653
No	245 (98.4)	37 (97.4)			
Yes	4 (1.6)	1 (2.6)			
N/A	4	1			
Narcotic Substances			1.073	1	0.300
No	248 (99.2)	37 (97.4)			
Yes	2 (0.8)	1 (2.6)			
N/A	3	1			
Assisted Fertilization			4.683	1	0.030
No	209 (83.9)	36 (97.3)			
Yes	40 (16.1)	1 (2.7)			
N/A	4	2			
Past Perinatal Psychiatric Disorders			9.882	1	0.002
No	236 (93.7)	29 (78.4)			
Yes	16 (6.3)	8 (21.6)			
N/A	1	2			
Pregnancy Complications			0.052	1	0.819
No	183 (73.2)	27 (75.0)			
Yes	67 (26.8)	9 (25.0)			
N/A	3	3			
Rest period			0.003	1	0.955
No	191 (76.1)	28 (75.7)			
Yes	60 (23.9)	9 (24.3)			
N/A	2	12			
Hospitalization During Pregnancy			0.767	1	0.381
No	237 (93.7)	36 (97.3)			
Yes	16 (6.3)	1 (2.7)			
N/A	-	2			
Partner's Support			1.526	1	0.217
No	14 (5.6)	4 (10.8)			
Yes	238 (94.4)	33 (89.2)			
N/A	1	2			
Family's Support			2.604	1	0.107
No	52 (20.6)	12 (32.4)			
Yes	200 (79.4)	25 (67.6)			
N/A	1	2			
Stressful Events			0.065	1	0.799
No	136 (54.8)	20 (52.6)			
Yes	112 (45.2)	18 (47.4)			
N/A	5	1			
ISQ—T0			145.953	1	<0.001
No	240 (94.9)	8 (20.5)			
Yes	13 (5.1)	31 (70.5)			
ISQ—T1			7.528	1	0.006
No	42 (93.3)	2 (50.0)			
Yes	3 (6.7)	2 (50.0)			

Note. N/A: data not available.

Participants provided written informed consent, in accordance with all applicable regulatory and Good Clinical Practice guidelines and in full respect of the Ethical Principles for Medical Research Involving Human Subjects, as adopted by the 18th World Medical Association General Assembly (WMA GA), Helsinki, Finland, June 1964, and subsequently amended by the 64th WMA GA, Fortaleza, Brazil, October 2013. It was approved by the local ethics committees (Boards of the Sant'Andrea Hospital, Rome and San Pietro Fatebenefratelli Hospital, Rome, the ethics committee of Lazio 1, San Camillo-Forlanini Hospital, Rome, Italy; 4 December 2017 Nr 2471/CE Lazio1).

3. Procedure and Measures

Screening tools were administered by psychologists of the Psychiatry Unit. Women were evaluated through a sociodemographic, clinical, and obstetric data collection sheet (Perinatal Interview; PI), the Pittsburgh Sleep Quality Index (PSQI), the Edinburgh Postnatal Depression Scale (EPDS), the Zung Self-Rating Anxiety Scale (SAS), the Hypomania CheckList-32 (HCL-32), the Temperament Evaluation of the Memphis, Pisa, Paris and San Diego-Autoquestionnaire (TEMPS-A), and the Insomnia Symptom Questionnaire (ISQ).

Insomnia was diagnosed according to standard diagnostic criteria at the time of the evaluation by two psychiatrists, sleep medicine specialists who were blind to the screening scores, using the Mini International Neuropsychiatric Interview Version 7 for DSM-5 [32].

Included measures for the screening evaluation were the following:

- **Perinatal Interview (PI)** is a paper-and-pencil questionnaire to collect sociodemographic and clinical information, allowing us to investigate predictive and protective factors for the development of psychiatric disorders. Besides place and date of birth, nationality, educational level, job, and marital status, the PI investigates habits (i.e., eating, drinking, and weight control), voluptuary substance use (including coffee, tobacco, and alcohol), physiological rhythms (i.e., time to go to sleep, waking time, and sleeping hours), past surgery, past and current pharmacological treatment, gynecological and obstetric history, focusing on the current and past pregnancies, past and current personal and family psychiatric history and any psychiatric treatment, stressful life events, partner and family/friends' support during pregnancy, and partner data.
- **The Pittsburgh Sleep Quality Index** (PSQI) [27,28] is a retrospective self-report questionnaire that measures sleep quality and disturbances over the previous month. The PSQI assesses seven clinically derived components of subjective sleep quality: 1. *sleep quality*, 2. *sleep latency*, 3. *sleep duration*, 4. *habitual sleep efficiency*, 5. *sleep disturbance*, 6. *use of sleep medications*, and 7. *daytime dysfunction*. The PSQI yields a global score that represents the sum of the seven component scores that are rated on a 4-point Likert scale ranging from 0 to 3, where 3 reflects the negative extreme of the Likert scale. A global score of 5 or higher is considered as an indicator of prominent sleep disturbance in at least two components or of moderate difficulties in more than three components, distinguishing between "good" and "bad" sleepers. In the Italian validation study [28], the PSQI showed high internal consistency with a Cronbach's alpha of 0.84.
- **The Edinburgh Postnatal Depression Scale** (EPDS) [33] is a 10-item self-report questionnaire administered to screen for depressive symptoms in both the antenatal and postnatal periods [34,35]. We used the recommended score of 13 or more that indicates probable major depression in postnatal Italian-speaking women [36]. In the Italian validation study, the EPDS showed good internal consistency with a Cronbach's alpha of 0.79.
- **The Zung Self-Rating Anxiety Scale** (SAS) [37] is a 20-item self-report assessment tool built to measure state anxiety levels. Raw scores range from 20 to 80. The initial cutoff was 50 [38], but the best cutoff was later proposed to be 40 for clinical settings and 36 for screening purposes [39]. The instrument is suited to investigate anxiety disorders and showed strong correlations with other similar instruments [40,41]. In this study, we used the Italian version [42].

- The Hypomania CheckList-32 (HCL-32) [43] is a 32-item self-rating questionnaire investigating the lifetime history of hypomanic symptoms. Individuals scoring ≥ 14 potentially have bipolar disorder/diathesis and should be carefully interviewed. The ideal cutoff point of the Italian version is 12, with a sensitivity of 0.85 and a specificity of 0.61 [44].
- The Temperament Evaluation of the Memphis, Pisa, Paris and San Diego-Autoquestionnaire (TEMPS-A) [45], is a 110 item yes-or-no self-report questionnaire designed to assess affective temperament in psychiatric and healthy subjects. It consists of five temperament traits, i.e., depressive (D), cyclothymic (C), hyperthymic (H), irritable (I), and anxious (A). The prevailing temperament is considered the one on which the completer obtains the higher score. We used the validated Italian version [46].
- Insomnia Symptom Questionnaire (ISQ) [31] is a 13-item self-report instrument designed to assess respondents' perceptions about their daytime functioning, nighttime sleep, and identify insomnia. The ISQ items are based on DSM-IV criteria for primary insomnia [2] and are consistent with the American Academy of Sleep Medicine's (AASM) Research Diagnostic Criteria (RDC) [47]. Items 1, 2, or 5 (example item: *During the past month did you have difficulties falling asleep?*) are used to determine the presence, frequency, and duration of sleep symptom criteria (example: *How long did the symptom last?*; example answer: # *weeks/months/years*) and are rated on a 6-point Likert scale, ranging from 0 (*never*) to 5 (*always/5–7 times a week*). Items 6–13 are used to identify significant daytime consequences of the sleep complaint (example item: *During the past month have your sleep difficulties affected your work?*) and are rated on a 5-point Likert scale, ranging from 0 (*not at all*) to 4 (*extremely*). The final outcome of the ISQ is obtained through a dichotomous response (*yes/no*) to the three sleep criteria (*sleep symptom criterion* items 1, 2, or 5; *duration criterion* items 1, 2, or 5; *daytime impairment criterion* items 6–13), which results in the "presence" (3 yes answer) or "absence" of insomnia. In the validation study [31], the ISQ obtained a Cronbach's alpha of 0.89, indicating a high degree of internal consistency. In our sample, the ISQ obtained a Cronbach's alpha of 0.92, showing comparable if not higher internal consistency. The Italian translation of the ISQ was carried out through a direct and reverse translation process [48]. Specifically, a bilingual Italian/English psychiatrist translated the ISQ from English to Italian. Subsequently, another bilingual Italian/English researcher back-translated the scale.

After discussing any differences between the two translations, the scale was back-translated by a native speaker researcher, unaware of previous translations. The Italian version of the ISQ includes 13 items, rated as in the original version.

4. Data Analyses

Descriptive statistics of the two samples were analyzed using the Chi-squared test for categorical variables and ANOVAs for continuous variables. The convergent validity of the Italian version of the ISQ has been assessed by conducting point-biserial correlations (r_{pb}) between the ISQ and the PSQI global score. We also dichotomized the PSQI global score at two cutoffs (> 5 and > 10) reflecting the scores used in the original study [31]. Discriminant validity has been evaluated between the ISQ and EPDS, HCL-32, and SAS global scores. ISQ reliability was tested using Cronbach's alpha and test-retest reliability was assessed by examining the correlation between the total ISQ score in the antenatal (T0) and postnatal (T1) period for a subsample of participants ($N = 49$) who completed the ISQ both antenatally and six months postpartum. ISQ accuracy, sensitivity, specificity, and negative and positive predictive power were also investigated. Furthermore, to determine the best cutoff score of the PSQI that optimally detected cases defined by a presence or absence of a DSM-5 insomnia diagnosis, the receiver operating characteristic (ROC) curve analysis was run.

The IBM SPSS-25 statistical package (IBM Inc., Armonk NY, USA, 2017) was used for all analyses.

5. Results

5.1. Descriptive Statistics

5.1.1. No-Insomnia Sample

The No-Insomnia sample included 265 Italian-fluent adult women of the general population screened during their third trimester of pregnancy (T0). The final sample consisted of 253 women, aged 19–46 (*mean* = 33.13 years; *SD* = 5.11).

5.1.2. Insomnia Sample

The Insomnia sample included 39 women, screened during their third trimester of pregnancy (T0). Participants were aged 22–42 (*mean* = 34.10 years; *SD* = 4.60).

Statistically significant differences were found between the *No-Insomnia* and *Insomnia Samples* on TEMPS-A Depressive ($F_{(1248)}$ = 41.885; $p < 0.001$), Cyclothymic ($F_{(1248)}$ = 20.226; $p < 0.001$), Irritable ($F_{(1242)}$ = 26.140; $p < 0.001$), Anxious ($F_{(1242)}$ = 43.933; $p < 0.001$), and TEMPS-A Prevailing Temperament ($F_{(1245)}$ = 4.943; $p = 0.027$), on EPDS ($F_{(1289)}$ = 52.439; $p < 0.001$), on SAS ($F_{(1271)}$ = 31.315; $p < 0.001$), on HCL-32 ($F_{(1254)}$ = 8.674; $p = 0.004$), and on PSQI Global Score ($F_{(1276)}$ = 144.850; $p < 0.001$). Furthermore, statistically significant differences were found between the No-Insomnia and Insomnia Samples on Previous Psychopharmacological Therapy (χ^2 = 16.772; $p < 0.001$), Psychiatric Family History (χ^2 = 10.287; $p = 0.001$), Medically Assisted Reproduction (χ^2 = 4.683; $p = 0.030$), Past Perinatal Psychiatric Disorders (χ^2 = 9.882; $p = 0.002$), on ISQ at T0 (χ^2 = 145.953; $p < 0.001$), and ISQ at T1 (χ^2 = 7.528; $p = 0.006$). Table 1 presents descriptive statistics, including all characteristics considered in both samples.

5.2. Criterion Validity of the ISQ

The criterion validity of the ISQ was assessed by examining the diagnostic accuracy of ISQ (antenatal period—T0) outcomes referenced to dichotomized PSQI scores (antenatal period—T0) (Table 2).

Table 2. Cross-tabulations between PSQI global score (cut-off of >5 and >10) and ISQ (T0) classifications of subjects (No-Insomnia and Insomnia).

		PSQI Global Score		PSQI Global Score		Total
		≤5	>5	≤10	>10	
ISQ						
No-Insomnia		124	122	216	20	236
Insomnia		0	42	18	24	42
Score (Yes or No)		124	154	234	44	278

PSQI global score > 5: χ^2 = 39.837 $p < 0.001$. PSQI global score > 10: χ^2 = 63.391 $p < 0.001$.

The ISQ score (antenatal period—T0) was significantly correlated with all the scales employed (antenatal period—T0), which are indicative of adequate convergent and discriminant validity (Table 3).

Table 3. Correlations matrix between the ISQ (T0) total score and other scales (T0).

		ISQ	PSQI	SAS	EPDS	HCL-32
ISQ	r_{pb}	-	0.519	0.352	0.366	0.167
	p		<0.001	<0.001	<0.001	0.007
	N	292	278	273	291	256

Abbreviations: EPDS: Edinburgh Postnatal Depression Scale; HCL-32: Hypomania CheckList-32; ISQ: Insomnia Symptom Questionnaire; PSQI: Pittsburgh Sleep Quality Index; SAS: Zung Self-rating Anxiety Scale.

5.3. Reliability Statistic and Test–Retest Reliability

The entire ISQ scale showed excellent reliability with a Cronbach's alpha of 0.92. The φ correlation coefficients were calculated to assess the test–retest reliability of the ISQ for a subsample of participants ($N = 49$) who completed the ISQ antenatally (T0) and postnatally (6-months postdelivery; T1). The correlation for the ISQ scores was 0.491, $p < 0.001$.

Screening Accuracy of the ISQ

In line with the formulated hypothesis, the ISQ offers a good diagnostic accuracy within the collected sample, it correctly identified 80% of cases identified by the DSM-5. The ISQ total score showed a diagnostic accuracy of 93% with a sensitivity of 79.5%, a specificity of 94.9%, a positive predictive power (PPP) of 70.5%, and a negative predictive power (NPP) of 96.8% (Table 4).

Table 4. Cross-tabulations between DSM-5 diagnosis and ISQ classifications of subjects (No-Insomnia and Insomnia).

	DSM-5 Diagnosis		Total
	Insomnia	No-Insomnia	
ISQ			
Insomnia	31	13	44
No-Insomnia	8	240	248
Total	39	253	292

$\chi^2 = 145.95; p \leq 0.001$ Cramér's V = 0.707, $p \leq 0.001$.

Furthermore, PSQI global score showed a high diagnostic accuracy within the collected sample, with an AUC value of 0.934 ($SE = 0.018$) (Figure 1). Through the ROC curve, it is also possible to identify the *best cutoff*, i.e., the value of the test that maximizes the difference between true positives and false positives (Youden's index) [49]. In our case, the best cutoff for the PSQI is 8.5 which is associated with a sensitivity of 89% and a false positive rate of 17%.

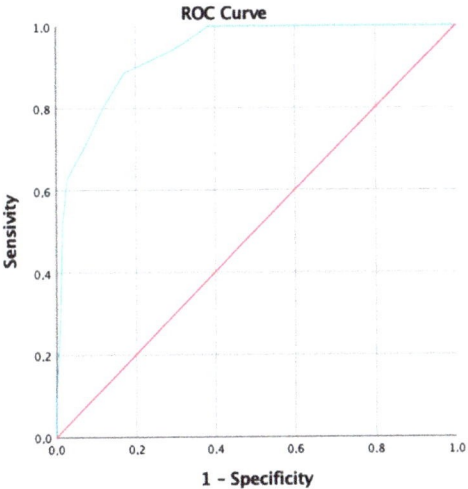

Figure 1. Graphical representation of receiver operator characteristic curve of the PSQI global score.

6. Discussion

Sleep disorders in pregnant women and new mothers are frequent. They may enhance distress levels [11] and expose them to postpartum depression [18]. Perinatal depression has a deep impact on mothers and their partners with significant consequences on the infant that includes increased risk for low birth weight and prematurity, impairment on the interaction between mother and child, infant malnutrition during the first year of life, as well as on the cognitive and emotional development of the child [50,51]. Suicidal behavior is the main maternal complication of perinatal depression and is the second most common cause of mortality in postpartum women [52]. Hence, there is a need to assess and monitor insomnia during the perinatal period. Specific instruments to rate insomnia during this period are few; the Insomnia Symptom Questionnaire [31] is short and easy-to-use, and validated to identify insomnia in late pregnancy but had not received heretofore validation in Italian. Our study investigated the psychometric properties of the Italian Version of the ISQ in pregnant women with and without DSM-5 insomnia disorder, investigating the validity, reliability, and convergent and discriminant validity of the tool during late pregnancy and 6-months postpartum according to the DSM-5 criteria. We used the Italian version of the ISQ and also investigated a set of variables that included assessments of temperament, depression, anxiety, and hypomania.

In agreement with the literature [53], results showed that women with psychiatric family history, past perinatal psychiatric disorders, and those with past and current psychopharmacological treatment, exhibited more sleep impairments throughout pregnancy and postpartum compared to women without any history of psychiatric disorder. Additionally, women with more sleep disturbances in mid and late pregnancy showed more depressive and anxiety symptoms than women with fewer sleep disturbances [54–56], and significantly higher mean score on HCL-32, indicating bipolar disorder/diathesis [57]. As reported in the literature and confirmed by our samples, anxious, cyclothymic, depressive, and irritable affective temperaments were related to more dysfunctional sleep patterns [12,58,59]. Further, it is not surprising that significantly more women undergoing assisted reproductive treatment were in our Insomnia Sample. Short sleep duration, excessive daytime sleepiness, and poor sleep quality are common in women undergoing in vitro fertilization (IVF), and sleep duration may be a mediator of important markers of IVF success [60].

The findings provided evidence for the very high internal consistency of the Italian version of ISQ (Cronbach's alpha of 0.92) with a better reliability coefficient compared to the original version [31]. Results also showed that the Italian version of the ISQ correlates strongly with established screening instruments, known to be sensitive to clinical insomnia such as the PSQI. The PSQI is used for subjective assessment of sleep quality and for identifying good and bad sleepers. However, it was not designed to assess insomnia based on diagnostic criteria or to investigate insomnia in the perinatal period. PSQI reliability and validity for identifying people who have difficulty initiating or maintaining sleep, necessary symptoms for the diagnosis of insomnia, may be improved by using a more stringent cutoff score than suggested (>5) [27,31,61,62]. Our results indicate that the best PSQI cutoff score to assess insomnia is 8.5 with a sensitivity of 89% and a false positive rate of 17%. In addition, the ISQ final score was significantly correlated with all the scales employed to investigate depression, anxiety, and hypomania, which indicates adequate convergent and discriminant validity.

The utility of this tool in pregnancy may be to identify women with persistent severe sleep problems. This may be clinically relevant given the emerging evidence that sleep disturbance increases the risk for adverse pregnancy outcomes.

It is curious that in our sample, only 44 pregnant women out of the final 292 included (15.07%) had insomnia. The literature generally reports higher prevalence rates in the third trimester of pregnancy, the time of our assessment, from 39.7% [9] to 42.4% [63]. It is possible that the different diagnostic methods used account for the discrepancy in findings.

7. Conclusions

Even though polysomnography is the most objective method for the assessment of most sleep disorders, the ICSD-3 and DSM-5 do not recommend it for the diagnosis of insomnia disorder due to its low feasibility. Subjective measures of sleep are a widespread issue in sleep research; however, daily fluctuations of sleep are hardly described by self-report questionnaires, such as the ISQ, which aims to investigate sleep quality over the past month. Furthermore, self-report estimates are very vulnerable to recall bias and overt or covert tendency to exaggerate the number and severity of symptoms [64]. A further possible limitation of the study could be related to the relatively small sample size to assess the test-retest reliability of the ISQ in a subsample of participants ($N = 49$). The fact that the original ISQ focused on the DSM-IV-TR, while we used the DSM-5, did not affect our results, inasmuch as the two diagnostic versions do not substantially modify insomnia diagnosis.

Future research should focus on the impact of maternal insomnia, as assessed through the ISQ, on future parenting style and child development, so as to identify methods to reduce it and ensure good maternal sleep in the perinatal period [65].

In conclusion, the results of the present study indicate that the ISQ is a useful, valid, and reliable tool for the assessment of perinatal insomnia also in the Italian language. The Italian version appears to be equivalent to the original version and to provide good and reliable discrimination between normal and pathological groups. The tool could be easily administered by obstetrics staff in everyday clinical practice.

Author Contributions: L.D.C., G.A., A.E.K. and M.B. designed the study; C.M. and E.R. designed and performed statistics, implemented the database, and performed literature searches, A.E.K., G.D.K., T.C. and L.D.C. searched the literature and provided the first draft, M.B., L.D.C., A.E.K. and G.A. saw and assessed patients; P.R., G.D.K., T.C. and G.A. supervised the writing of the manuscript and provided the final draft. All authors have accepted responsibility for the entire content of this manuscript, viewed, and approved its submission. All authors have read and agreed to the published version of the manuscript.

Funding: This study has received no funding.

Institutional Review Board Statement: This research, which involved human subjects only, complied with all relevant national regulations, institutional policies and is in accordance with the tenets of the Helsinki Declaration (as revised in 2013), and has been approved by the authors' Institutional Review Boards (Board of the Sant'Andrea Hospital, Rome) and ethics committee of Lazio 1, San Camillo-Forlanini Hospital, Rome, Italy (4/12/2017 Nr 2471/CE Lazio1).

Informed Consent Statement: Informed consent was obtained from all individuals included in this study.

Data Availability Statement: The dataset used and analyzed in the current study is available from the corresponding author upon reasonable request.

Acknowledgments: The authors gratefully acknowledge the contribution of Mimma Ariano, Ales Casciaro, Teresa Prioreschi, and Susanna Rospo, Librarians of the Sant'Andrea Hospital, School of Medicine and Psychology, Sapienza University, Rome, for rendering precious bibliographic material accessible.

Conflicts of Interest: The authors declare no conflict of interest.

References

1. American Psychiatric Association. *Diagnostic and Statistical Manual of Mental Disorders: Fifth Edition (DSM-5)*, 5th ed.; American Psychiatric Association: Arlington, VA, USA, 2013.
2. American Psychiatric Association. *Diagnostic and Statistical Manual of Mental Disorders, Fourth Edition, Text Revision (DSM-IV-TR)*, 4th ed.; American Psychiatric Association: Arlington, VA, USA, 2000; Volume 1, ISBN 9780890423349.
3. *International Classification of Sleep Disorders*, 3rd ed.; American Academy of Sleep Medicine (Ed.) American Academy of Sleep Medicine: Darien, IL, USA, 2014; ISBN 9780991543410.
4. Lee, K.A. Alterations in sleep during pregnancy and postpartum: A review of 30 years of research. *Sleep Med. Rev.* **1998**, *2*, 231–242. [CrossRef]
5. Mindell, J.A.; Cook, R.A.; Nikolovski, J. Sleep patterns and sleep disturbances across pregnancy. *Sleep Med.* **2015**, *16*, 483–488. [CrossRef] [PubMed]
6. Tomfohr, L.M.; Buliga, E.; Letourneau, N.L.; Campbell, T.S.; Giesbrecht, G.F. Trajectories of Sleep Quality and Associations with Mood during the Perinatal Period. *Sleep* **2015**, *38*, 1237–1245. [CrossRef] [PubMed]

7. Plancoulaine, S.; Flori, S.; Bat-Pitault, F.; Patural, H.; Lin, J.-S.; Franco, P. Sleep Trajectories among Pregnant Women and the Impact on Outcomes: A Population-Based Cohort Study. *Matern. Child Health J.* **2017**, *21*, 1139–1146. [CrossRef]
8. Sedov, I.D.; Cameron, E.E.; Madigan, S.; Tomfohr-Madsen, L.M. Sleep quality during pregnancy: A meta-analysis. *Sleep Med. Rev.* **2017**, *38*, 168–176. [CrossRef]
9. Sedov, I.D.; Anderson, N.J.; Dhillon, A.K.; Tomfohr-Madsen, L.M. Insomnia symptoms during pregnancy: A meta-analysis. *J. Sleep Res.* **2020**, *30*, e13207. [CrossRef] [PubMed]
10. Tochikubo, O.; Ikeda, A.; Miyajima, E.; Ishii, M. Effects of Insufficient Sleep on Blood Pressure Monitored by a New Multibiomedical Recorder. *Hypertension* **1996**, *27*, 1318–1324. [CrossRef] [PubMed]
11. Otchet, F. General health and psychological symptom status in pregnancy and the puerperium: What is normal? *Obstet. Gynecol.* **1999**, *94*, 935–941. [CrossRef]
12. Koukopoulos, A.; Mazza, C.; De Chiara, L.; Sani, G.; Simonetti, A.; Kotzalidis, G.D.; Armani, G.; Callovini, G.; Bonito, M.; Parmigiani, G.; et al. Psychometric Properties of the Perinatal Anxiety Screening Scale Administered to Italian Women in the Perinatal Period. *Front. Psychiatry* **2021**, *12*, 684579. [CrossRef]
13. Kamysheva, E.; Skouteris, H.; Wertheim, E.H.; Paxton, S.J.; Milgrom, J. A prospective investigation of the relationships among sleep quality, physical symptoms, and depressive symptoms during pregnancy. *J. Affect. Disord.* **2010**, *123*, 317–320. [CrossRef]
14. Hertenstein, E.; Feige, B.; Gmeiner, T.; Kienzler, C.; Spiegelhalder, K.; Johann, A.; Jansson-Fröjmark, M.; Palagini, L.; Rucker, G.; Riemann, D.; et al. Insomnia as a predictor of mental disorders: A systematic review and meta-analysis. *Sleep Med. Rev.* **2019**, *43*, 96–105. [CrossRef] [PubMed]
15. Alvaro, P.K.; Roberts, R.; Harris, J.K. A Systematic Review Assessing Bidirectionality between Sleep Disturbances, Anxiety, and Depression. *Sleep* **2013**, *36*, 1059–1068. [CrossRef]
16. Taylor, D.; Lichstein, K.L.; Durrence, H.H. Insomnia as a Health Risk Factor. *Behav. Sleep Med.* **2003**, *1*, 227–247. [CrossRef]
17. Taylor, D.J.; Lichstein, K.L.; Durrence, H.H.; Reidel, B.W.; Bush, A.J. Epidemiology of Insomnia, Depression, and Anxiety. *Sleep* **2005**, *28*, 1457–1464. [CrossRef] [PubMed]
18. Spoormaker, V.I.; Bout, J.V.D. Depression and anxiety complaints; relations with sleep disturbances. *Eur. Psychiatry* **2005**, *20*, 243–245. [CrossRef] [PubMed]
19. Emamian, F.; Khazaie, H.; Okun, M.L.; Tahmasian, M.; Sepehry, A.A. Link between insomnia and perinatal depressive symptoms: A meta-analysis. *J. Sleep Res.* **2019**, *28*, e12858. [CrossRef]
20. Okun, M.L. Sleep and postpartum depression. *Curr. Opin. Psychiatry* **2015**, *28*, 490–496. [CrossRef]
21. Okun, M.L. Disturbed Sleep and Postpartum Depression. *Curr. Psychiatry Rep.* **2016**, *18*, 1–7. [CrossRef] [PubMed]
22. Lawson, A.; Murphy, K.E.; Sloan, E.; Uleryk, E.; Dalfen, A. The relationship between sleep and postpartum mental disorders: A systematic review. *J. Affect. Disord.* **2015**, *176*, 65–77. [CrossRef]
23. González-Mesa, E.; Cuenca-Marín, C.; Suarez-Arana, M.; Tripiana-Serrano, B.; Ibrahim-Díez, N.; Gonzalez-Cazorla, A.; Blasco-Alonso, M. Poor sleep quality is associated with perinatal depression. A systematic review of last decade scientific literature and meta-analysis. *J. Périnat. Med.* **2019**, *47*, 689–703. [CrossRef]
24. MacLean, J.V.; Faisal-Cury, A.; Chan, Y.-F.; Menezes, P.R.; Winters, A.; Joseph, R.; Huang, H. The relationship between sleep disturbance in pregnancy and persistent common mental disorder in the perinatal period (sleep disturbance and persistent CMD). *J. Ment. Health* **2015**, *24*, 375–378. [CrossRef]
25. Harrison-Hohner, J.; Coste, S.; Dorato, V.; Curet, L.B.; McCarron, D.; Hatton, D. Prenatal calcium supplementation and postpartum depression: An ancillary study to a randomized trial of calcium for prevention of preeclampsia. *Arch. Women's Ment. Health* **2001**, *3*, 141–146. [CrossRef]
26. Reichner, C.A. Insomnia and sleep deficiency in pregnancy. *Obstet. Med.* **2015**, *8*, 168–171. [CrossRef] [PubMed]
27. Buysse, D.J.; Reynolds, C.F., III; Monk, T.H.; Berman, S.R.; Kupfer, D.J. The Pittsburgh sleep quality index: A new instrument for psychiatric practice and research. *Psychiatry Res.* **1989**, *28*, 193–213. [CrossRef]
28. Curcio, G.G.; Tempesta, D.; Scarlata, S.; Marzano, C.; Moroni, F.; Rossini, P.M.; Ferrara, M.; De Gennaro, L. Validity of the Italian Version of the Pittsburgh Sleep Quality Index (PSQI). *Neurol. Sci.* **2012**, *34*, 511–519. [CrossRef] [PubMed]
29. Bastien, C.H.; Vallieres, A.; Morin, C.M. Validation of the Insomnia Severity Index as an outcome measure for insomnia research. *Sleep Med.* **2001**, *2*, 297–307. [CrossRef]
30. Castronovo, V.; Galbiati, A.; Marelli, S.; Brombin, C.; Cugnata, F.; Giarolli, L.; Anelli, M.M.; Rinaldi, F.; Ferini-Strambi, L. Validation study of the Italian version of the Insomnia Severity Index (ISI). *Neurol. Sci.* **2016**, *37*, 1517–1524. [CrossRef]
31. Okun, M.L.; Kravitz, H.M.; Sowers, M.F.; Moul, D.E.; Buysse, D.J.; Hall, M. Psychometric Evaluation of the Insomnia Symptom Questionnaire: A Self-report Measure to Identify Chronic Insomnia. *J. Clin. Sleep Med.* **2009**, *5*, 41–51. [CrossRef]
32. Sheehan, D.V. *Mini International Neuropsychiatric Interview Version 7.0.2 for DSM-5*; Harm Research Institute: Tampa, FL, USA, 2016.
33. Cox, J.L.; Holden, J.M.; Sagovsky, R. Detection of Postnatal Depression. *Br. J. Psychiatry* **1987**, *150*, 782–786. [CrossRef]
34. Murray, D.; Cox, J.L. Screening for depression during pregnancy with the edinburgh depression scale (EDDS). *J. Reprod. Infant Psychol.* **1990**, *8*, 99–107. [CrossRef]
35. McBride, H.L.; Wiens, R.M.; McDonald, M.J.; Cox, D.W.; Chan, E.K.H. The Edinburgh Postnatal De-pression Scale (EPDS): A rieview of the reported validity evidence. In *Validity and Validation in Social, Behavioral, and Health Sciences*; Zumbo, B.D., Ed.; Springer: New York, NY, USA, 2014; pp. 157–174.

36. Benvenuti, P. The Edinburgh Postnatal Depression Scale: Validation for an Italian sample. *J. Affect. Disord.* **1999**, *53*, 137–141. [CrossRef]
37. Zung, W.W. A Rating Instrument For Anxiety Disorders. *Psychosomatics* **1971**, *12*, 371–379. [CrossRef]
38. Zung, W.W.K. The Measurement of Affects: Depression and Anxiety. In *Modern Trends in Pharma-Copsychiatry*; Pichot, P., Olivier-Martin, R., Eds.; Karger Publishers AG: Basilea, Switzerland, 1974; Volume 7, pp. 170–188. ISBN 9783805516303.
39. Dunstan, D.A.; Scott, N. Norms for Zung's Self-rating Anxiety Scale. *BMC Psychiatry* **2020**, *20*, 90. [CrossRef] [PubMed]
40. Dunstan, D.A.; Scott, N.; Todd, A.K. Screening for anxiety and depression: Reassessing the utility of the Zung scales. *BMC Psychiatry* **2017**, *17*, 329. [CrossRef] [PubMed]
41. Tanaka-Matsumi, J.; Kameoka, V.A. Reliabilities and concurrent validities of popular self-report measures of depression, anxiety, and social desirability. *J. Consult. Clin. Psychol.* **1986**, *54*, 328–333. [CrossRef] [PubMed]
42. Conti, L. The Zung Self-Rating Anxiety Scale (SAS). In *Repertorio Delle Scale di Valutazione in Psichiatria, Vol.1*; Conti, L., Ed.; SEE: Firenze, Italy, 1999; pp. 561–563.
43. Angst, J.; Adolfsson, R.; Benazzi, F.; Gamma, A.; Hantouche, E.; Meyer, T.D.; Skeppar, P.; Vieta, E.; Scott, J. The HCL-32: Towards a self-assessment tool for hypomanic symptoms in outpatients. *J. Affect. Disord.* **2005**, *88*, 217–233. [CrossRef]
44. Carta, M.G.; Hardoy, M.C.; Cadeddu, M.; Murru, A.; Campus, A.; Morosini, P.L.; Gamma, A.; Angst, J. The accuracy of the Italian version of the Hypomania Checklist (HCL-32) for the screening of bipolar disorders and comparison with the Mood Disorder Questionnaire (MDQ) in a clinical sample. *Clin. Pract. Epidemiol. Ment. Health* **2006**, *2*, 2. [CrossRef]
45. Akiskal, H.S.; Akiskal, K.K.; Haykal, R.F.; Manning, J.S.; Connor, P.D. TEMPS-A: Progress towards validation of a self-rated clinical version of the Temperament Evaluation of the Memphis, Pisa, Paris, and San Diego Autoquestionnaire. *J. Affect. Disord.* **2005**, *85*, 3–16. [CrossRef]
46. Pompili, M.; Girardi, P.; Tatarelli, R.; Iliceto, P.; De Pisa, E.; Tondo, L.; Akiskal, K.K.; Akiskal, H.S. TEMPS-A (Rome): Psychometric validation of affective temperaments in clinically well subjects in mid- and south Italy. *J. Affect. Disord.* **2008**, *107*, 63–75. [CrossRef]
47. Edinger, J.D.; Bonnet, M.H.; Bootzin, R.R.; Doghramji, K.; Dorsey, C.M.; Espie, C.A.; Jamieson, A.O.; McCall, W.; Morin, C.M.; Stepanski, E.J. Derivation of Research Diagnostic Criteria for Insomnia: Report of an American Academy of Sleep Medicine Work Group. *Sleep* **2004**, *27*, 1567–1596. [CrossRef] [PubMed]
48. Behling, O.; Law, K. *Translating Questionnaires and Other Research Instruments*; SAGE Publications, Inc.: Thousand Oaks, CA, USA, 2000; ISBN 9780761918240.
49. Youden, W.J. Index for Rating Diagnostic Tests. *Cancer* **1950**, *3*, 32–35. [CrossRef]
50. Hannigan, L.J.; Eilertsen, E.M.; Gjerde, L.C.; Reichborn-Kjennerud, T.; Eley, T.C.; Rijsdijk, F.; Ystrom, E.; A McAdams, T. Maternal prenatal depressive symptoms and risk for early-life psychopathology in offspring: Genetic analyses in the Norwegian Mother and Child Birth Cohort Study. *Lancet Psychiatry* **2018**, *5*, 808–815. [CrossRef]
51. Parsons, C.; Young, K.; Rochat, T.; Kringelbach, M.; Stein, A. Postnatal depression and its effects on child development: A review of evidence from low- and middle-income countries. *Br. Med Bull.* **2011**, *101*, 57–79. [CrossRef]
52. Lindahl, V.; Pearson, J.L.; Colpe, L. Prevalence of suicidality during pregnancy and the postpartum. *Arch. Women's Ment. Health* **2005**, *8*, 77–87. [CrossRef] [PubMed]
53. Coble, P.A.; Reynolds, C.F.; Kupfer, D.J.; Houck, P.R.; Day, N.L.; Giles, D.E. Childbearing in women with and without a history of affective disorder. II. Electroencephalographic sleep. *Compr. Psychiatry* **1994**, *35*, 215–224. [CrossRef]
54. Wolfson, A.R.; Crowley, S.J.; Anwer, U.; Bassett, J.L. Changes in Sleep Patterns and Depressive Symptoms in First-Time Mothers: Last Trimester to 1-Year Postpartum. *Behav. Sleep Med.* **2003**, *1*, 54–67. [CrossRef]
55. Osnes, R.S.; Roaldset, J.O.; Follestad, T.; Eberhard-Gran, M. Insomnia late in pregnancy is associated with perinatal anxiety: A longitudinal cohort study. *J. Affect. Disord.* **2019**, *248*, 155–165. [CrossRef] [PubMed]
56. Osnes, R.S.; Eberhard-Gran, M.; Follestad, T.; Kallestad, H.; Morken, G.; Roaldset, J.O. Mid-pregnancy insomnia is associated with concurrent and postpartum maternal anxiety and obsessive-compulsive symptoms: A prospective cohort study. *J. Affect. Disord.* **2020**, *266*, 319–326. [CrossRef]
57. Sharma, V.; Mazmanian, D. Sleep loss and postpartum psychosis. *Bipolar Disord.* **2003**, *5*, 98–105. [CrossRef]
58. Ottoni, G.L.; Lorenzi, T.M.; Lara, D.R. Association of temperament with subjective sleep patterns. *J. Affect. Disord.* **2011**, *128*, 120–127. [CrossRef]
59. Oniszczenko, W.; Rzeszutek, M.; Stanisławiak, E. Affective Temperaments, Mood, and Insomnia Symptoms in a Nonclinical Sample. *Behav. Sleep Med.* **2017**, *17*, 355–363. [CrossRef]
60. Goldstein, C.A.; Lanham, M.S.; Smith, Y.R.; O'Brien, L.M. Sleep in women undergoing in vitro fertilization: A pilot study. *Sleep Med.* **2016**, *32*, 105–113. [CrossRef]
61. Backhaus, J.; Junghanns, K.; Broocks, A.; Riemann, D.; Hohagen, F. Test–retest reliability and validity of the Pittsburgh Sleep Quality Index in primary insomnia. *Psychosomatics* **2002**, *53*, 737–740. [CrossRef]
62. Violani, C.; Devoto, A.; Lucidi, F.; Lombardo, C.; Russo, P.M. Validity of a Short Insomnia Questionnaire: The SDQ. *Brain Res. Bull.* **2004**, *63*, 415–421. [CrossRef] [PubMed]
63. Salari, N.; Darvishi, N.; Khaledi-Paveh, B.; Vaisi-Raygani, A.; Jalali, R.; Daneshkhah, A.; Bartina, Y.; Mohammadi, M. A systematic review and meta-analysis of prevalence of insomnia in the third trimester of pregnancy. *BMC Pregnancy Childbirth* **2021**, *21*, 284. [CrossRef] [PubMed]

64. Krystal, A.D.; Edinger, J.D. Measuring sleep quality. *Sleep Med.* **2008**, *9*, S10–S17. [CrossRef]
65. Adler, I.; Weidner, K.; Eberhard-Gran, M.; Garthus-Niegel, S. The Impact of Maternal Symptoms of Perinatal Insomnia on Social-emotional Child Development: A Population-based, 2-year Follow-up Study. *Behav. Sleep Med.* **2020**, *19*, 303–317. [CrossRef]

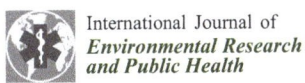

Opinion

Is Validating the Cutoff Score on Perinatal Mental Health Mood Screening Instruments, for Women and Men from Different Cultures or Languages, Really Necessary?

Stephen Matthey

Department of Clinical and Experimental Sciences, Faculty of Medicine and Surgery, Università degli Studi di Brescia, 25123 Brescia, Italy; travelresearch@hotmail.com

Abstract: *Background*: The most commonly used mood screening instrument in perinatal health is the Edinburgh Depression Scale. The screen-positive cut-off score on this scale, as for others, has been determined, via validation techniques, for over 20 languages/cultures, and for both women and men. While such validation appears to be considered essential, there are studies that could be interpreted to suggest that this is not an important consideration. *Methods*: Selective studies have been chosen to indicate these opposing points of view. *Results*: Examples of studies that support the notion of validating cut-off scores are described, as are examples of studies that appear not to support this point of view. *Conclusions*: (i) Clinical services and researchers need to be mindful of these opposing points of view, and openly discuss them when using screening cut-off scores for their respective populations. (ii) Researchers and Journals need to be more rigorous in ensuring this issue is correctly reported in studies, and/or openly discussed when relevant.

Keywords: perinatal; screening; validation; EPDS

Citation: Matthey, S. Is Validating the Cutoff Score on Perinatal Mental Health Mood Screening Instruments, for Women and Men from Different Cultures or Languages, Really Necessary? *IJERPH* **2022**, *19*, 4011. https://doi.org/10.3390/ijerph19074011

Academic Editor: Teodor T. Postolache

Received: 28 December 2021
Accepted: 17 March 2022
Published: 28 March 2022

Publisher's Note: MDPI stays neutral with regard to jurisdictional claims in published maps and institutional affiliations.

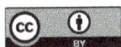

Copyright: © 2022 by the author. Licensee MDPI, Basel, Switzerland. This article is an open access article distributed under the terms and conditions of the Creative Commons Attribution (CC BY) license (https://creativecommons.org/licenses/by/4.0/).

1. Introduction

Validation of self-report mood screening questionnaires for the perinatal period, such as the Edinburgh Postnatal Depression Scale (EPDS) [1], is a practice that almost goes without question. Such validation produces an empirically derived cut-off score, or screen-positive score, that guides clinical services to decide when to refer a woman, or man, for further psychological assessment for the presence of whatever mood disorder the scale has been validated against (e.g., major depression; various anxiety disorders etc.). It also provides researchers with the validated cut-off score from which studies investigating issues such as prevalence, risk factors, and treatment effectiveness can be empirically explored.

The usual validation method is to compare the study sample's scores on the scale against the gold standard of diagnostic disorder status (e.g., DSM or ICD mental health disorders [2,3]), and to calculate its receiver operating characteristics (ROC). These ROC characteristics usually include the scale's sensitivity, specificity, and its positive predictive value (ppv), at all possible scores on the scale. The best desired mix of these is then chosen (sometimes based upon other resultant statistics) to determine the optimal screen-positive score for that sample, or population from which the sample was drawn.

Thus the EPDS has been translated, and validated, into many different languages, with reported optimum cut-off scores across cultures for depression, or depression and anxiety, currently varying from 4 or more [4] to 19 or more [5]. In addition, the optimal cut-off scores for men have been calculated in several different languages and/or cultures. Examples of such validation studies for women, with their recommended cut-off scores (which may be for different disorders, such as major or minor depression, or anxiety), include those in Ethiopia [6]: 6, 7, or 8 or more; Nigeria [7]: 9 or more; Vietnam [4]: 4 or more; Malta [8]: 14 or more; Denmark [9]: 11 or more, as well as the original English EPDS validation study [1]: 13 or more. For men, examples of such studies, with their recommended cut-off scores, include those in Vietnam [10]: 5 or more; England [11]: 11 or more; Saudi Arabia [12]: 9 or more; Sweden [13]: 12 or more; Australia [14]: 6 or more. and Italy [15]: 13 or more.

Some of the reasons investigators give as to why different optimal cut-off scores were obtained in their sample, compared to other cultural or gender groups, include that such groups may differ in their expression of depression or the actual symptoms experienced [4,9,10,12,16], as well as differences in the comprehension of the screening scale's items [4,6]. These reasons, as opposed to more procedural or psychometric reasons (e.g., different caseness criteria, or different gold-standard interviews, used across studies), would support the need to conduct validation studies in different populations to ensure any such emotional expressiveness, comprehension, or symptom experience differences are taken into account when screening women, and men, for possible emotional health difficulties.

All such validation studies thus inherently support the belief that the scale must be validated for each specific population, and that the optimal screen cut-off score should then be used in similar populations, both within research and clinical settings. The aim of this opinion piece is to create a critical debate in health professionals involved in the use of such screening scales, by describing studies that appear to support the opposite belief, that such scales do not need to be validated for different populations. This belief is either stated within the studies themselves, or can be inferred when a study has not used the previously validated cut-off score for that population without a reasonable rationale.

The purpose of this paper is therefore to question whether indeed such validations need to be done.

2. Materials and Methods

Selective studies will be reported that support the argument that screening scales, specifically the EPDS, should be validated regarding the optimal screen-positive cut-off score for each culture and/or gender (and sometimes for both pre and postnatal periods). Similarly, selective studies will be reported that appear to support, or could be interpreted to support, the counter argument—that there is now no need to validate the EPDS cut-off score for different cultures or genders, as a single cut-off score can be used for people from all cultures and/or genders. As some of what I say below may seem as criticism of various studies, I wish to emphasise that these are being used only as examples, and I do not exclude the fact I too may have made similar errors in my studies.

This methodology, of selectively reporting a number of studies to highlight the points being made, is considered by the author to be appropriate in the context of this being an opinion piece article, not a research study. This methodology has been used previously by the author [17] in a related discussion about emotional health screening with the EPDS.

The studies selected were chosen on the basis that (a) they provided examples which supported either position regarding whether or not validation of emotional screening scales needs to be undertaken across different populations; (b) the author was aware of these studies from his extensive reading of the literature over many years, and (c) sufficient numbers of such studies have been reported in this paper (approximately 22 for each side of the argument) to demonstrate that both sides of the argument are not simply supported by 'outlier' type studies (e.g., by just one or two studies).

3. Results

3.1. Studies Supporting the Validation of the EPDS across Cultures or Genders

The studies cited above, providing the optimal cut-off score on the EPDS for women or men in their specific culture or country, are by their very nature studies which clearly support the view that cross-cultural/gender validation studies need to be conducted if we wish to have empirical evidence guiding both clinical and research practice.

In addition some reviews also provide support for this argument. Gibson et al. [18], in their review of 37 EPDS validation studies across various cultures. concluded that their findings implied that "different cut-off scores should be used in different cultural groups"

(p. 359). Kozinsky and Dudas [19], in their review of 11 EPDS validation studies, also concluded this, stating "it is not advisable to use universal cut-off scores (on the EPDS), as there can be cultural differences . . . " (p. 101).

Housen et al. [20] stated that their study, validating various mental health instruments in India, showed "the importance of culturally adapting and validating screening instruments" (p. 361), while Heck et al. [21] commented that the EPDS may be culturally biased, and that its items need to be validated for conceptual equivalence in women from culturally diverse backgrounds.

Tran et al. [4], in studying the validity of the EPDS and other mood instruments for women in Vietnam (and on the EPDS for men), found much lower optimal cut-off scores than those for English-speaking western women and men. They gave as a possible reason for this finding that "Vietnamese people tend to report somatic symptoms more openly than psychiatric symptoms" (p. 286), and thus an instrument such as the EPDS, which does not include somatic symptoms, will result in a lower cut-off score being required to detect probably depressed people.

Harrington et al. [22] possibly best sum up this view, that one should not simply use a validated cut-off score from one culture with participants from another, or believe that an instrument developed for one culture is unquestionably valid in another culture, stating:

"Researchers and practitioners who use the EPDS (and PHQ-9) should be aware of the tools' limitations in their context and population . . . (and with) persons from diverse cultures whose conceptualizations and experiences of depression may not be fully assessed with Western-based screening tools even if validated quantitatively. New or adapted instruments that capture local linguistic and behavioral expressions of depression may need to be developed to improve accuracy of depression screening and diagnosis" (p. 958)

With respect to not just culture, but also the optimal cut-off scores on screening instruments for different perinatal time periods (antenatal/postnatal, or even different trimesters), Lau et al. [23] stated that "a cross-cultural understanding of the different cut-off points during different perinatal periods is crucial . . . " (p. 1141). They also stated that their findings of different cut-off scores being optimal for women from different areas of China, showed "the importance of proper validation for a psychiatric rating instrument in the different regions of China " (p. 1149).

3.2. Examples of Studies That Could Be Seen to Support the Argument That Screening Scales Do Not Need to Be Validated for Women, and Men, from Different Cultures or Countries

But in contrast to the above, there are an increasing number of studies that, for various reasons, either give the impression that the use of a validated cut-off score for a particular country, cultural group, or gender is not necessary, as a different one will suffice if it has been validated in a different group, or give the impression that one cut-off score could be used for all groups. The reasoning for these views seems to fall into five categories.

3.2.1. Continued Errors in Reading the Literature Regarding the Correct Validated Cutoff Scores

In 2006 I, with colleagues [17], reported on the frequent errors in reporting validated cut-off scores on the EPDS. Unfortunately, such errors continue. Examples where investigators have misinterpreted the original validation study's cut-off score for English-speaking postnatal women by Cox et al. [1] include those by [5,24–26]. In addition, Wroe et al. [27] incorrectly interpreted numerous studies when discussing the choice of the EPDS cut-off score for men, as explained by Matthey [28].

While incorrectly using a cut-off score of just one or two points difference from the validated score may seem to be negligible, Matthey et al. [17] demonstrated that not only can this have a major impact on reported rates of 'high scorers', but also—importantly— on the interpretation of whether or not rates of possible depression remain stable from pregnancy to postpartum.

3.2.2. Investigators Use a Validated Cutoff Score from a Different Cultural or Gender Group, Sometimes without Discussing the Possible Pitfalls of Doing This

Examples of such studies include:

Maleki et al. [29], in a study on Iranian fathers, used an EPDS cut-off score of 10 or more based upon that used in a study of principally Portuguese men [30]. They did not however give a rationale for using the same cut-off score for men from these two cultures, nor did they comment on the fact that the Portuguese study that they referred to had not given an empirical rationale for the cut-off score chosen for their men.

Do et al. [31] used a cut-off score of 12 or more for their Vietnamese female participants, without specifying why this was chosen, nor referring to an earlier study that had validated the EPDS for Vietnamese women against depression and some anxiety disorders, with a much lower cut-off score of 4 or more being optimal [4].

Affonso et al. [32] used the one cut-off score (of 10 or more) for women from nine different countries, across five continents. They chose this score as it was recommended by Cox et al. [1] in their original EPDS validation study with English-speaking women, but they did not discuss whether any of the other countries had had validation studies conducted (which in some cases there had been—e.g., Italy and Sweden), nor whether there could be an argument for questioning the use of an Anglo-score for women from very different cultures.

3.2.3. Investigators Choose to Use the Same Cutoff Score for Two or More Groups (e.g., Men and Women) or Different Cultures So That a Comparison Can Be Made Regarding Rates of Possible Depression, Even If They State That the Groups Have Different Validated Cutoff Scores

Examples of such studies include:

Afolabi et al. [16] used 13 or more on the EPDS for each of the three groups of mothers in their study: British mothers in the UK, immigrant Nigerian mothers in the UK, and Nigerian mothers in Nigeria. While they did however discuss how Nigerians can be less inclined to express distress through psychological, as opposed to physical or somatic symptoms, they did not discuss an earlier validation study on Nigerian women and the EPDS which had found a lower score was optimal [7].

Ramchandani et al. [33] used the same EPDS cut-off score for women and men, despite noting that the measure had been validated for men (who had a different optimal cut-off score to that for women). They stated "We therefore used the cut-off of >12 (13+) for both mothers and fathers for comparability" (p. 391).

Gonzalez-Mesa et al. [34] used 13 or more on the EPDS for both their Turkish and Spanish-speaking women, despite the fact that their reference regarding the Spanish version of the EPDS [35] reported that a different cut-off score, of 11 or more was found to be optimal.

Shakeel et al. [36] (2018) conducted a study using the EPDS in several cultural groups in Norway, with participants from Norway, Vietnam, Iran, Turkey, Pakistan, Sri Lanka, Eastern Europe, Africa south of the Sahara, East Asia, and South and Central America. They used a cut-off score of 10 or more for all of these groups, giving the rationale that this had been used in other epidemiolocal studies. While they report cultural differences with respect to perinatal traditions, and how this might be related to the obtained prevalence rates of possible depression, there is no discussion as to whether or not using the same cut-off score for such diverse groups is thus therefore the best approach.

3.2.4. Commonly Used/Internationally Recognized Cutoff Scores

Studies state that a certain cut-off score is now the internationally recognised one, though this seems to suggest that some International perinatal body has decreed this to be so, which to my knowledge is not the case. Those that state that a certain cut-off score is the one most commonly used are however often accurate, though this is usually because of two factors: (a) more studies have been conducted and published in English-speaking populations, which thus use the English-speaking validated EPDS cut-off score; (b) many studies from other cultures then also use these English-speaking validated cut-off sores, either inadvertently, or without fully justifying this, or not pointing out possible limitations of this approach (e.g., see Sections 3.2.2 and 3.2.3 above).

Examples of such studies include:

Afolabi et al. [16] (2017) state: " ... more recent studies have tended towards a general consensus for EPD cut-offs at 13 or more ... " (p. 429). Redinger et al. [37] state: "The internationally recognized threshold score for probable depression of ≥13 was used" (p. 31); Levis et al. [38] state " ... (scores on the on the EPDS) of 10 or higher and 13 or higher (are) typically used to identify women who might be depressed" (p. 1), and Eberhard-Gran et al. [39] state that a score of 10 or more "is frequently used in recent publications" (p. 114). Wesselhoeft et al. [40] used 13 or more for their samples of Danish, Vietnamese, and Tanzanian women, saying this score "is often used to identify women at risk for perinatal depression"(p. 59), citing English-speaking validation studies [1,41].

3.2.5. Meta-Analyses and Systematic Reviews Report Commonly Used Cutoff Scores or Report the Overall Optimal Cutoff Score on the EPDS by Aggregating Data from Different Studies

Examples of such studies include:

Levis et al. [38], using data from 58 studies across multiple cultures, concluded that 11 or more on the EPDS was the optimal screen-positive score when combining its sensitivity and specificity values. While they are clear that they are not recommending that services, or researchers, should simply use this cut-off score regardless of other factors (such as whether a service wishes to maximise sensitivity over specificity), and they are also clear that they were unable to do any cultural sub-group analyses, it is an interesting analysis that could lend weight to the argument that one cut-off score may suffice for all groups, rather than the need to consider different cut-off scores for different cultures.

Of note also is the meta-analysis of studies with men, by Cameron et al. [42]. These authors commented on the number of different EPDS cut-off scores used across the studies, making their analyses problematic. They thus stated "cut-off scores should be standardized (across measures) to ensure continuity in the literature" (p. 199). This difficulty, of using different cut-off scores to compare rates across cultures or groups, was also reported by Woody et al. [43] in their systematic review of perinatal depression in women. These views could be seen as a recommendation that one cut-off score should be agreed upon for use with men or women from all cultures, so as to allow comparisons in prevalence rates.

In addition, meta-analyses and reviews do not usually (if ever) have, as a stated criterion, that studies will only be included in their analyses if they have used the correct validated screening scale cut-off score for their population (or adequately discussed why they have not done so). This means that studies may be included in reviews or meta-analyses that have not used the empirically determined cut-off score for their sample, or not discussed potential limitations of this, thus lending weight to the argument that this is not a particularly important criterion.

4. Implementation in Clinical Practice

One could argue that validating a cut-off score is only really useful if is then used within clinical practice. If, however, services decide that it is too impractical to ensure women (or men) from different cultural backgrounds are screened using the validated cut-off score for their culture or gender, then having such validation studies is not clinically useful. Such impracticality could be for many reasons, including staff training difficulties, software modification difficulties, as well as the lack of specific research on when a migrant to a country is acculturated enough to warrant the use of the validated cut-off score on a scale for that country's 'indigenous' population, rather than from their 'home' country.

For example, in the health service where I work in Sydney, Australia, one cut-off score—the Anglo validated one (13 or more in pregnancy for possible minor depression)—is used for all women, regardless of culture. Brann et al. [26] also report a similar situation in Sweden. In Denmark, however, while the recent validation study [9] has led to the implementation of the validated Danish cut-off score in their clinical services, a group has been set-up to consider how the health service should implement the most appropriate cut-off score for non-Danish speaking women [44].

5. Discussion

Arguments, or implications, that validation studies are not warranted, appear to fall into various categories, as described above (Sections 3.2.1–3.2.5). I would argue that the research in this area would be greatly improved if investigators carefully consider, and justify, their use of screen-positive cut-off scores on whichever scale they are using in each of these categories. This is particularly important given the reports that different cultures or gender may express negative emotions differently (e.g., 4, 9, 10, 12), and hence screening scales need to be validated for each culture or gender group, and that these scores should thus be used, both in research and clinical practice.

Thus, studies that incorrectly cite a validated cut-off score (e.g., those similar to Section 3.2.1) need to be more diligent in their reading of the original source literature. Indeed, it is likely that many such errors are made because the investigators are only reading secondary literature, and they assume that this literature is accurate in the reporting of the primary source material, which unfortunately is often not the case.

If studies use a cut-off score that has not been validated for their population (e.g., those similar to Section 3.2.2), they should clearly state this, and discuss the implications of their decision. Similarly, those that choose to use the same cut-off score between different cultural or gender groups to facilitate comparisons, despite having explained that there are in fact different validated cut-off scores for their groups (e.g., those similar to Section 3.2.3), should discuss the implications of their decision, and how their findings would be different if they had used the validated score for each group.

Those that use a cut-off score based upon it being frequently used, or 'internationally recognised' (e.g., those similar to Section 3.2.4), should reference the body that states this, and should discuss the implications of whether or not women, or men, who are distressed may be missed if their group have been shown to require a lower cut-off score.

Finally, those studies that are similar to category Section 3.2.5, where they use aggregating techniques to determine which cut-off score can be used for all groups, should also discuss the implications of this strategy, with respect to the misclassification of the women or men from different cultural groups where their validated cut-off score is different to the one being proposed for all groups.

Journals could improve their evaluation of such studies by requiring authors to state that they have read the source material (and not just secondary material); that they have ascertained if a validated cut-off score exists, or does not exist, for their groups, and to give their rationale as to why they are choosing not to use this/these (if this is the case); and to discuss the implications of their findings if they had instead used the validated cut-off score if there is one (or different cut-off scores if more than one has been validated for that group). In particular, implications need to highlight whether the use of non-validated cut-off scores may therefore misclassify women, or men, as to their emotional health status (screen positive or screen negative).

6. Conclusions

There are many studies that determine the optimal screen-positive cut-off score for emotional health screening instruments, such as the EPDS, for women and men from different cultures or countries. These studies show that there is a great range of optimal scores depending upon the variables of culture and gender. There are also however a substantial number of studies which appear to indicate that validating cut-off scores for culture and gender is not considered that important, for a variety of reasons.

Clinical services and researchers need to be mindful of this difference in perspective or approach, and openly discuss this problematic issue when using screening instruments such as the EPDS.

Funding: This research received no external funding.

Institutional Review Board Statement: Ethical review and approval were waived for this study due to this being an Expert Opinion article, relying just on previously published papers and no new participant information.

Informed Consent Statement: Not applicable.

Data Availability Statement: Not applicable.

Acknowledgments: The author gratefully acknowledges the full contribution of IJERPH to the article-processing charges for this manuscript.

Conflicts of Interest: The author declares that in some of the cited papers he is an author or co-author. He has also conducted validation research in screening instruments for the perinatal period across cultures and genders, and has published a different type of screening measure due to his stated belief that ignoring cross-cultural issues, or gender issues, is a current weakness in our clinical and research practice.

References

1. Cox, J.; Holden, J.; Sagovsky, R. Detection of postnatal depression: Development of the 10 item Edinburgh Postnatal Depression Scale. *Brit. J. Psychiatry* **1987**, *150*, 782–786. [CrossRef] [PubMed]
2. American Psychiatric Association. *Diagnostic and Statistical Manual of Mental Disorders: DSM-5*, 5th ed.; American Psychiatric Publishing: Washington, DC, USA, 2013.
3. World Health Organization. *The ICD-10 Classification of Mental and Behavioural Disorders: Clinical Descriptions and Diagnostic Guidelines*; World Health Organization: Geneva, Switzerland, 1992; Volume 1.
4. Tran, T.D.; Tran, T.; La, B.; Lee, D.; Rosenthal, D.; Fisher, J. Screening for perinatal common mental disorders in women in the north of Vietnam: A comparison of three psychometric instruments. *J. Affect. Disord.* **2011**, *133*, 281–293. [CrossRef] [PubMed]
5. van der Westhuizen, C.; Brittain, K.; Koen, N.; Mare, K.; Zar, H.J.; Stein, D.J. Sensitivity and specificity of the SRQ-20 and the EPDS in diagnosing major depression ante- and postnatally in a South African birth cohort study. *Int. J. Ment. Health Addict.* **2018**, *16*, 175–186. [CrossRef]
6. Tesfaye, M.; Hanlon, C.; Wondimagegn, D.; Alem, A. Detecting postnatal mental disorders in Addis Ababa, Ethiopia: Validation of the Edinburgh Postnatal Depression Scale and Kessler Scales. *J. Affect. Disord.* **2010**, *122*, 102–108. [CrossRef]
7. Uwakwe, R. Affective (depressive) morbidity in puerperal Nigerian women: Validation of the Edinburgh postnatal depression scale. *Acta Psychiatr. Scand.* **2003**, *107*, 251–259. [CrossRef]
8. Felice, E.; Saliba, J.; Grech, V.; Cox, J. Validation of the Maltese version of the Edinburgh Postnatal Depression Scale. *Arch. Women's Ment. Health* **2006**, *9*, 75–80. [CrossRef]
9. Smith-Nielsen, J.; Matthey, S.; Lange, T.; Væver, M.S. Validation of the Danish Edinburgh Postnatal Depression Scale against DSM-5 and ICD-10 diagnostic criteria for depression. *BMC Psychiatry* **2018**, *18*, 393. [CrossRef]
10. Tran, T.D.; Tran, T.; Fisher, J. Validation of three psychometric instruments for screening for perinatal common mental disorders in men in the north of Vietnam. *J. Affect. Disord.* **2012**, *136*, 104–109. [CrossRef]
11. Edmondson, O.J.H.; Psychogiou, L.; Vlachos, H.; Netsi, E.; Ramchandani, P.G. Depression in fathers in the postnatal period: Assessment of the Edinburgh Postnatal Depression Scale as a screening measure. *J. Affect. Disord.* **2010**, *125*, 365–368. [CrossRef]
12. Shaheen, N.A.; AlAtiq, Y.; Thomas, A.; Alanazi, H.A.; AlZahrani, Z.E.; Younis, S.A.R.O.; Hussein, M.A. Paternal postnatal depression among fathers of newborn in Saudi Arabia. *Am. J. Men's Health* **2019**, *13*, 1557988319831219. [CrossRef]
13. Massoudi, P.; Hwang, C.P.; Wickberg, B. How well does the Edinburgh Postnatal Depression Scale identify depression and anxiety in fathers? A validation study in a population based Swedish sample. *J. Affect. Disord.* **2013**, *149*, 67–74. [CrossRef] [PubMed]
14. Matthey, S.; Barnett, B.E.W.; Kavanagh, D.J.; Howie, P. Validation of the Edinburgh Postnatal Depression Scale for men, and comparison of item endorsement with their partners. *J. Affect. Disord.* **2001**, *64*, 175–183. [CrossRef]
15. Loscalzo, Y.; Giannini, M.; Contena, B.; Gori, A.; Benvenuti, P. The Edinburgh Postnatal Depression Scale for Fathers: A contribution to the validation for an Italian sample. *Gen. Hosp. Psychiatry* **2015**, *37*, 251–256. [CrossRef]
16. Afolabi, O.; Bunce, L.; Lusher, J.; Banbury, S. Postnatal depression, maternal–infant bonding and social support: A cross-cultural comparison of Nigerian and British mothers. *J. Ment. Health* **2020**, *29*, 424–430. [CrossRef] [PubMed]
17. Matthey, S.; Henshaw, C.; Elliott, S.; Barnett, B. Variability in use of cut-off scores and formats on the Edinburgh Postnatal Depression Scale—Implications for clinical and research practice. *Arch. Women's Ment. Health* **2006**, *9*, 309–315. [CrossRef]
18. Gibson, J.; McKenzie-Mottarg, K.; Shakespeare, J.; Price, J.; Gray, R. A systematic review of studies validating the Edinburgh Postnatal Depression Scale in antepartum and postpartum women. *Acta Psychiatr. Scand.* **2009**, *119*, 350–364. [CrossRef]
19. Kozinszky, Z.; Dudas, R.B. Validation studies of the Edinburgh Postnatal Depression Scale for the antenatal period. *J. Affect. Disord.* **2015**, *176*, 95–105. [CrossRef]
20. Housen, T.; Lenglet, A.; Ariti, C.; Ara, S.; Shah, S.; Dar, M.; Hussain, A.; Paul, A.; Wagay, Z.; Viney, K.; et al. Validation of mental health screening instruments in the Kashmir Valley, India. *Transcult. Psychiatry* **2018**, *55*, 361–383. [CrossRef]

21. Heck, J.L. Screening for postpartum depression in American Indian/Alaska native women: A comparison of two instruments. *Am. Indian Alsk. Nativ. Ment. Health Res. (Online)* **2018**, *25*, 74–102. [CrossRef]
22. Harrington, B.J.; Klyn, L.L.; Ruegsegger, L.M.; Thom, A.; Jumbe, A.N.; Maliwichi, M.; Stockton, M.A.; Akiba, C.F.; Go, V.; Pence, B.W.; et al. Locally contextualizing understandings of depression, the EPDS, and PHQ-9 among a sample of postpartum women living with HIV in Malawi. *J. Affect. Disord.* **2021**, *281*, 958–966. [CrossRef]
23. Lau, Y.; Wang, Y.; Yin, L.; Chan, K.S.; Guo, X. Validation of the Mainland Chinese version of the Edinburgh Postnatal Depression Scale in Chengdu mothers. *Int. J. Nurs. Stud.* **2010**, *47*, 1139–1151. [CrossRef] [PubMed]
24. Jevitt, C.; Zapata, L.; Harrington, M.; Berry, E. Screening for perinatal depression with limited psychiatric resources. *J. Am. Psychiatri. Nurses Assoc.* **2006**, *11*, 359–363. [CrossRef]
25. Pakenham, K.I.; Smith, A.; Rattan, S.L. Applications of a stress and coping model to antenatal depressive symptomatology. *Psychol. Health Med.* **2007**, *12*, 266–277. [CrossRef]
26. Brann, E.; Fransson, E.; Wikman, A.; Kollia, N.; Nguyen, D.; Lilliecreutz, C.; Skalkidou, A. Who do we miss when screening for postpartum depression? A population-based study in a Swedish region. *J. Affect. Disord.* **2021**, *287*, 165–173. [CrossRef] [PubMed]
27. Wroe, J.; Campbell, L.; Fletcher, R.; McLoughland, C. "What am I thinking? Is this normal?" A cross-sectional study investigating the nature of negative thoughts, parental self-efficacy and psychological distress in new fathers. *Midwifery* **2019**, *79*, 102527. [CrossRef] [PubMed]
28. Matthey, S. Errors and omissions in reporting research using the Edinburgh Postnatal Depression Scale for fathers. *Midwifery* **2021**, *102*, 103071. [CrossRef] [PubMed]
29. Maleki, A.; Faghihzadeh, S.; Niroomand, S. The relationship between paternal prenatal depressive symptoms with postnatal depression: The PATH model. *Psychiatry Res.* **2018**, *269*, 102–107. [CrossRef]
30. Figueiredo, B.; Conde, A. Anxiety and depression symptoms in women and men from early pregnancy to 3-months postpartum: Parity differences and effects. *J. Affect. Disord.* **2011**, *132*, 146–157. [CrossRef]
31. Do, T.K.L.; Nguyen, T.T.H.; Pham, T.T.H. Postpartum Depression and Risk Factors among Vietnamese women. *BioMed Res. Int.* **2018**, *2018*, 4028913. [CrossRef]
32. Affonso, D.D.; De, A.K.; Horowitz, J.A.; Mayberry, L.J. An international study exploring levels of postpartum depressive symptomatology. *J. Psychosom. Res.* **2000**, *49*, 207–216. [CrossRef]
33. Ramchandani, P.G.; Stein, A.; O'Connor, T.G.; Heron, J.; Murray, L.; Evans, J. Depression in men in the postnatal period and later child psychopathology: A population cohort study. *J. Am. Acad. Child. Adolesc. Psychiatry* **2008**, *47*, 390–398. [CrossRef] [PubMed]
34. González-Mesa, E.; Kabukcuoglub, K.; Körükcüb, O.; Blascoc, M.; Ibrahimc, N.; Kavasd, T. Cultural factors influencing antenatal depression: A cross-sectional study in a cohort of Turkish and Spanish women at the beginning of the pregnancy. *J. Affect. Disord.* **2018**, *238*, 256–260. [CrossRef] [PubMed]
35. Garcia-Esteve, L.; Ascaso, C.; Ojuel, J.; Navarro, P. Validation of the Edinburgh Postnatal Depression Scale (EPDS) in Spanish mother. *J. Affect. Disord.* **2003**, *75*, 71–76. [CrossRef]
36. Shakeel, N.; Sletner, L.; Falk, R.S.; Slinning, K.; Martinsen, E.W.; Jenum, A.K.; Eberhard-Gran, M. Prevalence of postpartum depressive symptoms in a multiethnic population and the role of ethnicity and integration. *J. Affect. Disord.* **2018**, *241*, 49–58. [CrossRef] [PubMed]
37. Redinger, S.; Norris, S.A.; Pearson, R.M.; Richter, L.; Rochat, T. First trimester antenatal depression and anxiety: Prevalence and associated factors in an urban population in Soweto. *S. Afr. J. Dev. Orig. Health Dis.* **2018**, *9*, 30–40. [CrossRef] [PubMed]
38. Levis, B.; Negeri, Z.; Sun, Y.; Benedetti, A.; Thombs, B.D.; on behalf of the DEPRESsion Screening Data (DEPRESSD) EPDS Group. Accuracy of the Edinburgh Postnatal Depression Scale (EPDS) for screening to detect major depression among pregnant and postpartum women: Systematic review and meta-analysis of individual participant data. *BMJ* **2020**, *371*, m4022. [CrossRef]
39. Eberhard-Gran, M.; Eskild, A.; Tambs, K.; Opjordsmoen, S.; Samuelsen, S.O. Review of validation studies of the Edinburgh Postnatal Depression Scale. *Acta Psychiatr. Scandin.* **2001**, *104*, 243–249. [CrossRef]
40. Wesselhoeft, R.; Madsen, F.K.; Lichtenstein, M.B.; Sibbersen, C.; Manongi, R.; Mushi, D.L.; Nguyen, H.T.; Van, T.N.; Kyhl, H.; Bilenberg, N.; et al. Postnatal depressive symptoms display marked similarities across continents. *J. Affect. Disord.* **2020**, *261*, 58–66. [CrossRef]
41. Murray, L.; Carothers, A.D. The validation of the Edinburgh Post-natal Depression Scale on a community sample. *Brit. J. Psychiatry* **1990**, *157*, 288–290. [CrossRef]
42. Cameron, E.E.; Sedov, I.D.; Tomfohr-Madsen, L.M. Prevalence of paternal depression in pregnancy and the postpartum: An updated meta-analysis. *J. Affect. Disord.* **2016**, *206*, 189–203. [CrossRef]
43. Woody, C.A.; Ferrari, A.J.; Siskind, D.J.; Whiteford, H.A.; Harris, M.G. A systematic review and meta-regression of the prevalence and incidence of perinatal depression. *J. Affect. Disord.* **2017**, *219*, 86–92. [CrossRef] [PubMed]
44. Smith-Nielsen, J.; University of Copenhagen, Copenhagen K, Denmark. Personal communication, 10 December 2021.

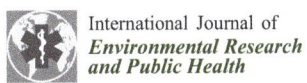

Review

Gender Transformative Interventions for Perinatal Mental Health in Low and Middle Income Countries—A Scoping Review

Archana Raghavan [1], Veena A. Satyanarayana [1,*], Jane Fisher [2], Sundarnag Ganjekar [1], Monica Shrivastav [3], Sarita Anand [3], Vani Sethi [4] and Prabha S. Chandra [1]

[1] National Institute of Mental Health and Neurosciences (NIMHANS), Bengaluru 530068, India
[2] School of Public Health and Preventive Medicine, University of Monash, Melbourne 3800, Australia
[3] ROSHNI-Centre of Women Collectives led Social Action, Lady Irwin College, New Delhi 110001, India
[4] United Nations Children's Fund (UNICEF) Regional Office for South Asia, Kathmandu 44600, Nepal
* Correspondence: veenas@nimhans.ac.in

Abstract: Perinatal mental health problems are linked to poor outcomes for mothers, babies and families. In the context of Low and Middle Income Countries (LMIC), a leading risk factor is gender disparity. Addressing gender disparity, by involving fathers, mothers in law and other family members can significantly improve perinatal and maternal healthcare, including risk factors for poor perinatal mental health such as domestic violence and poor social support. This highlights the need to develop and implement gender-transformative (GT) interventions that seek to engage with men and reduce or overcome gender-based constraints. This scoping review aimed to highlight existing gender transformative interventions from LMIC that specifically aimed to address perinatal mental health (partner violence, anxiety or depression and partner support) and identify components of the intervention that were found to be useful and acceptable. This review follows the five-stage Arksey and O'Malley framework and the Preferred Reporting Items for Systematic Reviews and Meta-Analyses extension for Scoping Reviews (PRISMA-ScR) checklist. Six papers that met the inclusion criteria were included in the review (four from Africa and two from Asia). Common components of gender transformative interventions across studies included couple-based interventions and discussion groups. Gender inequity and related factors are a strong risk for poor perinatal mental health and the dearth of studies highlights the strong need for better evidence of GT interventions in this area.

Keywords: perinatal mental health; gender transformative interventions; scoping review; LMIC

1. Introduction

Research and policies related to perinatal mental health have demonstrated how poor mental health both in pregnancy and postpartum is prevalent in the form of anxiety and depression, and may influence pregnancy outcomes and the health of the foetus and infant [1,2]. Untreated depression during pregnancy is also associated with a risk for suicide especially in those with a severe problem or when there is associated partner violence [2–4]. When studied through a socio-cultural context, women generally have reported high levels of anxiety, depression and higher levels of trauma during pregnancy as well as the postpartum period [5–7]. Rates of anxiety and depression in pregnancy from Low and Middle Income Countries (LMIC) range between 9–65% [8], indicating the importance of addressing mental health outcomes during pregnancy as well as post-pregnancy in the region [9].

Some of the well-established risk factors for poor perinatal mental health, particularly anxiety and depression, are related to gender inequity, especially in LMIC settings. These include partner violence (Intimate partner violence (IPV), Domestic violence

(DV) and Gender-based Violence (GBV)), younger age, poor social support, low education and male infant preference [10–12]. Other gender-based risk factors include low autonomy and decision-making power, lack of control over resources, low education and poverty [12], power dynamics within family [13], gender-based stigma and discrimination and inequitable spousal relationships [14,15]. Multiple reviews [16,17] and a recent report [7] using a decision tree analysis from 48 LMIC countries reported that gender-related factors play a strong role in perinatal mental health problems such as anxiety and depression, including in the South Asian context [18].

A few interventions for perinatal health in general that have addressed gender-related factors and focused on enhancing support systems for pregnant women or addressing gender inequity in the family have found improvement in rates of postpartum depression as well [19–21]. When specifically looking at interventions, literature suggests how addressing gender gaps with regards to perinatal health programs and policies can be an active agent of change in addressing low mobility, female genital mutilation, unintended pregnancy and increased preference for a male child [22].

Yet, different research reviews related to gender-based violence, and family and reproductive health have notably overlooked the practical ways of overcoming gender inequality to improve perinatal mental health [23]. Gender-based interventions in perinatal health may be gender intentional, gender accommodative or gender transformative. Gender intentional means identifying and understanding gender inequalities [24]. Gender-accommodating interventions seek to compensate for gender norms and ideally decrease *existing* inequalities; however, they are not aimed at role-reversal or changing gender norms [25]. Gender transformative interventions, on the other hand, are interventions that create opportunities for individuals to actively challenge gender norms and address power inequities between persons of different genders [26]. Principles of Gender Transformative Approach (GTA) go beyond improving healthcare systems and access for women alone but also include men, children and other family members to promote better health for communities, as a whole. However, while risk factors have been studied, gender-accommodative or transformative interventions have not been designed from a curative or a preventative lens [27]. Fathers have been involved at best as only one part of an intervention and these too have not addressed gender transformation [28–30]. Since gender transformative interventions aid in bridging the gender gap [26,27,31,32], it is necessary to develop interventions for perinatal mental health with a Gender Transformative (GT) lens, especially in countries with a large gender equity gap. This is especially true for the more prevalent perinatal mental health concerns such as depression and anxiety which are driven by a host of psychological and social risk factors.

Presently, there is meagre evidence based data on perinatal mental health interventions that are gender-transformative in LMIC countries. To examine available evidence as well as highlight the various components of the intervention and to encourage research in this area, this review attempts to (a) review the literature on GT interventions that have been implemented in LMIC, and have addressed perinatal mental health directly or indirectly, (b) describe components of these interventions and (c) based on this, provide a framework of action and recommendations for designing gender transformative intervention for perinatal mental health care, specifically for early identification and treatment of perinatal anxiety and depression in the community.

2. Method

This scoping review was conducted by utilising the framework developed by Arksey and O' Malley's [33] that included five stages, namely (1) identifying the research question that was broad in nature, (2) identifying relevant studies, a process that remains comprehensive and strategic, (3) select studies based on inclusion/exclusion criteria, based on familiarity with literature, (4) charting data related to key themes and issues and lastly, (5) collating, reporting and summarising the results which could be descriptive, thematic and/or numerical in nature [34]. The findings are reported according to the Preferred

Reporting Items for Systematic Reviews and Meta-Analyses extension for Scoping Reviews (PRISMA-ScR) checklist [35]. The sixth stage of a scoping review—stakeholder consultation—is an optional element and was not included in this review.

2.1. Identifying the Research Question

The research question for this scoping review was "what is known about gender transformative interventions that address perinatal mental health in Low and Middle Income Countries?" The specific research questions for the present reviews were as follows: (1) What are the objectives and purpose of developing gender transformative interventions for perinatal mental health in the context of the LMICs? (2) What are the components of these interventions (3) What are the kinds and contexts of male-involvement/engagement in these gender-transformative perinatal mental health interventions? and (4) What are the outcomes for perinatal mental health following these interventions?

2.2. Identifying Relevant studies

The following electronic databases were searched for English language publications between 2012 and present: PubMed, PsycInfo, Scopus, Web of Science. Journals were inclusive of Sage Publications, SpringerLink, Taylor and Francis, Wiley Online, and Oxford University Press. Other databases searched include Google Scholar. The authors also manually searched the reference lists of included papers, reports and other reviews to identify further eligible papers or studies.

A comprehensive search using keywords included Gender transformative interventions LMIC; Gender transformative interventions for maternal healthcare; Gender transformative interventions for perinatal healthcare and Gender transformative interventions for perinatal and maternal mental health. The specific search terms for studies included Perinatal OR mental health outcomes OR antenatal OR pregnancy OR childbirth OR postpartum OR postpartum depression OR maternal OR perinatal partner support OR involvement of fathers OR mental health outcomes OR perinatal IPV OR perinatal GBV [in title, abstract, keywords] AND male engagement interventions OR family interventions AND LMIC/Low and Middle income countries (in all).

2.3. Study Selection (Inclusion and Exclusion)

The inclusion and exclusion criteria were developed by the authors and are shown in Box 1. The search period ranged from studies published between the years of 2012–present. A longer time period was utilised to map the scope of literature owing to the limited number of studies that focused on gender transformative interventions that specifically focused on maternal or perinatal mental health and wellbeing. Moreover, to ensure a rigorous search, data from grey literature were also included. A quality assessment of the studies selected was carried out by two senior researchers (PS, VS). studies that developed gender transformative interventions inclusive of a component that targeted males or extended family members' involvement were reviewed.

Additionally, systematic reviews of interventions that targeted prevention or reduction of violence against women, girls or mothers were also included in the review. Since maternal and child's health and wellbeing are strong predictors of mental health [36,37], psychosocial interventions that were gender-transformative and addressed maternal health and care were also included. Inclusion criteria consisted of studies conducted in the LMIC region; countries belonging to LMIC were classified according to the Society for the Study of Human Biology [38]. For the current 2022 fiscal year, low-income economies are defined as those with a GNI per capita, calculated using the World Bank Atlas method, of USD 1045 or less in 2020 (World Bank Country and Lending Groups, 2020) [36]. The following exclusion criteria were applied: study location not in LMIC, not relating to perinatal period, not relating to mental health and not relating to maternal mental health.

Box 1. Inclusion and Exclusion criteria.

Inclusion criteria
1. Published in English
2. Programs designed and implemented in LMIC countries.
3. studies having any one of the three mental health outcomes in the perinatal period which include
a. Improvement in social support or better relationship with partner;
b. Decrease in depression, anxiety or any Common Mental Disorder;
c. Decrease in Domestic violence or Intimate Partner Violence.
4. Any study design—RCTs, Non Randomised Controlled studies, Case Control studies, pre post intervention studies.
5. Publication years 2007–2022.
Exclusion criteria
1. Study location not in LMIC.
2. studies not relating to perinatal period.
3. studies not relating to mental health or risk.
4. studies not relating to maternal mental health.

2.4. Charting the Data

Data were extracted according to the PRISMA-ScR [37,39] checklist [35]. The primary objectives, study characteristics (author, year, country/region and outcome measures), study population, components of interventions, primary outcomes and aspects of male engagement were tabulated in line with the research questions.

2.5. Reporting the Results

Using a narrative approach, these interventions were critically analysed by VS, AR and PC and reported in terms of intervention characteristics, risk of bias/methodological quality, categorisation of outcomes and identification of gaps in evidence as previously noted in scoping reviews that focused on GT interventions [40]. A total of 6 studies were then finalised and analysed descriptively to understand GT in perinatal care and GT in the context of LMIC.

3. Results

From the search process, 16 studies were identified since they met the inclusion criteria. However, 10 studies were excluded because 7 studies focused on gender but not on the gender "transformative" aspect and did not assess mental health outcomes and 3 studies did not assess perinatal mental health conditions. Figure 1 illustrates the PRISMA flowchart of our search strategy. Table 1 highlights the data summary obtained from the 6 studies and additionally displays the study characteristics, study population, components of interventions, primary outcomes and aspects of male engagement.

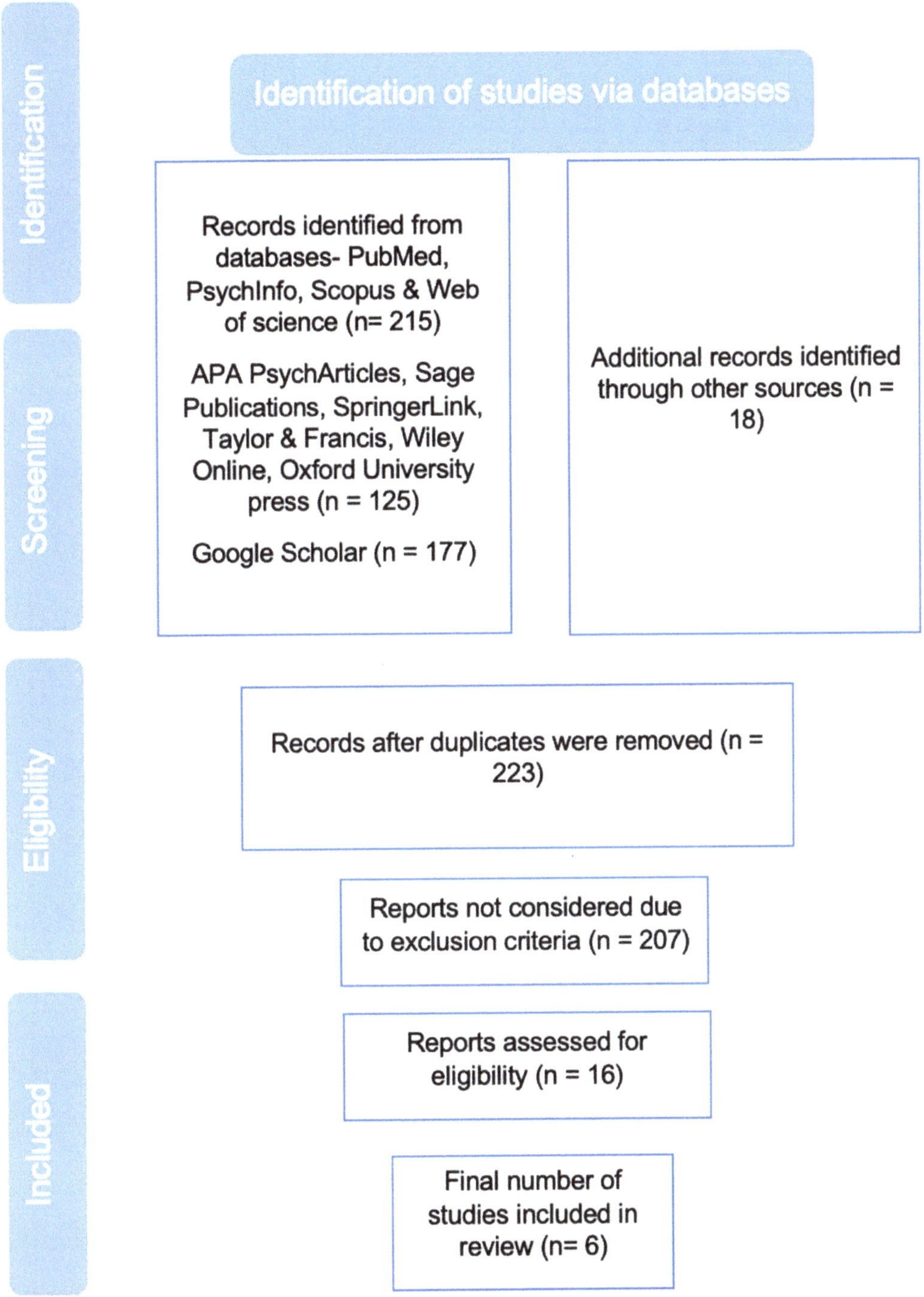

Figure 1. PRISMA flowchart of the search strategy.

Table 1. Description of study population and components of intervention.

S/No	Author, Year and Country	Target Population and Sample Size	Gender-Transformative Components	Aspect of Male Engagement	Primary Outcomes (With Data if Possible)
1	Santhya et al., 2008 [41] West Bengal and Gujarat, India	Women (pregnant and post-partum first time mothers), husbands and family members 2115 women	The First Time Parent project targeted young married women and their husbands as well as family members to modify gender norms and support prenatal as well as maternal healthcare behaviours.	Outreach workers interacted with husbands about pregnancy and delivery plans. Husbands received home visits from male outreach workers.	• Decision-making increased for married women in their household (61%). • More women adhered to egalitarian gender attitudes (38%) in Diamond Harbour; however, no difference was observed in Vadodara. • Positive change in women's perception about wife-beating and domestic violence (42%). • No significant differences between age and religion was found between the intervention and control group.
2	Comrie-Thomson, L. et al. (2015) [42] Bangladesh, Tanzania and Zimbabwe	Married men and their wives 237 males and females	Education and outreach were conducted with men's groups and individual men through designated gender equality champions, peer educators or role models. Dialogue, education and mobilisation were conducted with traditional and religious leaders, who have influence over community beliefs and behaviours. Integrated gender equality and male engagement messages delivered through a wide range of activities including community Theatre for Development (T4D), community radio (in Barguna), and community meetings.	Education and outreach were conducted with men's groups and individual men through designated gender equality champions, peer educators or role models.	• Male and female participants identified many benefits associated with male engagement in MNCH, including improved health outcomes for women, newborns and children. • Increased couple communication and improved couple relationships. • Increased maternal nutrition and rest during pregnancy. • Increased value of girl children. • Increased assistance of fathers in household chores (41.7%). • Assisting wives to access healthcare services (57.7%). • Increased couple communication and shared decision making.
3	Raj et al., 2016 [23] Yore et al., 2016 [43] Maharashtra, India	Married men and their wives 1081 Rural young husbands and their wives	The intervention involved three gender, culture and contextually-tailored family planning and gender equity (FP + GE) counseling sessions. A desk-sized CHARM flipchart was used by village health providers to provide men and couples with pictorial information on family planning options, barriers to family planning use including gender equity-related issues (e.g., son preference), the importance of healthy and shared family planning decision-making, and how to engage in respectful marital communication and interactions (inclusive of no spousal violence in the men's sessions).	Counseling Husbands to Achieve Reproductive Health and Marital Equity (CHARM) intervention, a multi-session intervention delivered to males alone, but included a session with their wives.	• Findings document that women from the CHARM condition, relative to controls, reported increased contraceptive use at 9-month follow-up (55.7%). • They were less likely to report physical IPV at 18-month follow-up (48%). • Men in the CHARM condition were less likely to report attitudes accepting of sexual IPV (51%). • No significant time by treatment effects were seen for sexual IPV between the control and intervention group.

Table 1. *Cont.*

S/No	Author, Year and Country	Target Population and Sample Size	Gender-Transformative Components	Aspect of Male Engagement	Primary Outcomes (With Data if Possible)
4	Doyle et al., 2018 [44] Rwanda	Expectant/current fathers and their partners (pregnant women) 575 couples and 1123 men	The Bandebereho couples' intervention engaged men and their partners in participatory, small group sessions of critical reflection and dialogue. In Rwanda, the MenCare+ program was known as Bandebereho, or "role model", as it aimed to transform norms around masculinity by demonstrating positive models of fatherhood.	Transform norms around masculinity by demonstrating positive models of fatherhood. Sessions addressed: gender and power; fatherhood; couple communication and decision-making; IPV; caregiving; child development; and male engagement in reproductive and maternal health.	• Compared to the control group, pregnant women in the intervention group reported: less past-year physical and sexual IPV, greater attendance and male accompaniment at antenatal care (61.17%). • Pregnant women (79.15%) and men (57.71%) in the intervention group reported: less child physical punishment. • Women reported greater modern contraceptive use and less dominance of men in decision-making (56.08%). However men's level of participation in childcare between the intervention group and control group remained the same.
5	Bapolisi et al., 2020 [45] Democratic Republic of Congo	Husbands and wives 800 men and women	The "Mawe tatu" program, links Village Savings and Loans Associations (VSLA) for women with men-to-men sensitisation to transform gender-inequitable norms and behaviours for the empowerment of women. Comprehensive sexuality education for young people, which includes gender and rights themes, is offered as well.	Developing "positive masculinity" by engaging men, if possible spouses of VSLA's members, towards women's rights using a peer-to-peer approach.	• The primary outcomes are to engage men for more gender equality, expecting a positive effect of this combined intervention on the household economy, on child nutritional status, on the use of reproductive health services including family planning, and on reducing sexual and gender-based violence (SGBV). • Note: Data on the study are not yet published.

Table 1. *Cont.*

S/No	Author, Year and Country	Target Population and Sample Size	Gender-Transformative Components	Aspect of Male Engagement	Primary Outcomes (With Data if Possible)
6	Comrie-Thomson et al., 2022 [46] Manicaland, Zimbabwe	Women and male co-parents 433 women (Pregnant and post-partum mothers up to 2 years post-pregnancy) and 273 men	Women participated in Participatory learning action (PLA) cycles conducted through monthly one-hour group discussions. Discussions explored MNCH services and home care practices recommended during pregnancy and between zero and two years of age, including services for the prevention of mother-to-child transmission of HIV (PMTCT). The +Men component was delivered by a trained male OPHID staff member who was also a nurse and midwife with substantial community development experience, targeting men. Men participated in monthly one-hour group discussions. Discussions explored similar health topics to those addressed in women's groups and the same flip chart was used to present information.	Men participated in monthly one-hour group discussions, facilitated by the male project staff member in men's workplaces or a central community location.	• Primary outcomes of interest reported • Decreased symptoms of depression and anxiety (63%). • Increased women's participation in decision-making (68.7%). • Improved men's gender attitudes, and couple relationship dynamics (88.7%). • Increased practical support provided by men (78.4%). • No effect was detected on the proportion of men participating in antenatal care consultations, supporting childbirth by providing money or goods, contributing to household chores during pregnancy or after childbirth, encouraging their pregnant coparent to rest, or settling their baby at night.

3.1. Article Characteristics

The six finalised studies ranged primarily between 2015–2022, although the study attempted to include studies over a period of 15 years (refer to Table 1). Only one study was conducted in 2008 [41]. The results were further indicative of how there were very few studies that focused on understanding perinatal mental health by implementing gender transformative interventions. All the six studies included men and women/husbands and wives. One study focused on women and husbands as well as extended family members [41]. All the interventions included a male engagement component in the intervention. All the interventions were mostly conducted in rural or semi-urban areas.

Most of the identified studies utilised group discussions as the basis to facilitate critical dialogue and awareness regarding gender roles and mental health. In the Bandebereho couples' intervention, from Rwanda, small groups of critical reflection and dialogues were initiated with couples and men [44]. Similarly, the Counseling Husbands to Achieve Reproductive Health and Marital Equity (CHARM) intervention implemented in Maharashtra, India, also involved sessions based on gender and culture for individuals to explore how gender roles influenced wellbeing for mothers [23]. Two studies in Zimbabwe and Congo [42,45] addressed how developing positive models of masculinity can decrease gender disparity by initiating men's groups and engaging in group discussions. Study designs ranged from randomised controlled trials [23,42,44,45] to pre and post evaluation designs [23,44]. In the following sections studies are presented thematically based on their objectives and primary outcomes. Overall, the studies highlighted the need to address perinatal mental health concerns through the involvement of other family members or husbands through a gender-transformative lens.

3.2. Program Evaluation

This section reports practical aspects of the interventions (Table 2) and important components of GT interventions that were designed, namely, to decrease gender-based violence, improve maternal mental health, and improve couples' relationships.

A successful couples' intervention designed by Doyle et al. [44], implemented in Rwanda, focused on engaging men and their partners in a participatory group session consisting of critical reflection and dialogue. Addressing power relations in the community demonstrated substantial improvements with respect to marriages and modern contraceptive uses. Therefore, while it did not address perinatal healthcare directly, the couple-focused interventions had longer term implications with respect to perinatal and maternal mental health [47]. The intervention induced a significant positive impact on maternal health by reducing instances of physical and sexual IPV. It also increased male accompaniment to antenatal care and decreased dominance of men in decision-making challenging existing gender norms. Components of intervention involved training community volunteers (local fathers) to co-facilitate sessions on pregnancy, family planning and marital communication. Sessions involved ice-breakers, group activities, games and media such as cartoons and short films [48] However, the research was implemented only for 12 months, leading to an unsustainable effect. This explains why despite greater male involvement, women's time spent on labour at home remained the same. Moreover, since behavioural changes were self-reported there is a risk of participants (both men and women) providing desirable answers.

A similar and older study from India targeted young married women, their husbands as well as family members to address and modify gender norms [41]. The study attempted to address communication and decision-making in the family by empowering women and creating supportive social structures by providing interventions to husbands and mother-in-laws through the First Time Parent Project in rural West-Bengal and Gujarat. Components of intervention included education and counselling sessions for young married women, training, outreach programs and workshops for husbands and mothers-in-law as well as developing support groups for women. While the study did not address maternal mental health directly, it addressed risk factors for poor maternal mental health since primary outcomes involved decreased gender-based violence and improving support in homecare practices. The study did not however ensure follow-ups and therefore, the effectiveness of the intervention remains unclear. The study however provided insightful recommendations that included allying influential members of a family within the interventions as well as creating a support network for different groups of mothers, such as those trying to conceive, delay the first pregnancy and new mothers.

Raj et al. [23] conducted a randomised controlled trial evaluation in India, across 50 geographic clusters in rural Maharashtra, which primarily focused on gender equity and family planning for men and couples. Based on the baseline scores of contraceptive behaviours and IPV attitudes, a CHARM intervention, comprising three sessions of family planning, gender-equity for couples was utilised. Sessions involved discussing gender-equity through pictorial flipcharts that addressed family planning, barriers to family planning and respectful marital communication. Results indicated that contraceptive communication increased and decreased intimate partner violence amongst couples was reported at an 18-month follow-up. While GT interventions have shown their efficacy across countries, in LMIC, since resources are low, it is imperative to note that investment interventions such as home visiting programs need to be maximised to prevent IPV or child maltreatment [48].

Another intervention that was targeted for women, children and men/fathers/co-parents in Mutasa district, Zimbabwe, used community-based training and discussion groups that addressed services for mothers, HIV transmissions and engaging in problem-solving therapy. Results indicated that addressing gender inequality improved maternal mental health [46]. The interesting aspect of this program included creating and implementing educational and outreach programs that encouraged "male champions". Separate tools were prepared for men and women participants. Interventions for women were delivered by local female village health workers through Participatory and Learning Action (PLA) cycles. For men, interventions involved male project members discussing gendered-division of labour, safe sex and men's contribution in care-seeking behaviour. The intervention successfully integrated gender equality and male engagement, leading to increased couples communication, reduced maternal workload and increased nutrition during pregnancy, another paramount implication included increased value of girl children.

Along the lines of men's involvement, the study by Bapolisi et al. [45] focused on investigating the impact of men's involvement on women's health and child nutrition. The primary focus in this study was to engage men for more gender equality, expecting a positive effect of this combined intervention on the household economy, on child nutritional status, on the use of reproductive health services including family planning, and on reducing sexual and gender-based violence (SGBV). The intervention in the aforementioned study involved developing positive masculinity by engaging men using a peer-based approach. Reflective conversations were conducted through Gender-Dialogue Groups (GDGs) facilitated by both one male and one female, trained as gender-based violence field agent and economic recovery field agent. Men were encouraged to adopt attitudes and behaviours that promoted women's economic empowerment as well as reduced gender-based violence. The study provided insightful implications regarding gender-power dynamics on both household as well as community levels. It can further be noted that through participatory interventions, mental health services inclusive of antenatal care, maternity and family planning can be improved through male-involvement.

Table 2. Details of the facilitators and recipients of the intervention.

S/No	Study Design (Format)	Male Engagement Intervention	Individual/Couple/Group Intervention	Facilitators	Inclusion of Other Family Members
1	Randomised controlled trial	MenCare+ program	Couple based intervention. Men along with their current partners (pregnant women) were included. Men alone were invited for 15 sessions and with their partners were invited for 8 sessions.	Sex-matched interviewers from Laterite, who had no involvement in the intervention, conducted the interviews. Community volunteers (local fathers) met with the same group of 12 men/couples on a weekly basis. The volunteers received a two-week training, material support, and refresher training. Local nurses and police officers co-facilitated the sessions on pregnancy, family planning, and local laws, respectively.	No
2	Cluster randomised controlled trial	CHARM gender-equity (GE) counselling in family planning (FP) services. The intervention involved three gender, culture and contextually-tailored family planning and gender equity (FP + GE) counselling sessions delivered by trained male village health care providers to married men (sessions 1 and 2) and couples (session 3) in a clinical setting.	Couple-based intervention	CHARM providers were allopathic (n = 9) and non-allopathic (n = 13) village health care providers trained over three days on FP counselling, GE and IPV issues, and CHARM implementation. All VHPs in the study villages were male; 22 VHPs were trained for delivery.	No
3	Qualitative study	Focus-group discussions and in-depth interviews	Men-only counselling Couples counselling	Male community workers engaged in men-only education group sessions.	No
4	Cluster-randomised, longitudinal intervention study	Positive masculinity groups	Only men peer-to-peer discussion groups	Information not given	No
5	A cluster-randomised controlled pragmatic trial	+Men component	Only men discussion groups Men and women were assessed separately for baseline scores.	Trained male Public Health Interventions and Development (OPHID) staff members.	No
6	A quasi-experimental research design	First-time Parents Project	Women-only sessions from female outreach workers. Husbands received home-visits from male outreach workers.	Same-sex facilitators conducted interventions.	Yes. Mothers and mother-in-law were included for home-visit based interventions (family sessions).

A recent study that contributed towards the current limited literature, was Comrie-Thomson et al.'s [46] trial on implementing a gender-synchronised intervention. Gender-synchronised interventions are conceptualised as programs that employ multiple strategies to change community norms related to gender as well as engage men to achieve gender equality and improve health [49]. As a part of the intervention, women participated in PLA cycles conducted through monthly one hour group discussions, facilitated by female village health workers in a central community location. Men, on the other hand, participated in monthly one-hour group discussions, facilitated by the male project staff member in men's workplaces or a central community location. Group discussions rooted in problem-solving therapy, focused on topics such as home care practices during pregnancy along with various gender-related challenges women faced. Results indicated that women reported decreased postnatal depression scores and care-seeking as well as relationships significantly improved.

However, the aforementioned GT interventions particularly focused on prenatal, maternal care and personal empowerment. Alternatively, it is indicative of how programs and interventions should focus more intentionally on postnatal mental health care, particularly gender-intentional postpartum family planning interventions to ensure antenatal and intrapartum care that were earlier provided remained sustainable and effective. By implementing these interventions, it can be inferred that perinatal mental health will significantly improve eventually decreasing mental health concerns such as anxiety and depression. Possible adverse events that have to be considered includes increased tension in parent relationships and familial relationships due to changed expectations and behaviours [50]. Therefore, developing GT interventions to explicitly address power dynamics, values and norms throughout perinatal, prenatal and postnatal maternal health as well as mental health remain a necessity to improve quality of care sustainably.

4. Discussion

Due to limited studies, the review could not identify major contexts in which GT interventions were designed. However, it was vastly noted that GT interventions had multifold implications with respect to improvement on mental health, maternal mental health, decreased IPV and GBV and improved couples' relationships and homecare practices. It was previously noted that gender related factors seem to play a strong role in mental health problems in pregnancy and the postpartum especially in the LMIC region [51]. Therefore, this review specifically identified key program components that may have contributed to positive mental health outcomes as well as improvement in social and partner support and decrease in IPV or DV, factors that have a strong link with depression and anxiety in the perinatal period.

Similar to previous reviews and studies, the results in the present paper indicate how main components of interventions to improve maternal mental health consist of quality time with the infant, group sessions with husbands or family members, counselling sessions and psychoeducational sessions [2,52]. Interventions are further indicative of how addressing gender disparities can significantly lead to positive outcomes. Moreover, apart from addressing maternal care specific to infant care, it also becomes necessary to address the general wellbeing of mothers through empowering GT interventions. These results demonstrate how development of gender transformative interventions is necessary to improve mental health outcomes long term, amongst mothers [53].

In programs that focused on fatherhood, targeting men, fathers and husbands, interventions mostly focused on educational sessions on gender-roles [44,54] indicating that addressing gender roles and norms was an important component of GT interventions as highlighted by studies previously [30,51]. Recent studies have highlighted the necessity of male engagement in maternal and perinatal healthcare [25,44]. Moreover, findings accordingly highlighted that GT interventions which focused on fatherhood helped in transforming harmful masculine norms which underpin gender-based violence. While these interventions aim for men to increase their involvement in their partner's pregnancies and accompany them to health services, it is necessary to note that increasing male engagement as a strategy should include ethical considerations to ensure men do not assume the stance of "protecting" and "looking after" women which in turn can cause power imbalance and gender disparities.

Furthermore, fatherhood programs when designed from a systemic lens can significantly support and protect women, families and children from violence. In support, a systematic review of male engagement in GT interventions for women in the community highlighted that 11 out of 12 GT interventions revealed a significant change in men's attitudes towards gender norms, establishing gender equality [31]. This is suggestive of the need to develop and design more GT interventions that focus increasingly on the aspect of male engagement. However, this study did not focus on women in the perinatal period.

Further, the aforementioned studies do not acknowledge the structural norms that influence masculinity and how norms related to masculinity are also changing [31]. Moreover, while the results are indicative of group education, community outreach and mass-media campaigns are all effective program interventions, none of the studies focus on evaluating long-term change. It remains unclear how family members, caregivers, and men will continue to succeed in sustaining their short-term change in the absence of contextual and structural changes.

To achieve long-term, sustainable change, community-level interventions need to be accompanied by policies that support the changes men undergo through GT interventions. Future recommendations for gender transformative interventions include taking a more relational perspective that attempts to integrate men and boys with efforts to empower women without adapting the attitude of "saving women and families" since it was noted that many men engaging in activism for equality or trials that promote equality are not disconnected from an inherent saviour complex [51].

Studies could also focus on developing strategies that address change at the level of families and communities leading to sustainable changes through involvement of other family members, which also result in sustainable and lasting effects. Additionally, future studies could focus on programmatic efforts on gender barriers that accompany life stages, that range from helping newly married couples with no children to delay in their first pregnancy. Developing GT interventions for specific groups such as those facing perinatal loss and adolescent mothers is needed. GT studies need to provide more information about how men were encouraged to participate in these trials and stay engaged through the course of multiple sessions, which components were preferred by the groups and whether the gender of the facilitators made a difference and if groups should be men only or combined. This information will enable future researchers to help in better planning of future GT intervention studies for perinatal mental health including deciding the "dose" of the intervention in addition to the methods.

Moreover, some reports [55,56] focusing on male engagement in perinatal mental health, from High Income Countries, have used technology such as SMS and other online tools. Countries in the LMIC region also reported using technology to improve perinatal mental health [57–59]; however, the interventions did not include a male engagement component. It is possible that technology-based interventions can increase accessibility as well as be useful in involving difficult-to-engage men.

5. Limitations

It is necessary to remain cautious while interpreting the findings of this review because the evidence is limited due to the small number of studies that were identified. Moreover, since the synthesised studies were not methodologically similar, the findings of the current review cannot be generalised. Our findings and recommendations are partially informed by the studies and their limitations, also accounted for, in our analysis. Moreover, given the sensitivity and stigmatised nature of these issues, consideration must be given to the presence of social desirability bias which may have influenced disclosure and involvement of participants in the programs. Future research may examine the dose or the optimum length of the intervention itself and on whether treatment gains are maintained over longer follow-up periods.

6. Conclusions

Our review has highlighted a need for GT interventions that focus on male engagement, family members and community as a whole. Our review also highlights the methodological strengths and deficits in existing interventions, paving the way for future research to address these limitations and mindfully develop programs that yield effective maternal health outcomes. Lastly, by emphasising programs implemented in the LMIC region, our review addresses the need to develop shared goals that address gender-based violence, cultural norms and family dynamics since perinatal and maternal mental health outcomes cannot be improved in isolation.

Author Contributions: Conceptualisation, P.S.C. and V.A.S.; methodology, P.S.C. and A.R.; validation, P.S.C., V.A.S. and S.G.; formal analysis, A.R.; investigation, A.R.; resources, P.S.C.; data curation, A.R.; writing—original draft preparation, A.R. and V.A.S.; writing—review and editing, J.F., S.G., M.S., S.A. and V.S.; visualisation, J.F. and P.S.C.; supervision, P.S.C. and V.A.S.; project administration, P.S.C.; funding acquisition, P.S.C. All authors have read and agreed to the published version of the manuscript.

Funding: This work was supported by the United Nations Children's Fund (UNICEF) [UNICEF/Nutrition/ 2021 07/09, 2021].

Institutional Review Board Statement: IRB approval was not applicable since this is a review paper.

Informed Consent Statement: Not applicable.

Data Availability Statement: Not applicable.

Conflicts of Interest: The authors declare no conflict of interest.

References

1. Mitchell, J.; Goodman, J. Comparative effects of antidepressant medications and untreated major depression on pregnancy outcomes: A systematic review. *Arch. Womens Ment. Health* **2018**, *21*, 505–516. [CrossRef] [PubMed]
2. Howard, L.M.; Khalifeh, H. Perinatal mental health: A review of progress and challenges. *World Psychiatry* **2020**, *19*, 313–327. [CrossRef] [PubMed]
3. Shiva, L.; Desai, G.; Satyanarayana, V.A.; Venkataram, P.; Chandra, P.S. Negative Childbirth Experience and Post-traumatic Stress Disorder-A Study Among Postpartum Women in South India. *Front. Psychiatry* **2021**, *12*, 640014. [CrossRef]
4. Huschke, S.; Murphy-Tighe, S.; Barry, M. Perinatal mental health in Ireland: A scoping review. *Midwifery* **2020**, *89*, 102763. [CrossRef] [PubMed]
5. Fawcett, E.J.; Fairbrother, N.; Cox, M.L.; White, I.R.; Fawcett, J.M. The prevalence of anxiety disorders during pregnancy and the postpartum period: A multivariate Bayesian meta-analysis. *J. Clin. Psychiatry* **2019**, *80*, 1181. [CrossRef]
6. Slomian, J.; Honvo, G.; Emonts, P.; Reginster, J.Y.; Bruyère, O. Consequences of maternal postpartum depression: A systematic review of maternal and infant outcomes. *Womens Health* **2019**, *15*, 1745506519844044. [CrossRef]
7. Coll, C.V.; Santos, T.M.; Devries, K.; Knaul, F.; Bustreo, F.; Gatuguta, A.; Houvessou, G.M.; Barros, A. Identifying the women most vulnerable to intimate partner violence: A decision tree analysis from 48 low and middle-income countries. *EClinicalMedicine* **2021**, *42*, 101214. [CrossRef]
8. Bachani, S.; Sahoo, S.M.; Nagendrappa, S.; Dabral, A.; Chandra, P. Anxiety and depression among women with COVID-19 infection during childbirth—Experience from a tertiary care academic center. *AJOG Glob. Rep.* **2022**, *2*, 100033. [CrossRef]
9. McNab, S.E.; Dryer, S.L.; Fitzgerald, L.; Gomez, P.; Bhatti, A.M.; Kenyi, E.; Somji, A.; Khadka, N.; Stalls, S. The silent burden: A landscape analysis of common perinatal mental disorders in low-and middle-income countries. *BMC Pregnancy Childbirth* **2022**, *22*, 342. [CrossRef]
10. Halim, N.; Beard, J.; Mesic, A.; Patel, A.; Henderson, D.; Hibberd, P. Intimate partner violence during pregnancy and perinatal mental disorders in low and lower middle income countries: A systematic review of literature, 1990–2017. *Clin. Psychol. Rev.* **2018**, *66*, 117–135. [CrossRef]
11. Greene, C.A.; Chan, G.; McCarthy, K.J.; Wakschlag, L.S.; Briggs-Gowan, M.J. Psychological and physical intimate partner violence and young children's mental health: The role of maternal posttraumatic stress symptoms and parenting behaviors. *Child Abus. Negl.* **2018**, *77*, 168–179. [CrossRef] [PubMed]
12. Ojha, J.; Bhandari, T.R. Associated Factors of Postpartum Depression in Women Attending a Hospital in Pokhara Metropolitan, Nepal. *Indian J. Obstet. Gynecol. Res.* **2019**, *6*, 369–373. [CrossRef]

13. Patel, V.; Rodrigues, M.; DeSouza, N. Gender, poverty, and postnatal depression: A study of mothers in Goa, India. *Am. J. Psychiatry* **2002**, *159*, 43–47. [CrossRef] [PubMed]
14. Atif, N.; Krishna, R.N.; Sikander, S.; Lazarus, A.; Nisar, A.; Ahmad, I.; Raman, R.; Fuhr, D.C.; Patel, V.; Rahman, A. Mother-to-mother therapy in India and Pakistan: Adaptation and feasibility evaluation of the peer-delivered Thinking Healthy Programme. *BMC Psychiatry* **2017**, *17*, 79. [CrossRef]
15. Pradhananga, P.; Mali, P.; Poudel, L.; Gurung, M. Prevalence of Postpartum Depression in a Tertiary Health Care. *JNMA J. Nepal Med. Assoc.* **2020**, *58*, 137. [CrossRef] [PubMed]
16. Khanna, T.; Garg, P.; Akhtar, F.; Mehra, S. Association between gender disadvantage factors and postnatal psychological distress among young women: A community-based study in rural India. *Glob. Public Health* **2021**, *16*, 1068–1078. [CrossRef]
17. Insan, N.; Weke, A.; Forrest, S.; Rankin, J. Social determinants of antenatal depression and anxiety among women in South Asia: A systematic review & meta-analysis. *PLoS ONE* **2022**, *17*, e0263760. [CrossRef]
18. Rahman, A.; Creed, F. Outcome of prenatal depression and risk factors associated with persistence in the first postnatal year: Prospective study from Rawalpindi, Pakistan. *J. Affect. Disord.* **2007**, *100*, 115–121. [CrossRef]
19. Rath, S.; Nair, N.; Tripathy, P.K.; Barnett, S.; Rath, S.; Mahapatra, R.; Gope, R.; Bajpai, A.; Sinha, R.; Prost, A. Explaining the impact of a women's group led community mobilisation intervention on maternal and newborn health outcomes: The Ekjut trial process evaluation. *BMC Int. Health Hum. Rights* **2010**, *10*, 25. [CrossRef]
20. Jat, T.R.; Deo, P.R.; Goicolea, I.; Hurtig, A.K.; Sebastian, M.S. Socio-cultural and service delivery dimensions of maternal mortality in rural central India: A qualitative exploration using a human rights lens. *Glob. Health Action* **2015**, *8*, 24976. [CrossRef]
21. Singh, K.; Bloom, S.; Brodish, P. Gender equality as a means to improve maternal and child health in Africa. *Health Care Women Int.* **2015**, *36*, 57–69. [CrossRef]
22. Harsha, G.T.; Acharya, M.S. Trajectory of perinatal mental health in India. *Indian J. Soc. Psychiatry* **2019**, *35*, 47.
23. Raj, A.; Ghule, M.; Ritter, J.; Battala, M.; Gajanan, V.; Nair, S.; Dasgupta, A.; Silverman, J.G.; Balaiah, D.; Saggurti, N. Cluster randomized controlled trial evaluation of a gender equity and family planning intervention for married men and couples in rural India. *PLoS ONE* **2016**, *11*, e0153190. [CrossRef] [PubMed]
24. Harrison, S.; McKague, K.; Musoke, J. *Gender Intentional Strategies to Enhance Health Social Enterprises in Africa: A toolkit*; Bluefish Publishing: Burgess Hill, UK, 2020.
25. Kraft, J.M.; Wilkins, K.G.; Morales, G.J.; Widyono, M.; Middlestadt, S.E. An evidence review of gender-integrated interventions in reproductive and maternal-child health. *J. Health Commun.* **2014**, *19* (Suppl. S1), 122–141. [CrossRef]
26. Greene, M.E.; Levack, A. *Synchronizing Gender Strategies: A Cooperative Model for Improving Reproductive Health and Transforming Gender Relations*; Agency for International Development: Washington, DC, USA, 2010.
27. Iyengar, U.; Jaiprakash, B.; Haitsuka, H.; Kim, S. One year into the pandemic: A systematic review of perinatal mental health outcomes during COVID-19. *Front. Psychiatry* **2021**, *12*, 674194. [CrossRef]
28. Doherty, W.J.; Erickson, M.F.; LaRossa, R. An intervention to increase father involvement and skills with infants during the transition to parenthood. *J. Fam. Psychol.* **2006**, *20*, 438. [CrossRef] [PubMed]
29. Nair, S.; Chandramohan, S.; Sundaravathanam, N.; Rajasekaran, A.B.; Sekhar, R. Father involvement in early childhood care: Insights from a MEL system in a behavior change intervention among rural Indian parents. *Front. Public Health* **2020**, *8*, 516. [CrossRef] [PubMed]
30. Williams, K.L.; Wahler, R.G. Are mindful parents more authoritative and less authoritarian? An analysis of clinic-referred mothers. *J. Child Fam. Stud.* **2010**, *19*, 230–235. [CrossRef]
31. Dworkin, S.L.; Fleming, P.J.; Colvin, C.J. The promises and limitations of gender-transformative health programming with men: Critical reflections from the field. *Cult. Health Sex.* **2015**, *17* (Suppl. S2), 128–143. [CrossRef]
32. Levy, J.K.; Darmstadt, G.L.; Ashby, C.; Quandt, M.; Halsey, E.; Nagar, A.; Greene, M.E. Characteristics of successful programmes targeting gender inequality and restrictive gender norms for the health and wellbeing of children, adolescents, and young adults: A systematic review. *Lancet Glob. Health* **2020**, *8*, e225–e236. [CrossRef]
33. Arksey, H.; O'Malley, L. Scoping studies: Towards a methodological framework. *Int. J. Soc. Res. Methodol.* **2005**, *8*, 19–32. [CrossRef]
34. Daudt, H.M.; van Mossel, C.; Scott, S.J. Enhancing the scoping study methodology: A large, inter-professional team's experience with Arksey and O'Malley's framework. *BMC Med. Res. Methodol.* **2013**, *13*, 48. [CrossRef]
35. Tricco, A.C.; Lillie, E.; Zarin, W.; O'Brien, K.K.; Colquhoun, H.; Levac, D.; Moher, D.; Peters, M.D.; Horsley, T.; Weeks, L.; et al. PRISMA extension for scoping reviews (PRISMA-ScR): Checklist and explanation. *Ann. Intern. Med.* **2018**, *169*, 467–473. [CrossRef] [PubMed]
36. World Bank Country and Lending Groups. Country Classification. 2022. Available online: https://datahelpdesk.worldbank.org/knowledgebase/articles/906519-world-bank-country-and-lending-groups (accessed on 25 July 2022).
37. Harris, M.W.; Barnett, T.; Bridgman, H. Rural Art Roadshow: A travelling art exhibition to promote mental health in rural and remote communities. *Arts Health* **2018**, *10*, 57–64. [CrossRef]
38. The Society for the Study of Human Biology, SSHB. Low or Middle Income Country LMIC. 2022. Available online: https://www.sshb.org/lmic/# (accessed on 25 June 2022).
39. Powell, N.; Dalton, H.; Perkins, D.; Considine, R.; Hughes, S.; Osborne, S.; Buss, R. Our healthy Clarence: A community-driven wellbeing initiative. *Int. J. Environ. Res. Public Health* **2019**, *16*, 3691. [CrossRef] [PubMed]

40. Ruane-McAteer, E.; Gillespie, K.; Amin, A.; Aventin, Á.; Robinson, M.; Hanratty, J.; Khosla, R.; Lohan, M. Gender-transformative programming with men and boys to improve sexual and reproductive health and rights: A systematic review of intervention studies. *BMJ Glob. Health* **2020**, *5*, e002997. [CrossRef]
41. Santhya, K.G.; Haberland, N.; Das, A.; Ram, F.; Sinha, R.K.; Ram, U.; Mohanty, S.K. Empowering Married Young Women and Improving Their Sexual and Reproductive Health: Effects of the First-Time Parents Project. 2008. Available online: https://knowledgecommons.popcouncil.org/cgi/viewcontent.cgi?article=1234&context=departments_sbsr-pgy (accessed on 29 March 2022).
42. Comrie-Thomson, L.; Tokhi, M.; Ampt, F.; Portela, A.; Chersich, M.; Khanna, R.; Luchters, S. Challenging gender inequity through male involvement in maternal and newborn health: Critical assessment of an emerging evidence base. *Cult. Health Sex.* **2015**, *17* (Suppl. S2), 177–189. [CrossRef]
43. Yore, J.; Dasgupta, A.; Ghule, M.; Battala, M.; Nair, S.; Silverman, J.; Saggurti, N.; Balaiah, D.; Raj, A. CHARM, a gender equity and family planning intervention for men and couples in rural India: Protocol for the cluster randomized controlled trial evaluation. *Reprod. Health* **2016**, *13*, 14. [CrossRef]
44. Doyle, K.; Levtov, R.G.; Barker, G.; Bastian, G.G.; Bingenheimer, J.B.; Kazimbaya, S.; Nzabonimpa, A.; Pulerwitz, J.; Sayinzoga, F.; Sharma, V.; et al. Gender-transformative Bandebereho couples' intervention to promote male engagement in reproductive and maternal health and violence prevention in Rwanda: Findings from a randomized controlled trial. *PLoS ONE* **2018**, *13*, e0192756. [CrossRef]
45. Bapolisi, W.A.; Ferrari, G.; Blampain, C.; Makelele, J.; Kono-Tange, L.; Bisimwa, G.; Merten, S. Impact of a complex gender-transformative intervention on maternal and child health outcomes in the eastern Democratic Republic of Congo: Protocol of a longitudinal parallel mixed-methods study. *BMC Public Health* **2020**, *20*, 51. [CrossRef]
46. Comrie-Thomson, L.; Webb, K.; Patel, D.; Wata, P.; Kapamurandu, Z.; Mushavi, A.; Nicholas, M.A.; Agius, P.A.; Davis, J.; Luchters, S. Engaging women and men in the gender-synchronised, community-based Mbereko+ Men intervention to improve maternal mental health and perinatal care-seeking in Manicaland, Zimbabwe: A cluster-randomised controlled pragmatic trial. *J. Glob. Health* **2022**, *12*, 04042. [CrossRef]
47. Chatterji, S.; Heise, L. Examining the bi-directional relationship between intimate partner violence and depression: Findings from a longitudinal study among women and men in rural Rwanda. *SSM-Ment. Health* **2021**, *1*, 100038. [CrossRef]
48. Bacchus, L.J.; Colombini, M.; Contreras Urbina, M.; Howarth, E.; Gardner, F.; Annan, J.; Ashburn, K.; Madrid, B.; Levtov, R.; Watts, C. Exploring opportunities for coordinated responses to intimate partner violence and child maltreatment in low and middle income countries: A scoping review. *Psychol. Health Med.* **2017**, *22* (Suppl. S1), 135–165. [CrossRef]
49. Bartel, D.; Greene, M.E. Involving Everyone in Gender Equality by Synchronizing Gender Strategies. Resource Handbook. 2018. Available online: https://www.prb.org/resources/involving-everyone-in-gender-equality-by-synchronizing-gender-strategies/ (accessed on 1 June 2022).
50. Oram, S.; Fisher, H.L.; Minnis, H.; Seedat, S.; Walby, S.; Hegarty, K.; Rouf, K.; Angénieux, C.; Callard, F.; Chandra, P.S.; et al. The Lancet Psychiatry Commission on intimate partner violence and mental health: Advancing mental health services, research, and policy. *Lancet Psychiatry* **2022**, *9*, 487–524. [CrossRef]
51. Kulkarni, M.; Jain, R. (Eds.) *Global Masculinities: Interrogations and Reconstructions*; Taylor & Francis: Abingdon, UK, 2018.
52. Bodnar, D.; Ryan, D.; Smith, J.E. (Eds.) *Self-Care Program for Women with Postpartum Depression and Anxiety*; BC Women's Hospital & Health Centre: Vancouver, BC, Canada, 2004.
53. Cole, S.M.; Kaminski, A.M.; McDougall, C.; Kefi, A.S.; Marinda, P.A.; Maliko, M.; Mtonga, J. Gender accommodative versus transformative approaches: A comparative assessment within a post-harvest fish loss reduction intervention. *Gend. Technol. Dev.* **2020**, *24*, 48–65. [CrossRef]
54. Bill and Melinda Gates Foundation. Gender and MNCH: A Review of the Evidence. 2020. Available online: https://www.gatesgenderequalitytoolbox.org/wp-content/uploads/BMGF_Gender-MNCH-Report_Hi-Res.pdf (accessed on 25 June 2022).
55. White, B.K.; Giglia, R.C.; Scott, J.A.; Burns, S.K. How new and expecting fathers engage with an app-based online forum: Qualitative analysis. *JMIR mHealth Uhealth* **2018**, *6*, e9999. [CrossRef]
56. Bonifácio, L.P.; Franzon, A.C.A.; Zaratini, F.S.; Vicentine, F.B.; Barbosa-Júnior, F.; Braga, G.C.; Sanchez, J.A.C.; Oliveira-Ciabati, L.; Andrade, M.S.; Fernandes, M.; et al. PRENACEL partner-use of short message service (SMS) to encourage male involvement in prenatal care: A cluster randomized controlled trial. *Reprod. Health* **2020**, *17*, 45. [CrossRef]
57. Johnson, D.; Juras, R.; Riley, P.; Chatterji, M.; Sloane, P.; Choi, S.K.; Johns, B. A randomized controlled trial of the impact of a family planning mHealth service on knowledge and use of contraception. *Contraception* **2017**, *95*, 90–97. [CrossRef]
58. Maslowsky, J.; Frost, S.; Hendrick, C.E.; Cruz, F.O.T.; Merajver, S.D. Effects of postpartum mobile phone-based education on maternal and infant health in Ecuador. *Int. J. Gynecol. Obstet.* **2016**, *134*, 93–98. [CrossRef]
59. Unger, J.A.; Ronen, K.; Perrier, T.; DeRenzi, B.; Slyker, J.; Drake, A.L.; Mogaka, D.; Kinuthia, J.; John-Stewart, G. Short message service communication improves exclusive breastfeeding and early postpartum contraception in a low-to middle-income country setting: A randomised trial. *BJOG Int. J. Obstet. Gynaecol.* **2018**, *125*, 1620–1629. [CrossRef]

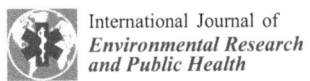

Review

Treatment of Peripartum Depression with Antidepressants and Other Psychotropic Medications: A Synthesis of Clinical Practice Guidelines in Europe

Sarah Kittel-Schneider [1], Ethel Felice [2], Rachel Buhagiar [3], Mijke Lambregtse-van den Berg [4], Claire A. Wilson [5,6], Visnja Banjac Baljak [7], Katarina Savic Vujovic [8], Branislava Medic [8], Ana Opankovic [9], Ana Fonseca [10] and Angela Lupattelli [11,*]

1. Department of Psychiatry, Psychotherapy and Psychosomatics, University Hospital of Würzburg, D-97080 Würzburg, Germany; Kittel_S@ukw.de
2. Department of Psychiatry, Faculty of Medicine & Surgery Msida, University of Malta, 2080 Majjistral, Malta; ethelfelice@gmail.com
3. Health-Mental Health Services, 2080 Majjistral, Malta; rachel.buhagiar@gov.mt
4. Departments of Psychiatry and Child & Adolescent Psychiatry, Erasmus University Medical Center, 3015 GD Rotterdam, The Netherlands; mijke.vandenberg@erasmusmc.nl
5. Section of Women's Mental Health, King's College London, London SE5 8AF, UK; claire.1.wilson@kcl.ac.uk
6. South London and Maudsley NHS Foundation Trust, Bethlem Royal Hospital Monks Orchard Road, Beckenham BR3 3BX, UK
7. Clinic of Psychiatry, University Clinical Center of the Republic of Srpska, 78000 Banjaluka, Bosnia and Herzegovina; visnjab76@hotmail.com
8. Department of Pharmacology, Clinical Pharmacology and Toxicology, Faculty of Medicine, University of Belgrade, P.O. Box 38, 11129 Belgrade, Serbia; katarinasavicvujovic@gmail.com (K.S.V.); brankicamedic@gmail.com (B.M.)
9. Clinic for Psychiatry, University Clinical Center, 11000 Belgrade, Serbia; ana.opankovic@gmail.com
10. Center for Research in Neuropsychology and Cognitive-Behavioral Intervention, University of Coimbra, 3000-115 Coimbra, Portugal; ana.fonseca77@gmail.com
11. PharmacoEpidemiology and Drug Safety Research Group, Department of Pharmacy, PharmaTox Strategic Research Initiative, Faculty of Mathematics and Natural Sciences, University of Oslo, 0316 Oslo, Norway
* Correspondence: angela.lupattelli@farmasi.uio.no

Abstract: This study examined (1) the availability and content of national CPGs for treatment of peripartum depression, including comorbid anxiety, with antidepressants and other psychotropics across Europe and (2) antidepressant and other psychotropic utilization data as an indicator of prescribers' compliance to the guidelines. We conducted a search using Medline and the Guidelines International Network database, combined with direct e-mail contact with national Riseup-PPD COST ACTION members and researchers within psychiatry. Of the 48 European countries examined, we screened 41 records and included 14 of them for full-text evaluation. After exclusion of ineligible and duplicate records, we included 12 CPGs. Multiple CPGs recommend antidepressant initiation or continuation based on maternal disease severity, non-response to first-line non-pharmacological interventions, and after risk-benefit assessment. Advice on treatment of comorbid anxiety is largely missing or unspecific. Antidepressant dispensing data suggest general prescribers' compliance with the preferred substances of the CPG, although country-specific differences were noted. To conclude, there is an urgent need for harmonized, up-to-date CPGs for pharmacological management of peripartum depression and comorbid anxiety in Europe. The recommendations need to be informed by the latest available evidence so that healthcare providers and women can make informed, evidence-based decisions about treatment choices.

Keywords: clinical practice guideline; depression; anxiety; antidepressant; psychotropic medications; peripartum

1. Introduction

Peripartum or perinatal depression, which is depression arising in the period between the start of a pregnancy and the end of the first postpartum year, to use a broad definition, affects approximately one in eight women [1]. Peripartum and perinatal depression are used interchangeably, although the former term relates more specifically to the woman. The disorder often persists throughout the peripartum period, with as many as 47% of women with postnatal depression having experienced an antenatal episode [2]. In many cases, depression concurs with anxiety, and this adds a substantial mental health burden to the woman [3]. One recent study has proposed multiple subtypes of perinatal depression, which differ in terms of symptom dimension and time of onset [4]. Women may, therefore, need tailored treatment strategies, including pharmacotherapy, depending on their individual depression course, timing of onset, and prominent symptom typology.

Perinatal depression is associated with a spectrum of obstetric and long-term negative outcomes in the offspring [5,6], including possible adverse impacts on the mother-infant relationship [7,8]. It also substantially affects women's well-being and functioning, and it can even lead to suicide [9]. In moderate to severe cases or after non-response to first-line psychotherapy, pharmacotherapy with antidepressants is often needed [10]. Pooled results from 40 cohort studies [11] indicate that selective serotonin reuptake inhibitors (SSRIs) are the most commonly used antidepressants, with a population prevalence of filled prescriptions ranging from 3.5% before pregnancy to 3.0% during gestation and 4.7% in the first year postpartum. Augmentation with antipsychotics or adjuvant pharmacotherapy with benzodiazepines or sedative antihistamines may be needed in some cases [10]. Nevertheless, pregnancy remains a major driver for discontinuation of antidepressants, and 49% of those individuals who chose to continue have low antidepressant adherence [12,13].

The decision-making process about antidepressant treatment during pregnancy or lactation is complex, as it involves weighing the possible risk of exposure in utero or in breast milk against the potential adverse effects of sub-optimally treated maternal peripartum depression to both the mother and child. Clinical practice guidelines (CPGs) for peripartum depression management may facilitate this decision-making process. However, many countries have not established CPGs for peripartum depression, and for those available, the recommendations are not always uniform [14]. In 2018, one systematic review evaluated the content of the available CPGs, and it was found that only four countries recommend continuation into pregnancy of a pre-existing antidepressant treatment [14]. This prior work extracted only recommendations from CPGs adhering to the quality criteria of the Appraisal of Guidelines for Research and Evaluation (AGREE) instrument. Thus, there are still knowledge gaps on current clinical practices from CPGs not meeting such quality criteria. Furthermore, the extent to which national CPGs are followed in relation to antidepressant and other psychotropic prescribing remains unknown.

Therefore, the aim of this review was to examine the availability of national CPGs for treatment of peripartum depression with antidepressants across Europe and review their content and recommendations for the pregnancy and postpartum periods. We further evaluate antidepressant utilization data in women during the perinatal period as an indicator of compliance to the guidelines. To shed additional light on mental disorder co-morbidity, we evaluated whether CPGs for peripartum depression provide guidance on psychopharmacological treatment for co-morbid anxiety, along with prescription fill data for other psychotropics (i.e., antipsychotics and benzodiazepines) and sedative antihistamines during pregnancy and postpartum.

2. Materials and Methods

2.1. Search and Selection Criteria for Clinical Practice Guidelines

We conducted an extensive search of CPGs for treatment of peripartum depression in 48 countries in Europe, including member countries of the European Union, Schengen states, and other European countries. San Marino and the Holy See, both located geographically in Italy, were not included, as the former follows guidelines in Italy and the latter was not relevant. We combined multiple search strategies. First, we searched the literature in the Medline database (via PubMed) from inception to 31 August 2021 using the free text terms "antidepressant, peripartum, perinatal, pregnancy, postpartum, antenatal period, prenatal period, postnatal period, depression, mental health, psychiatric" and applied the filter for guidelines only. Second, we searched the Guidelines International Network (GIN) database using the terms "depression, peripartum, perinatal, pregnancy" on 31 August 2021. Third, we contacted directly via email the national members of Riseup-PPD COST ACTION (CA18138–Research Innovation and Sustainable Pan-European Network in Peripartum Depression Disorder) with an inquiry about the existence of a CPG for peripartum depression in the country. Last, we contacted researchers within peripartum psychiatry in various countries. No exclusion criteria were employed based on language. In the searches in Medline and GIN, we did not include published CPGs from countries outside Europe. We did not restrict the search to CPGs meeting the quality criteria of the AGREE instrument, as we aimed to gather as much information as possible about current clinical practices. Case reports and animal studies were excluded. We excluded CPGs on depression or mental health in adults which did not cover or mention peripartum depression within them and CPGs on peripartum depression that did not mention pharmacotherapy interventions. Clinical recommendations without clear references or without a description of the process that led to the recommendation were also excluded. The literature searches and abstract screenings were performed by a single author. The selection of the CPGs eligible for inclusion were agreed upon by all authors.

Data abstraction was performed by one author depending on the relevant language and, thereafter, quality-checked by another author. We extracted recommendations regarding (1) initiation, continuation or discontinuation, and switching of the antidepressant for both new and preexisting depression in pregnancy or postpartum, (2) preferred and non-preferred antidepressants in pregnancy and while breastfeeding, (3) compatibility of antidepressants with breastfeeding, (4) antidepressant level monitoring or dose adjustment, and (5) recommendations for pharmacological treatment of comorbid anxiety in pregnancy and postpartum.

2.2. Search and Selection Criteria for Antidepressant and Psychotropic Utilization Studies

We searched the literature in the Medline database (via PubMed) from inception to 31 August 2021 using the free text terms "antidepressant, psychotropic, antipsychotic, anxiolytic, "medication use", "drug use", peripartum, perinatal, pregnancy, postpartum, antenatal period, prenatal period, postnatal period, depression, mental health, psychiatric". We extracted the most complete or recent antidepressant drug utilization studies among those published in the last 10–15 years originating from countries in Europe. We applied no restriction as to the way antidepressant use in pregnancy and postpartum was measured in the studies (e.g., based on self-reporting, prescription fills, or medical records). The outcome criteria were prevalence estimates for antidepressant use before, during, and after pregnancy. The same criteria applied to the search and data extraction for other psychotropic medications. If available, we extracted prevalence estimates from more than one study.

2.3. Ethics Statement

No ethics approval was sought, as this review evaluated existing clinical practice guidelines. No informed consent was collected, as the study did not involve patients. The synthesis was not registered in PROSPERO.

3. Results
3.1. Identified Clinical Practice Guidelines

Figure 1 describes the flow diagram of the various search strategies to achieve the final sample of CPGs included in the study. Across the 48 countries examined, we were unable to identify a contact person or did not receive a response in 22 (45.8%) of the countries.

We received a response or identified a CPG in the literature search for 26 countries in Europe, of which 10 (38.5%) (i.e., Austria, Bulgaria, Croatia, Cyprus, France, Greece, Iceland, Portugal, Turkey, and Bosnia and Herzegovina) did not have a national CPG for intervention strategies of peripartum depression or mental health, either specific or broader for the adult population, with mention of the peripartum population. In Ireland, we could only retrieve an information leaflet on peripartum depression for women, which is not classified as a CPG. In Ukraine (personal communication), the criteria for treatment of peripartum depression were reported to be in place, which included pharmacotherapy interventions with amitriptyline, phenazepam, relanium, frenolone, and with vitamins (e.g., ascorbic acid). However, no further information was obtained. Belgium and Sweden used protocols or guidelines for screening and treatment of peripartum depression based on international guidelines (NICE). However, pharmacotherapy interventions are not mentioned [15,16]. Of the searches in PubMed and the GIN database, we screened three CPGs from Spain, Poland, and the UK, which were duplicates of the ones obtained via the contact persons in these countries. We included and fully evaluated 12 CPGs. In the CPG from Latvia, recommendations on pharmacological interventions were only provided for the postpartum period.

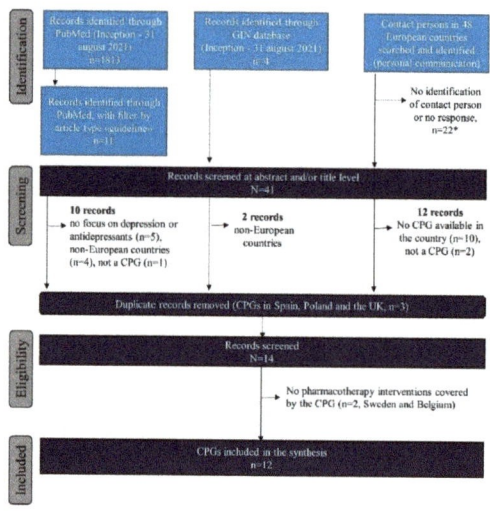

Figure 1. Flow chart of the review process for the clinical practice guideline synthesis. Abbreviations: CPG = clinical practice guideline; GIN = Guidelines International Network. * No response or identification in Albania, Andorra, Armenia, Azerbaijan, Belarus, Croatia, Czech Republic, Estonia, Georgia, Hungary, Kazakhstan, Kosovo, Liechtenstein, Luxembourg, Moldova, Montenegro, North Macedonia, Romania, Russia, Slovakia, Slovenia, and Switzerland.

3.2. Pharmacological Interventions for Treatment of Antenatal Depression

Table 1 shows that most CPGs advise initiation of antidepressants in women with new onset or moderate-to-severe antenatal depression. This treatment should be undertaken after an individualized risk–benefit evaluation and following non-response to psychotherapy. In contrast, the CPG in Poland discourages the use of antidepressants in the first trimester and states that this medication should be discontinued before delivery. All the CPGs seem unanimous in recommending or mentioning the possibility to continue antidepressants in pregnancy for preexisting moderate-to-severe depression (Table 1). In the UK CPG, monotherapy (if possible) and the lowest effective dose are advised in the context of both initiation and continuation of the antidepressant. On the basis of filled prescription and drug utilization data, there was a decrease in the prevalence of antidepressant use from preconception (range: 1.6–9.6%) into pregnancy (range: 0.3–4.1%), with SSRI being the most commonly prescribed group in most countries (Table 1). For many countries in Eastern Europe, no such utilization data were available.

There is general agreement between the CPGs in evaluating individual drug response in the period prior to pregnancy in the decision making about antidepressant continuation during pregnancy. The CPGs provide less uniform guidance regarding switching antidepressants during pregnancy (Table 1). In the CPGs of Malta and Norway, switching is discouraged unless the drug is ineffective. The CPG in the Netherlands considers switching from paroxetine to a preferred antidepressant but before pregnancy. Multiple CPGs (Finland, Germany, Italy, and Serbia) do not provide guidance on switching. Likewise, information on antidepressant level monitoring in serum or plasma and on dosage adjustment is missing for the CPGs in Italy and Denmark.

Multiple CPGs mention sertraline and citalopram as preferred antidepressants in pregnancy, whereas others (i.e., Finland, Serbia, and Spain) list the class of SSRIs. Paroxetine was mentioned as not a preferred antidepressant in most CPGs, except for Serbia, the UK, and Norway. In the two latter countries, the CPGs advise basing the choice of the antidepressant on maternal prior response and its safety profile. Generally, the antidepressants recommended in the CPGs were also the ones most often used in gestation, except in Denmark (for fluoxetine), the Netherlands and Spain (for paroxetine), and Germany (for amitriptyline). Paroxetine ranked among the most commonly used antidepressants in pregnancy in specific countries (i.e., Italy, the Netherlands, or Spain).

3.3. Pharmacological Interventions for Treatment of Postpartum Depression

Table 2 summarizes the content and recommendations of the CPGs for the postpartum period. Most CPGs ($n = 11$) recommend initiation or continuation of antidepressant medications in women suffering from depression in the postpartum period. Nearly all CPGs suggest an individual risk–benefit evaluation of the antidepressant treatment in the case of breastfeeding. Recommendations about breastfeeding compatibility with maternal antidepressant use were not specified in three GPGs (Spain, Serbia, and Norway). The CPGs in the Netherlands, Italy, and Finland state that antidepressant use does not prevent breastfeeding, whereas the UK and Denmark advise closely monitoring the exposed breastfed infant for potential adverse effects, such as weight gain. The Maltese CPG advises that only healthy and full-term infants should be breastfed when mothers are taking antidepressants. The Polish CPG gives a detailed recommendation about the timing of antidepressant intake and breastfeeding (i.e., to take one daily dose before the longest sleep of the child and breastfeed directly before that). Recommendations about switching antidepressants are either unspecified ($n = 5$) in the CPG or discouraged, especially if it affects the woman. The prevalence estimates of antidepressant use postpartum were greater than in the antenatal period and generally returned to the magnitude seen pre-pregnancy. For most of the countries included in this work, no antidepressant utilization data postpartum are available.

Table 1. Overview of recommendations in the CPGs about antidepressant treatment in women with antenatal depression, with prevalence estimates of antidepressant and other psychotropic medication use in the country.

Country, Publication Year, Type	New Depression, Initiate AD	Preexisting Depression, Continue AD	AD Dose Adjustment and Monitoring	Switching AD	Preferred or Not Preferred AD	AD Use before vs during Pregnancy (%)	Most Common ADs Used during Pregnancy	Treatment of Co-Morbid Anxiety	Other Psychotropics during Pregnancy (%)
Denmark [17] PMH-S	Yes, if severe and no response to psychotherapy	Yes	NS	Yes, if effective for woman's depression	Sertraline, citalopram / Paroxetine, fluoxetine	2.0 vs. 1.9–4.1 [18,19]	Citalopram, sertraline, fluoxetine [19]	NS	BZD: 0.6 [20] AP: 0.4 [21] Quetiapine: 0.2 [21]
Finland [22] N-PPD	NS	Yes, in moderate-to-severe cases Psychotherapy first line	Monitoring of response is important	NS	SSRIs / Paroxetine, fluoxetine, tricyclics	1.6–4.0 [23] vs. 3.6* [24]	NA	NS	BZD: 1.2* [25] AP: 0.8 [21] Quetiapine: 0.9 [21]
Germany [26] N-PPD	Yes, after individual risk benefit evaluation, individual disease history, preference and availability of alternative treatments	Yes, in moderate-to-severe cases. Abrupt discontinuation is discouraged. Psychotherapy first line	Monotherapy if possible, lowest effective dose Continuous measurement of plasma levels	NS	Sertraline, citalopram / Paroxetine, fluoxetine	4.0 [27] vs. 0.4 (unpublished data)	Amitriptyline, (es)citalopram, sertraline (unpublished data)	NS	BZD: 3.3 [25] AP: 0.3 [21] Quetiapine: 0.2 [21]
Italy [28] PMH-S	Yes, after individual risk–benefit assessment	Yes, after individual risk–benefit assessment	NS	NS	NS	3.3–4.4 [29] vs. 1.2–1.6 [29]	Paroxetine, sertraline, citalopram [29]	Yes, BZD can be used	BZD: 1.4 [30] AP: 0.8 [31] Quetiapine: NA SAH: 0.4* [24]
Malta [32] PMH-S	Yes, after individual risk–benefit assessment; drug choice based on lowest risk, monotherapy if possible and at the lowest effective dose	Yes, after individual risk–benefit assessment; drug choice based on lowest risk, monotherapy if possible and at the lowest effective dose; previous response is considered	NS	If possible, switch paroxetine to other SSRI	Sertraline ¥; Fluoxetine / Paroxetine	NA	Sertraline, fluoxetine (unpublished data)	BZD only short term for extreme anxiety or agitation; BZD should be avoided in late pregnancy	BZD: NA AP: NA Quetiapine: NA
The Netherlands [33] PMH-S	Yes, after individual risk–benefit assessment	Yes, if woman is stable with medication	Yes, lowest effective dose; paroxetine preferably not >20 mg/day	If possible, switch paroxetine to other SSRI but pre-pregnancy	Sertraline ¥ / Paroxetine ¥	3.9 vs. 2.1 [34]	Sertraline, paroxetine, citalopram [34]	NS	BZD: 1.1 [25,35] AP: NA Quetiapine: NA

184

Table 1. Cont.

Country, Publication Year, Type	New Depression, Initiate AD	Preexisting Depression, Continue AD	AD Dose Adjustment and Monitoring	Switching AD	Preferred or Not Preferred AD	AD Use before vs during Pregnancy (%)	Most Common ADs Used during Pregnancy	Treatment of Co-Morbid Anxiety	Other Psychotropics during Pregnancy (%)
Norway [6] PMH-S	Yes, if severe and with non-pharmacological therapy	Yes, after individual risk-benefit assessment. Psychotherapy first line. Abrupt discontinuation is discouraged.	Yes, serum concentration	No	Choice based on prior drug response and its safety profile	2.0 vs. 1.5 [37]	(Es)citalopram, sertraline, venlafaxine [19]	NS	BZD: 0.9 [38] AP: 1.2 [21] Quetiapine: 0.3 [21] SAH: 1.0 [24] *
Poland [39] PMH-S	If severe depression or ongoing mild-to-moderate symptoms, AD should be considered. Gradual discontinuation if mild symptoms with psychotherapy. **As for new depression.	Individual risk-benefit assessment to be made. **AD in 1 trimester should be avoided, and AD should be discontinued before delivery	Monotherapy, lowest effective dose	Yes, switching an AD which is effective and offers fewer adverse effects	NS / Paroxetine	- vs. 0.3 [24] *	NA	Yes, but do not offer BZD except for the short-term treatment of severe anxiety and agitation	BZD: 0.2–14.0 [24,25] * AP: NA Quetiapine: NA SAH: 0.4 [24] *
Serbia [40] N-PPD	Yes, if severe after individual risk-benefit assessment	Yes, after individual risk-benefit assessment	Yes, serum concentration	NS	Fluoxetine, citalopram, fluvoxamine, paroxetine, sertraline / TCA	- vs. 0.3 [24] *	(Es)citalopram, sertraline, mirtazapine, duloxetine (unpublished data)	Yes, BZD	BZD: 0.2–14.0 [24,25] * AP: NA Quetiapine: NA SAH: 0.4 [24] *
Spain [41] PMH-S	Yes, after individual risk-benefit assessment	Yes, after individual risk-benefit assessment and based on individual drug response	Monotherapy if possible, lowest effective dose; continuous measurement of plasma levels due to fluctuations in pregnancy is recommended	Yes, if lower risk to child and effective in mothers	SSRIs / Paroxetine, tricyclics, fluoxetine	- vs. 0.5–0.8 [42,43]	Paroxetine, citalopram, fluoxetine44	Yes, but for acute symptoms for maximum 4 weeks	BZD: 1.9 [42] AP: 0.1 [43] Quetiapine: NA

Table 1. Cont.

Country, Publication Year, Type	New Depression, Initiate AD	Preexisting Depression, Continue AD	AD Dose Adjustment and Monitoring	Switching AD	Preferred or Not Preferred AD	AD Use before vs during Pregnancy (%)	Most Common ADs Used during Pregnancy	Treatment of Co-Morbid Anxiety	Other Psychotropics during Pregnancy (%)
United Kingdom [44,45] PMH-S	Yes, particularly for moderate-to-severe depression, after discussing with the woman the risk–benefit assessment of AD; drug choice based on lowest risk, monotherapy if possible and at the lowest effective dose	Yes, particularly for moderate-to-severe depression, after discussing with the woman the risk–benefit assessment of AD; monotherapy if possible and at the lowest effective dose	Yes, dosages may need to be adjusted in pregnancy	Option to be discussed with the woman but aim is to expose fetus to as few drugs as possible	Unspecified, choice based on prior drug response and its safety profile	8.8–9.6 vs. 3.7 [29]	Fluoxetine, citalopram [29]	Yes, with ADs. Do not offer BZD except for the short-term treatment of severe anxiety and agitation.	BZD: 1.2 * [25] AP: 0.3–4.6 [21,46] Quetiapine: 0.4 [21]

AD = antidepressant; BZD = benzodiazepines; AP = antipsychotics; SAH = sedative antihistamines; PMH-S = peripartum mental health-specific; N-PPD = not specific to peripartum depression, but pregnant women are dealt with within the guideline for adult depression. Estimates of sedative antihistamines are only shown when available. As such, data are lacking for most countries. * Average estimate for the region at aggregated level (non-country specific) or for the specific country within the meta-analysis. ¥ Applies to first episode in pregnancy, when the woman starts on a new medication.

Table 2. Overview of recommendations in the CPGs about antidepressant treatment in women with postnatal depression, with prevalence estimates of antidepressants and other psychotropic medication use in the country.

Country, Publication Year, Type	Depression, Initiate or Continue AD	AD Intake by Time of BF	Switching AD	Preferred or Not Preferred AD	AD Use Postpartum (%)	Most Common ADs Postpartum	Treatment Co-Morbid Anxiety	Other Psychotropic Postpartum (%)
Denmark [17] PMH-S	NS	No, but weight gain in infant should be monitored. Formula can be considered.	No, if the AD is effective and was taken in pregnancy	Sertraline, paroxetine / Fluoxetine, (es)citalopram, fluvoxamine, venlafaxine	4.1 [29]	NA	NS	BZD: 1.3 [20] AP: NA Quetiapine: NA
Finland [22] N-PPD	As for non-pregnant adults, psychotherapy is recommended for mild symptoms	No, use of SSRI does not prevent BF	NS	SSRIs / Fluoxetine	NA	NA	NS	BZD: 0.7–3.2 [47] AP: NA Quetiapine: NA

Table 2. *Cont.*

Country, Publication Year, Type	Depression, Initiate or Continue AD	AD Intake by Time of BF	Switching AD	Preferred or Not Preferred AD	AD Use Postpartum (%)	Most Common ADs Postpartum	Treatment Co-Morbid Anxiety	Other Psychotropic Postpartum (%)
Germany [26] N-PPD	Yes, after risk–benefit analysis for mother and child and individual disease history, preference, and availability of alternative treatments	Yes, after risk–benefit analysis for mother and child	NS	SSRIs, tricyclics / NS	NA	NA	NS	BZD: NA AP: NA Quetiapine: NA
Italy [28] PMH-S	Yes, after risk–benefit analysis for mother and child	No, use of SSRI does not prevent BF	NS	NS / Fluoxetine	2.5–3.4 [29]	NA	Yes, short-term acting BZD	BZD: NA AP: NA Quetiapine: NA
Latvia [48] PMH-S	Yes, after risk–benefit analysis for mother and child in case of BF. For initiation of AD, start with lowest effective dose.	Assess whether dosage and regimen are compatible with BF	NS	SSRIs, sertraline / Fluoxetine	NA	NA	Yes, mirtazapine or atypical AP; quetiapine for augmentation therapy. Olanzapine only at low doses. BZD should be avoided.	BZD: NA AP: NA Quetiapine: NA
Malta [32] PMH-S	Yes, after individual risk–benefit assessment; drug choice based on lowest risk, monotherapy if possible and at the lowest effective dose	Yes, after individual risk–benefit assessment; drug choice based on lowest risk, monotherapy if possible, and at the lowest effective dose, previous response is considered	NS	Iimipramine, nortriptyline, sertraline / Citalopram, fluoxetine	NA	SSRIs e.g., sertraline, paroxetine (unpublished data)	Short-term BZD (caution in BF). Close monitoring of babies exposed to BZD via breastmilk. Diazepam should not be used while BF.	BZD: NA AP: NA Quetiapine: NA
The Netherlands 33 PMH-S	Yes, continue SSRI after delivery	Yes, BF is recommended	No, no evidence for switching	Paroxetine, sertraline / Fluoxetine, citalopram	3.1 [34]	Paroxetine, citalopram, sertraline [34]	NS	BZD: NA AP: NA Quetiapine: NA
Norway [36] PMH-S	Yes, if severe after individual risk–benefit assessment	NS	No	Sertraline, paroxetine / Doxepin, fluoxetine, citalopram	1.0 [37]	NA	NS	BZD: 0.8 [37] AP: 0.2 [37] Quetiapine: NA
Poland [39] PMH-S	Yes, initiate if severe and continue to prevent relapse. If history of severe depression or ongoing mild-to-moderate symptoms, AD should be considered.	Yes, AD in one daily dose before the child's longest sleep, and BF is recommended just before AD intake	No, same treatment pattern should be used after delivery	Sertraline, citalopram / Fluoxetine	NA	NA	NA	BZD: NA AP: NA Quetiapine: NA

Table 2. Cont.

Country, Publication Year, Type	Depression, Initiate or Continue AD	AD Intake by Time of BF	Switching AD	Preferred or Not Preferred AD	AD Use Postpartum (%)	Most Common ADs Postpartum	Treatment Co-Morbid Anxiety	Other Psychotropic Postpartum (%)
Serbia [40] N-PPD	Yes, if severe after individual risk–benefit assessment	NS	No	Fluoxetine	NA	Paroxetine (data unpublished)	NS	BZD: NA AP: NA Quetiapine: NA
Spain [41] PMH-S	Yes, if severe after individual risk–benefit assessment	NS	NS	Nortriptyline, sertraline, paroxetine / Citalopram, fluoxetine	NA	NA	NS	BZD: NA AP: NA Quetiapine: NA
United Kingdom [44,45] PMH-S	Yes, particularly for moderate-to-severe depression after discussing with the woman of the risk-benefit assessment of AD; drug choice based on lowest risk, monotherapy if possible and at the lowest effective dose.	Consider risks and benefits of BF, which should generally be encouraged, but monitor baby for any adverse effects.	Option to be discussed with the woman, but aim is to expose the breastfed infant to as few drugs as possible.	Unspecified, choice based on prior drug response and its safety profile in breastfeeding.	5.5–12.9 [29,46]	SSRI [49]	Yes, but do not offer BZD except for the short-term treatment of severe anxiety. BZD best avoided in BF if possible; use drug with shortest half-life.	BZD: NA AP: 0.4 [46] Quetiapine: NA

NA = not available; NS = not specified; AD = antidepressant; BF = breastfeeding; BZD = benzodiazepines; AP = antipsychotics; SAH = sedative antihistamines; PMH-S = peripartum mental health specific.

The specific substances recommended and not recommended vary considerably between the CPGs, but taken together, sertraline (8/12 CPGs) and paroxetine (5/12 CPGs) are the ones most commonly preferred, while fluoxetine is not preferred in most CPGs (8/12 CPGs) due to its very long half-life with the risk of accumulation in the infant. Paroxetine, citalopram, sertraline, or SSRI in general are also the antidepressants most commonly taken by women postpartum. Fluoxetine does not rank high in drug utilization studies in the postpartum period.

3.4. Pharmacological Interventions for Antenatal or Postpartum Comorbid Anxiety and Use of Other Psychotropics

Treatment recommendations for comorbid anxiety are largely missing for both the antenatal and the postpartum period (Tables 1 and 2). Only seven GPGs state that benzodiazepines can be offered in the case of severe anxiety during pregnancy but only for short-term treatment. In Malta, benzodiazepines are recommended only as needed, and the treatment of choice is augmentation with quetiapine, both during pregnancy and postpartum. During the latter period, sedative antihistamines represent a treatment option. In the UK, it is advised to treat comorbid anxiety with antidepressants during pregnancy or short-term benzodiazepines, and the latter medication is discouraged at postpartum in case of breastfeeding. The CPG in Latvia recommends treatment of comorbid anxiety postpartum with mirtazapine or atypical antipsychotics, including olanzapine at a low dose, while benzodiazepines should be avoided.

Prenatal use data for benzodiazepines, antipsychotics, and quetiapine specifically are lacking for some countries, and for sedative antihistamines, data are very sparse. During pregnancy, benzodiazepines are often used to a larger extent than antidepressants in specific countries (i.e., Germany, Poland, Serbia, and Spain), while in Norway, the use of benzodiazepine and sedative antihistamines is comparable (about 1%). With regard to the use of other psychotropic medication (as an add-on) in the postpartum period, utilization data are largely unavailable, as only the Nordic countries and the UK report postpartum use of benzodiazepines and antipsychotics in the ranges of 0.8–3.2% and 0.2–0.4%, respectively.

4. Discussion

This review across European countries reports important gaps in the availability, agreement, and up-to-date evidence-based content of CPGs for the pharmacological treatment of peripartum depression. This may have implications in the decision making and uptake of effective treatment among perinatal women and consequently in reducing the pervasive costs of peripartum depression. Several of our findings are important for clinical practice and perinatal drug research at large. First, we identified a national CPG only in 12 out of the 48 countries in Europe, adding 6 guidelines to the latest synthesis by Molenaar et al. in 2018 [14]. Nevertheless, the absence of a CPG in most countries raises clear concerns about the pharmacological management of depression in pregnant women and new mothers [10], especially in countries where higher rates of peripartum depression [50,51] are paralleled by low use of antidepressants and greater use of benzodiazepines [24]. Second, we found general agreement within the CPGs in recommending psychotherapy as first-line intervention, as well as antidepressant initiation or continuation based on psychotherapy non-response or depression severity. However, the recommendations are sometimes unspecific and not uniform across guidelines. Third, emerging issues and questions that are met in the real-world practice are not covered with the latest available evidence (e.g., drug monitoring or dose adjustments, antidepressant switching and treatment augmentation, adjuvant strategies for comorbid anxiety, and compatibility of breastfeeding with antidepressant treatment). Finally, the unavailability of antidepressant and other psychotropic utilization data from pre-pregnancy through the end of the first postpartum year, especially in some countries, impedes the evaluation of prescribers' compliance to a CPG and calls for ad hoc perinatal drug utilization research.

The available evidence about antidepressant safety and antidepressant effectiveness in the context of continuation, discontinuation, or initiation is limited, especially for the pregnancy period [50,52–57]. It is now widely acknowledged that intrauterine exposure to SSRIs does not substantially increase the risk of congenital anomalies in offspring, while the risk for negative longer-term developmental outcomes is less clear [58–60]. However, only more recent studies have compared outcomes in offspring born to continuers versus discontinuers [61]. Antidepressant continuation in pregnancy was found to increase the risk of low birth weight, premature birth, or affective disorder diagnosis later in childhood [62–65]. Yet, the role of confounding by maternal disease severity remains an important concern in this research. Regarding antidepressant effectiveness, a recent meta-analysis [53] found a 74% increased risk of depression relapse during pregnancy with antidepressant discontinuation relative to continuation in pregnancy. The four included studies were, however, very heterogeneous and adopted an oversimplified definition of antidepressant continuation or discontinuation that did not reflect the treatment intensity, dose changes, or timing of exposure as in real-world settings [66–68].

No observational or randomized study to date has investigated the benefit of antidepressant initiation in pregnancy on relapse or remission of peripartum depression. The need for clinical drug trials in pregnant and postpartum women has never been greater [69]. The findings from the "stop or go" randomized trial indicated no significant difference in the risk of relapse of depression in women who tapered SSRIs with additional preventive cognitive therapy, relative to those who continued SSRIs [70]. However, the study included only 44 women, demonstrating the need for larger trials which also address the efficacy of antidepressant initiation in pregnancy. In 2019, the Food and Drug Administration in the US approved the first drug specifically for the treatment of postpartum depression: the GABA-A receptor modulator brexanolone. Brexanolone is not yet approved in the EU, but regulatory pathways have been initiated for future marketing authorization. This new drug constitutes an important therapeutic option for women with severe postpartum depression, but its difficult administration in terms of duration and form (i.e., intravenously) may limit its usage. Determining the comparative effectiveness and safety of brexanolone versus any other treatment for postnatal depression [54] will be crucial to inform clinical decisions involving CPGs at an international level. Similarly, more research is needed about the comparative effectiveness of different pharmacological interventions versus other therapeutic options, such as electroconvulsive therapy for treatment of severe perinatal depression.

There remains a need for more unified guidelines on the use of antidepressants to treat peripartum depression to guide clinical decision making. However, the decision to treat peripartum depression with antidepressants must always consider the individualized risk–benefit profile of the medication for each woman [54]. Most CPGs recommend an individualized risk–benefit assessment, which should consider the psychiatric history of the woman, her response to prior or ongoing antidepressants, mental health outcomes following prior attempts to discontinue the medication, the woman's treatment preference, and her desire to breastfeed. The antidepressant with the lowest known risk for breastfed children in the lowest effective dose and in the lowest effective drug serum concentration should be prescribed [60]. To the best of our knowledge, there is no evidence base to discourage breastfeeding of preterm or low birth weight infants. However, caution is needed due to the immature liver metabolic capacity in preterm infants, especially in combination with maternal fluoxetine use, which has a long half-life and increased risk of accumulation in the breastfed infant [60]. The decision making in pregnancy and while breastfeeding could be aided by further development of patient decision aid (PDA) tools. Early data suggest that they are acceptable to users and reduce decisional conflict [71,72].

Generally, there was satisfactory compliance in prescribing preferred antidepressants during pregnancy (e.g., sertraline and citalopram), although exceptions were noted. Paroxetine ranked among the most commonly used antidepressants in pregnancy in specific countries, despite being a non-preferred antidepressant. However, we could not corroborate whether this drug choice was derived from an individualized assessment based on maternal prior response to the drug or whether it reflects poor prescriber compliance to the CPG. One Dutch study [73] found that gynecologists and midwives were aware of the national CPG on antidepressants in pregnancy, yet only 13.9% of them adhered to its recommendations. Efforts are, therefore, necessary to facilitate the uptake of the CPG recommendations in routine clinical practice by all healthcare professionals involved in the care of women with peripartum depression.

One key finding is that guidance on intervention strategies for comorbid anxiety and advice on augmentation with antipsychotics are largely missing across the examined CPGs, and when present, it is too unspecific with regard to drug selection and maximum permissible doses. Indeed, we observed important country-specific fluctuations in the utilization of benzodiazepines that need to be addressed. Uniform, specific recommendations for this problem are needed for multiple reasons: (1) some women manifest active depressive symptoms despite antidepressant treatment, and clinicians need evidence-based guidance to treat them; (2) anxiety is a prominent symptom of severe peripartum depression [4]; and (3) benzodiazepines should be used only sporadically during pregnancy or postpartum, and alternative interventions are necessary for protracted treatments [60]. Yet, to date, evidence does not exist to help make recommendations for the perinatal population, which calls for urgent population-based perinatal drug research.

Strengths and Limitations

Several strengths and limitations need mentioning. One of the main strengths of this synthesis is that we provided a global view of the existing CPGs across Europe. We applied multiple search strategies, our search was not restricted to CPGs meeting the AGREE instrument, and we applied no language restrictions, which enabled us to gather as many CPGs as possible, including current clinical practices. Direct contact with representatives of the COST network and experts in psychiatry and psychology allowed us to examine CPG availability in low- and middle-income countries in Europe, which are unlikely to publish national CPGs. Our review did not include consensus statements or expert opinion articles, as these items only reflect individuals' perspectives or practices. In addition, we extracted psychotropic utilization data from the literature as a proxy of prescribers' compliance to their national CPGs. However, such a proxy is not ideal, and specific field studies are necessary to accurately measure prescribers' adherence to the CPGs [73]. Identification of CPGs eligible for inclusion in the review was performed by a single author, but the final decision for inclusion or exclusion was agreed upon by all authors. We did not assess the quality of the included CPGs based on the AGREE instrument, and therefore, we could not assess the degree of the evidence upon which the different CPG recommendations were based. Lastly, our review was restricted to European countries, and so our results are not generalizable to countries outside Europe.

5. Conclusions

Many countries in Europe do not have a CPG for pharmacological treatment of peripartum depression, and where present, recommendations are not fully uniform and not up to date with the latest available evidence. This review expresses the urgent need for a harmonized, up-to-date CPG for pharmacological management of peripartum depression and comorbid anxiety in Europe. Treatment recommendations need to be informed by the latest available evidence and cover emerging issues that are met in the current clinical practice. Our work is only the first step in facilitating the complex decision making in pharmacological treatment of women with peripartum depression. Women across Europe should be empowered to make informed, evidence-based decisions about their treatments during pregnancy and while breastfeeding.

Author Contributions: All authors participated in the conceptualization, methodology, review, and editing; formal analysis, A.L.; writing—original draft preparation, A.L., S.K.-S., E.F., R.B., M.L.-v.d.B., C.A.W., V.B.B., K.S.V., B.M., A.F. and A.O.; data curation, A.L.; project administration, A.L. All authors have read and agreed to the published version of the manuscript.

Funding: This paper was supported by COST under COST Action Riseup-PPD CA18138 www.cost.eu (access date 30 September 2021). A.L. was supported by the Norwegian Research Council (grant number 288696). C.A.W. was funded by the UK's National Institute for Health Research (NIHR). The funders had no role in the analyses, interpretation of results, or the writing of this manuscript.

Institutional Review Board Statement: Not applicable.

Informed Consent Statement: Not applicable.

Data Availability Statement: All data are available online in Medline (via PubMed).

Acknowledgments: We are grateful to all national members of Riseup-PPD COST ACTION and the researchers and clinicians that supported our search for clinical practice guidelines. This paper is based upon work from the COST Action Riseup-PPD CA 18138 and was supported by COST under COST Action Riseup-PPD CA18138 www.cost.eu (access date 30 September 2021).

Conflicts of Interest: The authors declare no conflict of interest.

References

1. Woody, C.A.; Ferrari, A.J.; Siskind, D.J.; Whiteford, H.A.; Harris, M.G. A systematic review and meta-regression of the prevalence and incidence of perinatal depression. *J. Affect. Disord.* **2017**, *219*, 86–92. [CrossRef]
2. Underwood, L.; Waldie, K.; D'Souza, S.; Peterson, E.R.; Morton, S. A review of longitudinal studies on antenatal and postnatal depression. *Arch. Womens Ment. Health* **2016**, *19*, 711–720. [CrossRef] [PubMed]
3. Falah-Hassani, K.; Shiri, R.; Dennis, C.L. The prevalence of antenatal and postnatal co-morbid anxiety and depression: A meta-analysis. *Psychol. Med.* **2017**, *47*, 2041–2053. [CrossRef] [PubMed]
4. Putnam, K.T.; Wilcox, M.; Robertson-Blackmore, E.; Sharkey, K.; Bergink, V.; Munk-Olsen, T.; Deligiannidis, K.M.; Payne, J.; Altemus, M.; Newport, J.; et al. Clinical phenotypes of perinatal depression and time of symptom onset: Analysis of data from an international consortium. *Lancet Psychiatry* **2017**, *4*, 477–485. [CrossRef]
5. Stein, A.; Pearson, R.M.; Goodman, S.H.; Rapa, E.; Rahman, A.; McCallum, M.; Howard, L.M.; Pariante, C.M. Effects of perinatal mental disorders on the fetus and child. *Lancet* **2014**, *384*, 1800–1819. [CrossRef]
6. Slomian, J.; Honvo, G.; Emonts, P.; Reginster, J.-Y.; Bruyère, O. Consequences of maternal postpartum depression: A systematic review of maternal and infant outcomes. *Womens Health* **2019**, *15*, 1745506519844044. [CrossRef] [PubMed]
7. Grigoriadis, S.; VonderPorten, E.H.; Mamisashvili, L.; Tomlinson, G.; Dennis, C.L.; Koren, G.; Steiner, M.; Mousmanis, P.; Cheung, A.; Radford, K.; et al. The impact of maternal depression during pregnancy on perinatal outcomes: A systematic review and meta-analysis. *J. Clin. Psychiatry* **2013**, *74*, e321–e341. [CrossRef]
8. Gordon, H.; Nath, S.; Trevillion, K.; Moran, P.; Pawlby, S.; Newman, L.; Howard, L.M.; Molyneaux, E. Self-Harm, Self-Harm Ideation, and Mother-Infant Interactions: A Prospective Cohort Study. *J. Clin. Psychiatry* **2019**, *80*, 18m12708. [CrossRef]
9. Cantwell, R.; Clutton-Brock, T.; Cooper, G.; Dawson, A.; Drife, J.; Garrod, D.; Harper, A.; Hulbert, D.; Lucas, S.; McClure, J.; et al. Saving Mothers' Lives: Reviewing maternal deaths to make motherhood safer: 2006–2008. The Eighth Report of the Confidential Enquiries into Maternal Deaths in the United Kingdom. *BJOG* **2011**, *118* (Suppl. 1), 1–203. [CrossRef]
10. Hendrick, V. *Psychiatric Disorders in Pregnancy and the Postpartum: Principles and Treatment*; Humana Press: Totowa, NJ, USA, 2006.
11. Molenaar, N.M.; Bais, B.; Lambregtse-van den Berg, M.P.; Mulder, C.L.; Howell, E.A.; Fox, N.S.; Rommel, A.S.; Bergink, V.; Kamperman, A.M. The international prevalence of antidepressant use before, during, and after pregnancy: A systematic review and meta-analysis of timing, type of prescriptions and geographical variability. *J. Affect. Disord.* **2020**, *264*, 82–89. [CrossRef]
12. Lupattelli, A.; Spigset, O.; Bjornsdottir, I.; Hameen-Anttila, K.; Mardby, A.C.; Panchaud, A.; Juraski, R.G.; Rudolf, G.; Odalovic, M.; Drozd, M.; et al. Patterns and factors associated with low adherence to psychotropic medications during pregnancy—A cross-sectional, multinational web-based study. *Depress. Anxiety* **2015**, *32*, 426–436. [CrossRef]
13. Petersen, I.; Gilbert, R.E.; Evans, S.J.; Man, S.L.; Nazareth, I. Pregnancy as a major determinant for discontinuation of antidepressants: An analysis of data from The Health Improvement Network. *J. Clin. Psychiatry* **2011**, *72*, 979–985. [CrossRef]
14. Molenaar, N.M.; Kamperman, A.M.; Boyce, P.; Bergink, V. Guidelines on treatment of perinatal depression with antidepressants: An international review. *Aust. N. Z. J. Psychiatry* **2018**, *52*, 320–327. [CrossRef] [PubMed]
15. Van Damme, R.; Van Parys, A.S.; Vogels, C.; Roelens, K.; Lemmens, G.M.D. A mental health care protocol for the screening, detection and treatment of perinatal anxiety and depressive disorders in Flanders. *J. Psychosom. Res.* **2020**, *128*, 109865. [CrossRef]
16. Swedish National Board of Health and Welfare. National Guidelines for Care for Depression and Anxiety Syndrome—Support for Control and Management. Available online: https://www.socialstyrelsen.se/globalassets/sharepoint-dokument/artikelkatalog/nationella-riktlinjer/2017-12-1.pdf (accessed on 30 March 2021).
17. Middelboe, T.; Wøjdemann, K.; Bjergager, M.; Klindt Poulsen, B. *Anvendelse af Psykofarmaka Ved Graviditet Og Amning—Kliniske Retningslinjer*; Dansk Psykiatrisk Selskab; Dansk Selskab for Obstetrik og Gynækologi; Dansk Pædiatrisk Selskab og Dansk Selskab for Klinisk Farmakologi: Rønde, Denmark, 27 October 2014. Available online: https://www.dpsnet.dk/wp-content/uploads/2021/02/anvendelse_af_psykofarmaka_okt_2014.pdf (accessed on 3 February 2022).

18. Jimenez-Solem, E.; Andersen, J.T.; Petersen, M.; Broedbaek, K.; Andersen, N.L.; Torp-Pedersen, C.; Poulsen, H.E. Prevalence of antidepressant use during pregnancy in Denmark, a nation-wide cohort study. *PLoS ONE* **2013**, *8*, e63034. [CrossRef]
19. Zoega, H.; Kieler, H.; Norgaard, M.; Furu, K.; Valdimarsdottir, U.; Brandt, L.; Haglund, B. Use of SSRI and SNRI Antidepressants during Pregnancy: A Population-Based Study from Denmark, Iceland, Norway and Sweden. *PLoS ONE* **2015**, *10*, e0144474. [CrossRef] [PubMed]
20. Bais, B.; Munk-Olsen, T.; Bergink, V.; Liu, X. Prescription patterns of benzodiazepine and benzodiazepine-related drugs in the peripartum period: A population-based study. *Psychiatry Res.* **2020**, *288*, 112993. [CrossRef] [PubMed]
21. Reutfors, J.; Cesta, C.E.; Cohen, J.M.; Bateman, B.T.; Brauer, R.; Einarsdottir, K.; Engeland, A.; Furu, K.; Gissler, M.; Havard, A.; et al. Antipsychotic drug use in pregnancy: A multinational study from ten countries. *Schizophr. Res.* **2020**, *220*, 106–115. [CrossRef] [PubMed]
22. Current Clinical Care—Depression. Finnish Medical Association's Duodecim and the Finnish Psychiatric Association. Available online: https://www.kaypahoito.fi/hoi50023#s13 (accessed on 30 June 2021).
23. Gissler, M.; Artama, M.; Ritvanen, A.; Wahlbeck, K. Use of psychotropic drugs before pregnancy and the risk for induced abortion: Population-based register-data from Finland 1996–2006. *BMC Public Health* **2010**, *10*, 383. [CrossRef]
24. Lupattelli, A.; Spigset, O.; Twigg, M.J.; Zagorodnikova, K.; Mardby, A.C.; Moretti, M.E.; Drozd, M.; Panchaud, A.; Hameen-Anttila, K.; Rieutord, A.; et al. Medication use in pregnancy: A cross-sectional, multinational web-based study. *BMJ Open* **2014**, *4*, e004365. [CrossRef]
25. Bais, B.; Molenaar, N.M.; Bijma, H.H.; Hoogendijk, W.J.G.; Mulder, C.L.; Luik, A.I.; Lambregtse-van den Berg, M.P.; Kamperman, A.M. Prevalence of benzodiazepines and benzodiazepine-related drugs exposure before, during and after pregnancy: A systematic review and meta-analysis. *J. Affect. Disord.* **2020**, *269*, 18–27. [CrossRef] [PubMed]
26. *German S3 Guideline/National Health Care Guideline. Unipolar Depression*; ÄZQ—Redaktion Nationale VersorgungsLeitlinien: Berlin, Germany, Peripartum Depression 2017; Chapter 3.9.1; pp. 151–159.
27. Lewer, D.; O'Reilly, C.; Mojtabai, R.; Evans-Lacko, S. Antidepressant use in 27 European countries: Associations with sociodemographic, cultural and economic factors. *Br. J. Psychiatry* **2015**, *207*, 221–226. [CrossRef]
28. Anniverno, R.; Bramante, A.; Petrilli, G.; Mencacci, C. *Prevenzione, Diagnosi E Trattamento Della Psicopatologia Perinatale: Linee Guida Per Professionisti Della Salute*; Osservatorio Nazionale sulla Salute della Donna: Milano, Italy, 2010.
29. Charlton, R.A.; Jordan, S.; Pierini, A.; Garne, E.; Neville, A.J.; Hansen, A.V.; Gini, R.; Thayer, D.; Tingay, K.; Puccini, A.; et al. Selective serotonin reuptake inhibitor prescribing before, during and after pregnancy: A population-based study in six European regions. *BJOG* **2015**, *122*, 1010–1020. [CrossRef] [PubMed]
30. Lupattelli, A.; Picinardi, M.; Cantarutti, A.; Nordeng, H. Use and Intentional Avoidance of Prescribed Medications in Pregnancy: A Cross-Sectional, Web-Based Study among 926 Women in Italy. *Int. J. Environ. Res. Public Health* **2020**, *17*, 3830. [CrossRef] [PubMed]
31. Barbui, C.; Conti, V.; Purgato, M.; Cipriani, A.; Fortino, I.; Rivolta, A.L.; Lora, A. Use of antipsychotic drugs and mood stabilizers in women of childbearing age with schizophrenia and bipolar disorder: Epidemiological survey. *Epidemiol. Psychiatr. Sci.* **2013**, *22*, 355–361. [CrossRef]
32. Agius, R.; Felice, E.; Buhagia, R. Women with Mental Health Problems—During Pregnancy, Birth and the Postnatal Period. Malta. *unpublished*.
33. Federatie Medisch Specialisten. SSRI-Gebruik en Zwangerschap. Available online: https://richtlijnendatabase.nl/richtlijn/ssri_en_zwangerschap/ssri-gebruik_en_zwangerschap_-_startpagina.html (accessed on 23 June 2021).
34. Molenaar, N.M.; Lambregtse-van den Berg, M.P.; Bonsel, G.J. Dispensing patterns of selective serotonin reuptake inhibitors before, during and after pregnancy: A 16-year population-based cohort study from the Netherlands. *Arch. Womens Ment. Health* **2020**, *23*, 71–79. [CrossRef]
35. Radojcic, M.R.; El Marroun, H.; Miljkovic, B.; Stricker, B.H.C.; Jaddoe, V.W.V.; Verhulst, F.C.; White, T.; Tiemeier, H. Prenatal exposure to anxiolytic and hypnotic medication in relation to behavioral problems in childhood: A population-based cohort study. *Neurotoxicol. Teratol.* **2017**, *61*, 58–65. [CrossRef]
36. Thorbjørn, B.S.; Eberhard-Gran, M.; Nordeng, H.; Nerum, H.; Lyng, S. Mental Helse i Svangerskapet. Veileder i Fødselshjelp 2020. Available online: https://www.legeforeningen.no/foreningsledd/fagmed/norsk-gynekologisk-forening/veiledere/veileder-i-fodselshjelp/ (accessed on 26 October 2020).
37. Engeland, A.; Bjorge, T.; Klungsoyr, K.; Hjellvik, V.; Skurtveit, S.; Furu, K. Trends in prescription drug use during pregnancy and postpartum in Norway, 2005 to 2015. *Pharmacoepidemiol. Drug Saf.* **2018**, *27*, 995–1004. [CrossRef]
38. Riska, B.S.; Skurtveit, S.; Furu, K.; Engeland, A.; Handal, M. Dispensing of benzodiazepines and benzodiazepine-related drugs to pregnant women: A population-based cohort study. *Eur. J. Clin. Pharmacol.* **2014**, *70*, 1367–1374. [CrossRef] [PubMed]
39. Samochowiec, J.; Rybakowski, J.; Galecki, P.; Szulc, A.; Rymaszewska, J.; Cubala, W.J.; Dudek, D. Recommendations of the Polish Psychiatric Association for treatment of affective disorders in women of childbearing age. Part I: Treatment of depression. *Psychiatr. Pol.* **2019**, *53*, 245–262. [CrossRef]
40. Milasinovic, G.; Vukicevic, D. *Nacionalni Vodic Dobre Klinicke Orakse Za Djagnostikovanje i Lecenje Depresije*; Ministarstvo zdravlja Republike Srbije: Belgrade, Serbia, 2011.

41. García-Herrera, P.B.J.M.; Nogueras Morillas, E.V.; Muñoz Cobos, F.; Morales Asencio, J.M. *Guía de Práctica Clínica Para el Tratamiento de la Depresión en Atención Primaria*; Distrito Sanitario Málaga-UGC Salud Mental Hospital Regional Universitario "Carlos Haya": Málaga, Spain, 2011.
42. Lendoiro, E.; Gonzalez-Colmenero, E.; Concheiro-Guisan, A.; de Castro, A.; Cruz, A.; Lopez-Rivadulla, M.; Concheiro, M. Maternal hair analysis for the detection of illicit drugs, medicines, and alcohol exposure during pregnancy. *Ther. Drug Monit.* **2013**, *35*, 296–304. [CrossRef] [PubMed]
43. De Las Cuevas, C.; de la Rosa, M.A.; Troyano, J.M.; Sanz, E.J. Are psychotropics drugs used in pregnancy? *Pharmacoepidemiol. Drug Saf.* **2007**, *16*, 1018–1023. [CrossRef] [PubMed]
44. NICE—National Institute for Health and Care Excellence. Antenatal and Postnatal Mental Health: Clinical Management and Service Guidance. 11 February 2020. Available online: https://www.nice.org.uk/guidance/cg192 (accessed on 31 August 2021).
45. McAllister-Williams, R.H.; Baldwin, D.S.; Cantwell, R.; Easter, A.; Gilvarry, E.; Glover, V.; Green, L.; Gregoire, A.; Howard, L.M.; Jones, I.; et al. British Association for Psychopharmacology consensus guidance on the use of psychotropic medication preconception, in pregnancy and postpartum 2017. *J. Psychopharmacol.* **2017**, *31*, 519–552. [CrossRef] [PubMed]
46. Margulis, A.V.; Kang, E.M.; Hammad, T.A. Patterns of prescription of antidepressants and antipsychotics across and within pregnancies in a population-based UK cohort. *Matern. Child Health J.* **2014**, *18*, 1742–1752. [CrossRef] [PubMed]
47. Raitasalo, K.; Holmila, M.; Autti-Ramo, I.; Martikainen, J.E.; Sorvala, V.M.; Makela, P. Benzodiazepine use among mothers of small children: A register-based cohort study. *Addiction* **2015**, *110*, 636–643. [CrossRef]
48. Slimību Profilakses un Kontroles Centrs. Klīniskie Algoritmi un Pacientu Ceļi. Available online: https://www.spkc.gov.lv/lv/kliniskie-algoritmi-un-pacientu-celi (accessed on 23 June 2021).
49. Petersen, I.; Peltola, T.; Kaski, S.; Walters, K.R.; Hardoon, S. Depression, depressive symptoms and treatments in women who have recently given birth: UK cohort study. *BMJ Open* **2018**, *8*, e022152. [CrossRef]
50. Lupattelli, A.; Twigg, M.J.; Zagorodnikova, K.; Moretti, M.E.; Drozd, M.; Panchaud, A.; Rieutord, A.; Juraski, R.G.; Odalovic, M.; Kennedy, D.; et al. Self-reported perinatal depressive symptoms and postnatal symptom severity after treatment with antidepressants in pregnancy: A cross-sectional study across 12 European countries using the Edinburgh Postnatal Depression Scale. *Clin. Epidemiol.* **2018**, *10*, 655–669. [CrossRef]
51. Wachs, T.D.; Black, M.M.; Engle, P.L. Maternal Depression: A Global Threat to Children's Health, Development, and Behavior and to Human Rights. *Child Dev. Perspect.* **2009**, *3*, 51–59. [CrossRef]
52. Molyneaux, E.; Telesia, L.A.; Henshaw, C.; Boath, E.; Bradley, E.; Howard, L.M. Antidepressants for preventing postnatal depression. *Cochrane Database Syst. Rev.* **2018**, *4*, CD004363. [CrossRef]
53. Bayrampour, H.; Kapoor, A.; Bunka, M.; Ryan, D. The Risk of Relapse of Depression During Pregnancy After Discontinuation of Antidepressants: A Systematic Review and Meta-Analysis. *J. Clin. Psychiatry* **2020**, *81*, 19r13134. [CrossRef]
54. Wilson, C.A.; Robertson, L.; Brown, J.V.; Ayre, K.; Khalifeh, H. Brexanolone and related neurosteroid GABA(A) positive allosteric modulators for postnatal depression. *Cochrane Database Syst. Rev.* **2021**, *5*, CD014624. [CrossRef]
55. Swanson, S.A.; Hernandez-Diaz, S.; Palmsten, K.; Mogun, H.; Olfson, M.; Huybrechts, K.F. Methodological considerations in assessing the effectiveness of antidepressant medication continuation during pregnancy using administrative data. *Pharmacoepidemiol. Drug Saf.* **2015**, *24*, 934–942. [CrossRef] [PubMed]
56. Yonkers, K.A.; Gotman, N.; Smith, M.V.; Forray, A.; Belanger, K.; Brunetto, W.L.; Lin, H.; Burkman, R.T.; Zelop, C.M.; Lockwood, C.J. Does antidepressant use attenuate the risk of a major depressive episode in pregnancy? *Epidemiology* **2011**, *22*, 848–854. [CrossRef] [PubMed]
57. Cohen, L.S.; Altshuler, L.L.; Harlow, B.L.; Nonacs, R.; Newport, D.J.; Viguera, A.C.; Suri, R.; Burt, V.K.; Hendrick, V.; Reminick, A.M.; et al. Relapse of major depression during pregnancy in women who maintain or discontinue antidepressant treatment. *JAMA* **2006**, *295*, 499–507. [CrossRef] [PubMed]
58. Grigoriadis, S.; VonderPorten, E.H.; Mamisashvili, L.; Roerecke, M.; Rehm, J.; Dennis, C.L.; Koren, G.; Steiner, M.; Mousmanis, P.; Cheung, A.; et al. Antidepressant exposure during pregnancy and congenital malformations: Is there an association? A systematic review and meta-analysis of the best evidence. *J. Clin. Psychiatry* **2013**, *74*, e293–e308. [CrossRef] [PubMed]
59. Grigoriadis, S.; VonderPorten, E.H.; Mamisashvili, L.; Eady, A.; Tomlinson, G.; Dennis, C.L.; Koren, G.; Steiner, M.; Mousmanis, P.; Cheung, A.; et al. The effect of prenatal antidepressant exposure on neonatal adaptation: A systematic review and meta-analysis. *J. Clin. Psychiatry* **2013**, *74*, e309–e320. [CrossRef] [PubMed]
60. Spigset, O.; Nordeng, H. Safety of Psychotropic Drugs in Pregnancy and Breastfeeding. In *Pharmacovigilance in Psychiatry*; Spina, E., Trifirò, G., Eds.; Springer International Publishing: Cham, Switzerland, 2016; pp. 299–319. [CrossRef]
61. Rommel, A.S.; Bergink, V.; Liu, X.; Munk-Olsen, T.; Molenaar, N.M. Long-Term Effects of Intrauterine Exposure to Antidepressants on Physical, Neurodevelopmental, and Psychiatric Outcomes: A Systematic Review. *J. Clin. Psychiatry* **2020**, *81*. [CrossRef]
62. Park, M.; Hanley, G.E.; Guhn, M.; Oberlander, T.F. Prenatal antidepressant exposure and child development at kindergarten age: A population-based study. *Pediatr. Res.* **2021**, *89*, 1515–1522. [CrossRef]
63. Rommel, A.S.; Momen, N.C.; Molenaar, N.M.; Liu, X.; Munk-Olsen, T.; Bergink, V. Long-term prenatal effects of antidepressant use on the risk of affective disorders in the offspring: A register-based cohort study. *Neuropsychopharmacology* **2021**, *46*, 1518–1525. [CrossRef]
64. Wartko, P.D.; Weiss, N.S.; Enquobahrie, D.A.; Chan, K.C.G.; Stephenson-Famy, A.; Mueller, B.A.; Dublin, S. Association of Antidepressant Continuation in Pregnancy and Infant Birth Weight. *J. Clin. Psychopharmacol.* **2021**, *41*, 403–413. [CrossRef]

65. Wolgast, E.; Lilliecreutz, C.; Sydsjö, G.; Bladh, M.; Josefsson, A. The impact of major depressive disorder and antidepressant medication before and during pregnancy on obstetric and neonatal outcomes: A nationwide population-based study. *Eur. J. Obstet. Gynecol. Reprod. Biol.* **2021**, *257*, 42–50. [CrossRef] [PubMed]
66. Wood, M.E.; Lupattelli, A.; Palmsten, K.; Bandoli, G.; Hurault-Delarue, C.; Damase-Michel, C.; Chambers, C.D.; Nordeng, H.M.E.; van Gelder, M. Longitudinal Methods for Modeling Exposures in Pharmacoepidemiologic Studies in Pregnancy. *Epidemiol. Rev.* **2021**, *43*, 130–146. [CrossRef] [PubMed]
67. Lupattelli, A.; Mahic, M.; Handal, M.; Ystrom, E.; Reichborn-Kjennerud, T.; Nordeng, H. Attention-deficit/hyperactivity disorder in children following prenatal exposure to antidepressants: Results from the Norwegian mother, father and child cohort study. *BJOG* **2021**, *128*, 1917–1927. [CrossRef]
68. Trinh, N.T.; Nordeng, H.M.; Bandoli, G.; Eberhard-Gran, M.; Lupattelli, A. Antidepressant and mental health care utilization in pregnant women with depression and/or anxiety: An interrupted time-series analysis. *medRxiv* **2021**. [CrossRef]
69. Scaffidi, J.; Mol, B.W.; Keelan, J.A. The pregnant women as a drug orphan: A global survey of registered clinical trials of pharmacological interventions in pregnancy. *BJOG* **2017**, *124*, 132–140. [CrossRef] [PubMed]
70. Molenaar, N.M.; Brouwer, M.E.; Burger, H.; Kamperman, A.M.; Bergink, V.; Hoogendijk, W.J.G.; Williams, A.D.; Bockting, C.L.H.; Lambregtse-van den Berg, M.P. Preventive Cognitive Therapy With Antidepressant Discontinuation During Pregnancy: Results From a Randomized Controlled Trial. *J. Clin. Psychiatry* **2020**, *81*, 19l13099. [CrossRef]
71. Khalifeh, H.; Molyneaux, E.; Brauer, R.; Vigod, S.; Howard, L.M. Patient decision aids for antidepressant use in pregnancy: A pilot randomised controlled trial in the UK. *BJGP Open* **2019**, *3*, bjgpopen19X101666. [CrossRef]
72. Vigod, S.N.; Hussain-Shamsy, N.; Stewart, D.E.; Grigoriadis, S.; Metcalfe, K.; Oberlander, T.F.; Schram, C.; Taylor, V.H.; Dennis, C.L. A patient decision aid for antidepressant use in pregnancy: Pilot randomized controlled trial. *J. Affect. Disord.* **2019**, *251*, 91–99. [CrossRef]
73. Molenaar, N.M.; Brouwer, M.E.; Duvekot, J.J.; Burger, H.; Knijff, E.M.; Hoogendijk, W.J.; Bockting, C.L.H.; de Wolf, G.S.; Lambregtse-van den Berg, M.P. Antidepressants during pregnancy: Guideline adherence and current practice amongst Dutch gynaecologists and midwives. *Midwifery* **2018**, *61*, 29–35. [CrossRef]

MDPI
St. Alban-Anlage 66
4052 Basel
Switzerland
Tel. +41 61 683 77 34
Fax +41 61 302 89 18
www.mdpi.com

International Journal of Environmental Research and Public Health Editorial Office
E-mail: ijerph@mdpi.com
www.mdpi.com/journal/ijerph

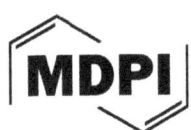